RN Mental Health Nursing
REVIEW MODULE EDITION 10.0

Contributors

Norma Jean E. Henry, MSN/Ed, RN

Mendy McMichael, DNP, MSN

Janean Johnson, MSN, RN, CNE

Agnes DiStasi, DNP, RN, CNE

Kellie L. Wilford, MSN, RN

Terri Lemon, DNP, MSN, RN

Consultants

Susan Adcock, RN, MS

Katherine McKinley, APRN, FNP-C, MSN

Sheri Stone, MSN, RN, APRN-AGCNS, CCRN, MICT

Deb Johnson-Schuh, RN, MSN, CNE

Lisa Kongable, MA, PMH-CNS, ARNP, CNE

Director of content review: Kristen Lawler

Director of development: Derek Prater

Project management: Janet Hines, Nicole Burke

Coordination of content review: Norma Jean E. Henry, Mendy McMichael

Copy editing: Kelly Von Lunen, Derek Prater

Layout: Spring Lenox, Randi Hardy

Illustrations: Randi Hardy

Online media: Morgan Smith, Ron Hanson, Nicole Lobdell, Brant Stacy

Cover design: Jason Buck

Interior book design: Spring Lenox

IMPORTANT NOTICE TO THE READER

User's Guide

Welcome to the Assessment Technologies Institute®
RN Mental Health Nursing Review Module Edition 10.0.
The mission of ATI's Content Mastery Series® Review
Modules is to provide user-friendly compendiums of
nursing knowledge that will:
- Help you locate important information quickly.
- Assist in your learning efforts.
- Provide exercises for applying your nursing knowledge.
- Facilitate your entry into the nursing profession as a
  newly licensed nurse.

This newest edition of the Review Modules has been
redesigned to optimize your learning experience. We've
fit more content into less space and have done so in a
way that will make it even easier for you to find and
understand the information you need.

ORGANIZATION

This Review Module is organized into units covering
foundations for mental health nursing, traditional
nonpharmacological therapies, psychobiologic disorders,
psychopharmacological therapies, specific populations, and
psychiatric emergencies. Chapters within these units conform
to one of four organizing principles for presenting the content.
- Nursing concepts
- Procedures
- Disorders
- Medications

Nursing concepts chapters begin with an overview
describing the central concept and its relevance to nursing.
Subordinate themes are covered in outline form to
demonstrate relationships and present the information in a
clear, succinct manner.

Procedures chapters include an overview describing the
procedure(s) covered in the chapter. These chapters provide
nursing knowledge relevant to each procedure, including
indications, nursing considerations, and complications.

Disorders chapters include an overview describing the
disorder. These chapters cover assessments, including risk
factors and expected findings, and patient-centered care,
including nursing care, medications, therapeutic procedures,
and interprofessional care.

Medications chapters include an overview describing a
disorder or group of disorders. Medications used to treat
these disorders are grouped according to classification.
A specific medication can be selected as a prototype or
example of the characteristics of medications in this
classification. These sections include information about
how the medication works and its therapeutic uses.
Next, you will find information about complications,
contraindications/precautions, and interactions, as well as
nursing interventions and client education to help prevent
and/or manage these issues. Finally, the chapter includes
information on nursing administration of the medication and
evaluation of the medication's effectiveness.

ACTIVE LEARNING SCENARIOS
AND APPLICATION EXERCISES

Each chapter includes opportunities for you to test your
knowledge and to practice applying that knowledge. Active
Learning Scenario exercises pose a nursing scenario
and then direct you to use an ATI Active Learning
Template (included at the back of this book) to record
the important knowledge a nurse should apply to the
scenario. An example is then provided to which you can
compare your completed Active Learning Template. The
Application Exercises include NCLEX-style questions, such
as multiple-choice and multiple-select items, providing
you with opportunities to practice answering the kinds of
questions you might expect to see on ATI assessments or
the NCLEX. After the Application Exercises, an answer key
is provided, along with rationales.

NCLEX® CONNECTIONS

To prepare for the NCLEX-RN, it is important to
understand how the content in this Review Module
is connected to the NCLEX-RN test plan. You can find
information on the detailed test plan at the National
Council of State Boards of Nursing's website, www.ncsbn.
org. When reviewing content in this Review Module,
regularly ask yourself, "How does this content fit into
the test plan, and what types of questions related to this
content should I expect?"

To help you in this process, we've included NCLEX
Connections at the beginning of each unit and with each
question in the Application Exercises Answer Keys. The
NCLEX Connections at the beginning of each unit point
out areas of the detailed test plan that relate to the content
within that unit. The NCLEX Connections attached to the
Application Exercises Answer Keys demonstrate how each
exercise fits within the detailed content outline.
These NCLEX Connections will help you understand how
the detailed content outline is organized, starting with
major client needs categories and subcategories and
followed by related content areas and tasks. The major
client needs categories are:
- Safe and Effective Care Environment
  - Management of Care
  - Safety and Infection Control
- Health Promotion and Maintenance
- Psychosocial Integrity
- Physiological Integrity
  - Basic Care and Comfort
  - Pharmacological and Parenteral Therapies
  - Reduction of Risk Potential
  - Physiological Adaptation

An NCLEX Connection might, for example, alert you that
content within a unit is related to:
- Psychosocial Integrity
  - Behavioral Interventions
    - Incorporate behavioral management techniques
      when caring for a client.

QSEN COMPETENCIES

As you use the Review Modules, you will note the integration of the Quality and Safety Education for Nurses (QSEN) competencies throughout the chapters. These competencies are integral components of the curriculum of many nursing programs in the United States and prepare you to provide safe, high-quality care as a newly licensed nurse. Icons appear to draw your attention to the six QSEN competencies.

Safety: The minimization of risk factors that could cause injury or harm while promoting quality care and maintaining a secure environment for clients, self, and others.

Patient-Centered Care: The provision of caring and compassionate, culturally sensitive care that addresses clients' physiological, psychological, sociological, spiritual, and cultural needs, preferences, and values.

Evidence-Based Practice: The use of current knowledge from research and other credible sources, on which to base clinical judgment and client care.

Informatics: The use of information technology as a communication and information-gathering tool that supports clinical decision-making and scientifically based nursing practice.

Quality Improvement: Care related and organizational processes that involve the development and implementation of a plan to improve health care services and better meet clients' needs.

Teamwork and Collaboration: The delivery of client care in partnership with multidisciplinary members of the health care team to achieve continuity of care and positive client outcomes.

ICONS

Icons are used throughout the Review Module to draw your attention to particular areas. Keep an eye out for these icons.

(N) This icon is used for NCLEX Connections.

(G) This icon indicates gerontological considerations, or knowledge specific to the care of older adult clients.

Qs This icon is used for content related to safety and is a QSEN competency. When you see this icon, take note of safety concerns or steps that nurses can take to ensure client safety and a safe environment.

Qpcc This icon is a QSEN competency that indicates the importance of a holistic approach to providing care.

Qebp This icon, a QSEN competency, points out the integration of research into clinical practice.

Qi This icon is a QSEN competency and highlights the use of information technology to support nursing practice.

Qqi This icon is used to focus on the QSEN competency of integrating planning processes to meet clients' needs.

Qtc This icon highlights the QSEN competency of care delivery using an interprofessional approach.

M◇ This icon appears at the top-right of pages and indicates availability of an online media supplement, such as a graphic, animation, or video. If you have an electronic copy of the Review Module, this icon will appear alongside clickable links to media supplements. If you have a hard copy version of the Review Module, visit www.atitesting.com for details on how to access these features.

FEEDBACK

ATI welcomes feedback regarding this Review Module. Please provide comments to comments@atitesting.com.

Table of Contents

When reviewing the following chapters, keep in mind the relevant topics and tasks of the NCLEX outline, in particular:

Client Needs: Management of Care

CLIENT RIGHTS: Advocate for client rights and needs.

COLLABORATION WITH INTERDISCIPLINARY TEAM: Collaborate with interprofessional members when providing client care.

CONFIDENTIALITY/INFORMATION SECURITY: Maintain client confidentiality and privacy.

ETHICAL PRACTICE: Practice in an manner consistent with a code of ethics for registered nurses.

LEGAL RIGHTS AND RESPONSIBILITIES: Report client conditions as required by law.

Client Needs: Safety and Infection Control

ACCIDENT/ERROR/INJURY PREVENTION: Identify factors that influence accident/injury prevention.

USE OF RESTRAINTS/SAFETY DEVICES: Monitor/evaluate the client's response to restraints/safety device.

Client Needs: Psychosocial Integrity

COPING MECHANISMS: Assess the client's ability to adapt to temporary/permanent role changes.

MENTAL HEALTH CONCEPTS: Recognize the client use of defense mechanisms.

THERAPEUTIC COMMUNICATION
Assess verbal and nonverbal client communication needs.

Evaluate the effectiveness of communications with the client.

THERAPEUTIC ENVIRONMENT: Provide a therapeutic environment for clients.

UNIT 1   FOUNDATIONS FOR MENTAL HEALTH NURSING

CHAPTER 1 # Basic Mental Health Nursing Concepts

Provision of care to clients in mental health settings is based on standards of care set by the American Nurses Association, the American Psychiatric Nurses Association, and the International Society of Psychiatric-Mental Health Nurses. Foundational to this care is the use of the nursing process.

Nurses working in mental health settings should use the nursing process, as well as a holistic approach (biological, social, psychological, and spiritual aspects) to care for clients.

Nurses should use various methods to assess clients. These methods include observation, interviewing, physical examination, and collaboration.

ASSESSMENT

Each encounter with a client involves an ongoing assessment.

PSYCHOSOCIAL HISTORY

- Perception of own health, beliefs about illness and wellness Qpcc
- Activity/leisure activities, how the client passes time
- Use of substances/substance use disorder
- Stress level and coping abilities: usual coping strategies, support systems

Cultural beliefs and practices

- Assess the client's cultural health care beliefs, practices, and values.
- Assess for cultural factors that can impact the client's care.

> For example: Does the client's diet consist of culture-specific foods? Does the client have specific beliefs or practices regarding health care? How is the client's diagnosis viewed in his culture?

- The nurse's awareness of culture alleviates stereotyping and stigmatizing
- Use a trained interpreter when needed.

Spiritual and religious beliefs

Spiritual and religious beliefs affect the way in which a client finds meaning, hope, purpose, and a sense of peace.
- Spirituality refers to a client's internal values, sense of morality, and how he views the purpose of life. The client might not connect these spiritual views with religion.
- Religion refers to a client's beliefs according to an organized set of patterns of worship and rituals.
- Assist client to identify support persons and resources.

MENTAL STATUS EXAMINATION (MSE)

Level of consciousness

Described using the following terms, and observed behavior included in documentation.

Alert: The client is responsive and able to fully respond by opening her eyes and attending to a normal tone of voice and speech. She answers questions spontaneously and appropriately.

Lethargic: The client is able to open her eyes and respond but is drowsy and falls asleep readily.

Stuporous: The client requires vigorous or painful stimuli (pinching a tendon or rubbing the sternum) to elicit a brief response. She might not be able to respond verbally.

Comatose: The client is unconscious and does not respond to painful stimuli.
- Abnormal posturing in the client who is comatose
  - **Decorticate rigidity:** Flexion and internal rotation of upper-extremity joints and legs
  - **Decerebrate rigidity:** Neck and elbow extension, wrist and finger flexion

Physical appearance

Examination includes assessment of personal hygiene, grooming, and clothing choice. Expected findings with regard to this assessment are that the client is well-kempt, clean, and dressed appropriately for the given environment.

Behavior

Examination includes assessment of voluntary and involuntary body movements, and eye contact.

Mood: A client's mood provides information about the emotion that she is feeling.

Affect: A client's affect is an objective expression of mood, such as a flat affect or a lack of facial expression.

Cognitive and intellectual abilities

- Assess the client's orientation to time, person, and place.
- Assess the client's memory, both recent and remote.
  - **Immediate:** Ask the client to repeat a series of numbers or a list of objects.
  - **Recent:** Ask the client to recall recent events, such as visitors from the current day, or the purpose of the current mental health appointment or admission.
  - **Remote:** Ask the client to state a fact from his past that is verifiable, such as his birth date or his mother's maiden name.
- Assess the client's level of knowledge. For example, ask him what he knows about his current illness or hospitalization.
- Assess the client's ability to calculate. For example, can he count backward from 100 in serials of 7?
- Assess the client's ability to think abstractly. For example, can he interpret a cliché such as, "A bird in the hand is worth two in the bush"? The ability to interpret this demonstrates a higher-level thought process.
- Perform an objective assessment of the client's perception of his illness.
- Assess the client's judgment based on his answer to a hypothetical question. For example, how would he answer the question, "What would you do if there were a fire in your room?" The client should provide a logical response.
- Assess the client's rate and volume of speech, as well as the quality of his language. His speech should be articulate and his responses meaningful and appropriate.

STANDARDIZED SCREENING TOOLS

Mini-mental state examination (MMSE)

This examination is used to objectively assess a client's cognitive status by evaluating the following: Q**EBP**
- Orientation to time and place
- Attention span and ability to calculate by counting backward by seven
- Registration and recalling of objects
- Language, including naming of objects, following of commands, and ability to write

Glasgow Coma Scale

This examination is used to obtain a baseline assessment of a client's level of consciousness, and for ongoing assessment. Eye, verbal, and motor response is evaluated, and a number value based on that response is assigned. The highest value possible is 15, which indicates that the client is awake and responding appropriately. A score of 7 or less indicates that the client is in a coma.

CONSIDERATIONS ACROSS THE LIFESPAN

Children and adolescents

Assessment includes temperament, social and environmental factors, cultural and religious concerns, and developmental level. Q**PCC**
- Mentally healthy children and adolescents trust others, view the world as safe, accurately interpret their environments, master developmental tasks, and use appropriate coping skills.
- Children and adolescents experience some of the same mental health problems as adults.
- Mental health and developmental disorders are not always easily diagnosed, potentially resulting in delayed or inadequate treatment interventions. Factors contributing to this include the following.
  - Lack of the ability or necessary skills to describe what is happening
  - A wide variation of "normal" behavior, especially in different developmental stages
- Assess for mood; anxiety; developmental, behavioral, and eating disorders; and risk for self-injury or suicide.
- Use the standardized assessment tool, Home environment, Education/employment, Activities, Drug and substance use, Sexuality, and Suicide/depression, Savagery (HEADSSS) psychosocial assessment, to evaluate risk factors in the adolescent. Q**EBP**
  - **Home environment:** What is the client's relationship like with his parents and other family members living in the home?
  - **Education/employment:** Is the client employed? How is the client's school performance?
  - **Activities:** Does the client participate in sports or other activities? How does the client interact with peers?
  - **Drug and substance use:** Does the client use substances such as alcohol, tobacco, or marijuana?
  - **Suicide/depression:** Is the client at risk for suicide or self-injury? Does the client have indications of depression?
  - **Savagery:** Is the client exposed to abuse in his home or violence in his neighborhood?

Older adults

- In addition to the aforementioned assessments, a comprehensive assessment of the older adult client includes the following:
    - Functional ability, such as the ability to independently get dressed or manage household tasks
    - Economic and social status
    - Environmental factors, such as stairways in the home, that can affect the client's well-being and lifestyle
    - Physical assessment
- Standardized assessment tools that are appropriate for the older adult population include the following.
    - Geriatric Depression Scale (short form) Ⓒ
    - Michigan Alcoholism Screening Test: Geriatric Version
    - MMSE
    - Pain assessments including visual analogue scales, Wong-Baker FACES Pain Rating Scale, the Faces Pain Scale-Revised, the McGill Pain Questionnaire (MPQ), and the Pain Assessment in Advanced Dementia (PAINAD) scale
- Conduct an assessment of all clients, including older adult clients in the following manner.
    - Use a private, quiet space with adequate lighting to accommodate for impaired vision and hearing.
    - Make an introduction, and determine the client's name preference.
    - Stand or sit at the client's level to conduct the interview, rather than standing over a client who is lying in bed or sitting in a chair.
    - Use touch to communicate caring as appropriate. However, respect the client's personal space if he does not wish to be touched.
    - Be sure to include questions relating to difficulty sleeping, incontinence, falls or other injuries, depression, dizziness, and loss of energy.
    - Include the family and significant others as appropriate.
    - Obtain a detailed medication history.
    - Following the interview, summarize and ask for feedback from the client.

MENTAL HEALTH DIAGNOSES

- The *Diagnostic and Statistical Manual of Mental Disorders*, 5th Edition (DSM-5), published by the American Psychiatric Association, is used as a diagnostic tool to identify mental health diagnoses. It is used by mental health professionals for clients who have mental health disorders.
- Nurses use the DSM-5 in the mental health setting to identify diagnoses and diagnostic criteria to guide assessment; to identify nursing diagnoses; and to plan, implement, and evaluate care. Ⓠ EBP

SERIOUS MENTAL ILLNESS

- Includes disorders classified as severe and persistent mental illnesses
- Clients often have difficulty with activities of daily living (ADLs)
- Can be chronic or recurrent

ROLE AND LIFE CHANGES

- Role transitions include loss of employment, divorce, retirement, grand-parenthood, widowhood, death of parent, and becoming a caregiver or recipient of care.
- Some role changes are predicted, such as an upcoming retirement. However, the client might find that others are unexpected, such as becoming the recipient of care due to a sudden illness or injury.
- Assessing the client's ability to adapt and cope includes the following.
    - Health status and functional abilities
    - Living arrangements and employability
    - Personality factors (e.g., attitudes)
    - Client, caregiver and family assessments
    - Levels of information (e.g., community programs)
    - Medication use and supplemental services
- Evaluating whether client has successfully adapted includes the following.
    - Able to state positive coping behaviors
    - Able to identify maladaptive coping behaviors
    - Able to participate in community resources
    - Able to list stress reduction techniques
    - Able to maintain housing and employment

THERAPEUTIC STRATEGIES IN THE MENTAL HEALTH SETTING

Counseling
- Using therapeutic communication skills
- Assisting with problem solving
- Crisis intervention
- Stress management

Milieu therapy
- Orienting the client to the physical setting
- Identifying rules and boundaries of the setting
- Ensuring a safe environment for the client
- Assisting the client to participate in appropriate activities

Promotion of self-care activities
- Offering assistance with self-care tasks
- Allowing time for the client to complete self-care tasks
- Setting incentives to promote client self-care

Psychobiological interventions
- Administering prescribed medications
- Providing teaching to the client/family about medications
- Monitoring for adverse effects and effectiveness of pharmacological therapy

Cognitive and behavioral therapies
- Modeling
- Operant conditioning
- Systematic desensitization

Health teaching: Teaching social and coping skills

Health promotion and health maintenance
- Assisting the client with cessation of smoking
- Monitoring other health conditions

Case management: Coordinating holistic care to include medical, mental health, and social services

Application Exercises

1. A charge nurse is discussing mental status examinations with a newly licensed nurse. Which of the following statements by the newly licensed nurse indicates an understanding of the teaching? (Select all that apply.)

   A. "To assess cognitive ability, I should ask the client to count backward by sevens."

   B. "To assess affect, I should observe the client's facial expression."

   C. "To assess language ability, I should instruct the client to write a sentence."

   D. "To assess remote memory, I should have the client repeat a list of objects."

   E. "To assess the client's abstract thinking, I should ask the client to identify our most recent presidents."

2. A nurse is planning care for a client who has a mental health disorder. Which of the following actions should the nurse include as a psychobiological intervention?

   A. Assist the client with systematic desensitization therapy.

   B. Teach the client appropriate coping mechanisms.

   C. Assess the client for comorbid health conditions.

   D. Monitor the client for adverse effects of medications.

3. A nurse in an outpatient mental health clinic is preparing to conduct an initial client interview. When conducting the interview, which of the following actions should the nurse identify as the priority?

   A. Coordinate holistic care with social services.

   B. Identify the client's perception of her mental health status.

   C. Include the client's family in the interview.

   D. Teach the client about her current mental health disorder.

4. A nurse is told during change-of-shift report that a client is stuporous. When assessing the client, which of the following findings should the nurse expect?

   A. The client arouses briefly in response to a sternal rub.

   B. The client has a Glasgow Coma Scale score less than 7.

   C. The client exhibits decorticate rigidity.

   D. The client is alert but disoriented to time and place.

5. A nurse is planning a peer group discussion about the *Diagnostic and Statistical Manual of Mental Disorders*, 5th Edition (DSM-5). Which of the following information is appropriate to include in the discussion? (Select all that apply.)

   A. The DSM-5 includes client education handouts for mental health disorders.

   B. The DSM-5 establishes diagnostic criteria for individual mental health disorders.

   C. The DSM-5 indicates recommended pharmacological treatment for mental health disorders.

   D. The DSM-5 assists nurses in planning care for client's who have mental health disorders.

   E. The DSM-5 indicates expected assessment findings of mental health disorders.

PRACTICE Active Learning Scenario

A nurse is admitting an older adult client who has depression to an acute mental health facility. Use the ATI Active Learning Template: Basic Concept to complete this item.

UNDERLYING PRINCIPLES

- Identify the standardized assessment tool the nurse should use to assess the older adult client's severity of depression.
- Identify at least four assessment/communication techniques the nurse should use when assessing the older adult client.

NURSING INTERVENTIONS: Identify at least three factors the nurse should assess to determine if role and life changes are contributing to the client's depression.

Application Exercises Key

1. A. **CORRECT:** Counting backward by 7s is an appropriate technique to assess a client's cognitive ability.

   B. **CORRECT:** Observing a client's facial expression is appropriate when assessing affect.

   C. **CORRECT:** Writing a sentence is an indication of language ability.

   D. Asking the client to repeat a list of objects is appropriate to assess immediate, rather than remote, memory.

   E. Asking the client to identify recent presidents is appropriate to assess cognitive knowledge rather than abstract thinking.

   Ⓝ *NCLEX® Connection: Psychosocial Integrity, Mental Health Concepts*

2. A. Assisting with systematic desensitization therapy is a cognitive and behavioral, rather than a psychobiological intervention.

   B. Teaching appropriate coping mechanisms is a counseling or health teaching, rather than a psychobiological intervention.

   C. Assessing for comorbid health conditions is health promotion and maintenance, rather than a psychobiological, intervention.

   D. **CORRECT:** Monitoring for adverse effects of medications is an example of a psychobiological intervention.

   Ⓝ *NCLEX® Connection: Psychosocial Integrity, Mental Health Concepts*

3. A. It is appropriate to coordinate holistic care for the client with social services as part of case management. However, it is not the highest priority action when using the nursing process approach to client care.

   B. **CORRECT:** Assessment is the priority action when using the nursing process approach to client care. Identifying the client's perception of her mental health status provides important information about the client's psychosocial history.

   C. If the client wishes, it is appropriate to include the client's family in the interview. However, it is not the highest priority action when using the nursing process approach to client care.

   D. It is appropriate to teach the client about her disorder. However, it is not the highest priority action when using the nursing process approach to client care.

   Ⓝ *NCLEX® Connection: Health Promotion and Maintenance, Health Screening*

4. A. **CORRECT:** A client who is stuporous requires vigorous or painful stimuli to elicit a response.

   B. A GCS score of less than 7 indicates a comatose, rather than stuporous, level of consciousness.

   C. Abnormal posturing is associated with a comatose, rather than stuporous, level of consciousness.

   D. A client who is stuporous is not alert.

   Ⓝ *NCLEX® Connection: Physiological Adaptation, Unexpected Response to Therapies*

5. A. The DSM-5 is used by mental health professionals. However, it does not include client education handouts.

   B. **CORRECT:** The DSM-5 establishes diagnostic criteria for mental health disorders.

   C. The DSM-5 does not indicate pharmacological treatment for mental health disorders.

   D. **CORRECT:** Nurses use the DSM-5 to plan, implement, and evaluate care for client's who have mental health disorders.

   E. **CORRECT:** The DSM-5 identifies expected findings for mental health disorders.

   Ⓝ *NCLEX® Connection: Psychosocial Integrity, Mental Health Concepts*

PRACTICE Answer

Using ATI Active Learning Template: Basic Concept

UNDERLYING PRINCIPLES
- Standardized assessment tool for depression: Geriatric Depression Scale
- Assessment/communication techniques
  - Use a private, quiet space with adequate lighting to accommodate for impaired vision and hearing.
  - Make an introduction, and determine the client's name preference.
  - Stand or sit at the client's level to conduct the interview.
  - Use touch to communicate caring as appropriate.
  - Include questions relating to difficulty sleeping, incontinence, falls or other injuries, depression, dizziness, and loss of energy.
  - Include the family and significant others as appropriate.
  - Obtain a detailed medication history.
  - Following the interview, summarize and ask for feedback from the client.

NURSING INTERVENTIONS: Assessment of role and life changes
- Recent role transitions and whether they were expected or unexpected
- Client's knowledge and use of positive coping behaviors
- Participation in community resources
- Client's knowledge and use of stress reduction techniques
- Ability to maintain housing or employment

Ⓝ *NCLEX® Connection: Psychosocial Integrity, Mental Health Concepts*

CHAPTER 2 *Legal and Ethical Issues*

A nurse who works in the mental health setting is responsible for practicing ethically, competently, safely, and in a manner consistent with all local, state, and federal laws.

Nurses must have an understanding of ethical principles and how they apply when providing care for clients in mental health settings.

Nurses are responsible for understanding and protecting client rights.

LEGAL RIGHTS OF CLIENTS IN THE MENTAL HEALTH SETTING

- Clients who have a mental health disorder diagnosis or who are receiving acute care for mental health disorder are guaranteed the same civil rights as any other citizen. These include the following.
  - The right to humane treatment and care, such as medical and dental care
  - The right to vote
  - The rights related to granting, forfeiture, or denial of a driver's license
  - The right to due process of law, including the right to press legal charges against another person
- Clients also have various specific rights, including the following.
  - Informed consent and the right to refuse treatment
  - Confidentiality
  - A written plan of care/treatment that includes discharge follow-up, as well as participation in the care plan and review of that plan
  - Communication with people outside the mental health facility, including family members, attorneys, and other health care professionals
  - Provision of adequate interpretive services if needed
  - Care provided with respect, dignity, and without discrimination
  - Freedom from harm related to physical or pharmacological restraint, seclusion, and any physical or mental abuse or neglect
  - A psychiatric advance directive that includes the client's treatment preferences in the event that an involuntary admission is necessary
  - Provision of care with the least restrictive interventions necessary to meet the client's needs without allowing him to be a threat to himself or others

- Some legal issues regarding health care are decided in court using a specialized civil category called a tort. A tort is a wrongful act or injury committed by an entity or person against another person or another person's property. Torts can be used to decide liability issues, as well as intentional issues that can involve criminal penalties, such as abuse of a client.
- State laws can vary greatly. The nurse is responsible for knowing specific laws regarding client care within the state or states in which the nurse practices.

ETHICAL ISSUES FOR CLIENTS IN THE MENTAL HEALTH SETTING

- In comparison to laws, statutes, and regulations (enacted by local, state, or federal government), ethical issues are philosophical ideas regarding right and wrong.
- Nurses are frequently confronted with ethical dilemmas regarding client care (bioethical issues).
- Because ethics are philosophical and involve values and morals, there is frequently no clear-cut, simple resolution to an ethical dilemma.
- The nurse must use ethical principles to decide ethical issues. These include the following:

Beneficence: The quality of doing good; can be described as charity

> Example: A nurse helps a newly admitted client who has a psychotic disorder to feel safe in the environment of the mental health facility.

Autonomy: The client's right to make her own decisions. But the client must accept the consequences of those decisions. The client must also respect the decisions of others.

> Example: Rather than giving advice to a client who has difficulty making decisions, a nurse helps the client explore all alternatives and arrive at a choice.

Justice: Fair and equal treatment for all

> Example: During a treatment team meeting, a nurse leads a discussion regarding whether or not two clients who broke the same facility rule were treated equally.

Fidelity: Loyalty and faithfulness to the client and to one's duty

> Example: A client asks a nurse to be present when he talks to his mother for the first time in a year. The nurse remains with the client during this interaction.

Veracity: Honesty when dealing with a client

> Example: A client states, "You and that other staff member were talking about me, weren't you?" The nurse truthfully replies, "We were discussing ways to help you relate to the other clients in a more positive way."

CONFIDENTIALITY

- The client's right to privacy is protected by the Health Insurance Portability and Accountability Act (HIPAA) Privacy Rule of 2003.
- It is important to gain an understanding of the federal law and of state laws as they relate to confidentiality in specific health care facilities.
- The nurse should share information about the client, either verbal or written, only with those who are responsible for implementing the client's treatment plan.
- Only if the client provides consent should the nurse share information with other persons not involved in the client treatment plan.
- Specific mental health issues include disclosing HIV status, the duty to warn and protect third parties, and the reporting of child and vulnerable adult abuse.
- If the nurse becomes aware that a client's right to privacy is being violated, for example if a conversation in the elevator is overheard, he should immediately take action to stop the violation.

RESOURCES FOR SOLVING ETHICAL CLIENT ISSUES

- Code of Ethics for Nurses, found at http://nursingworld.org
- Patient Care Partnership, found at www.aha.org
- The nurse practice act of a specific state
- Legal advice from attorneys
- Facility policies
- Other members of the health care team, including facility bioethics committee (if available)
- Members of the clergy and other spiritual or ethical counselors

TYPES OF ADMISSION TO A MENTAL HEALTH FACILITY

Voluntary admission: The client or client's guardian chooses admission to a mental health facility in order to obtain treatment. A voluntarily admitted client has the right to apply for release at any time. This client is considered competent, and so has the right to refuse medication and treatment.

Temporary emergency admission: The client is admitted for emergent mental health care due to the inability to make decisions regarding care. The medical healthcare provider may initiate the admission which is then evaluated by a mental healthcare provider. The length of the temporary admission varies by the client's need and state laws but often is not to exceed 15 days.

Involuntary admission: The client enters the mental health facility against her will for an indefinite period of time. The admission is based on the client's need for psychiatric treatment, the risk of harm to self or others, or the inability to provide self-care. **Qs**

- The number of physicians, which is usually two, required to certify that the client's condition requires commitment varies from state to state. This may be imposed by a family member, legal guardian, primary care provider, or a mental health provider.
- The client can request a legal review of the admission at any time.
- An involuntary admission is limited to 60 days at which time a psychiatric and legal review of the admission is required.
- Clients admitted under involuntary commitment are still considered competent and have the right to refuse treatment, including medication. The client who has been judged incompetent has a temporary or permanent guardian, usually a family member if possible, appointed by the court. The guardian can sign informed consent for the client. The guardian is expected to consider what the client would want if he were still competent.

Long-term involuntary admission: A type of admission that is similar to temporary commitment but must be imposed by the courts. Time of commitment varies, but is usually 60 to 180 days. Sometimes, there is no set release date.

CLIENT RIGHTS REGARDING SECLUSION AND RESTRAINT

- Nurses must know and follow federal/state/facility policies that govern the use of restraints.
- Use of seclusion rooms and/or restraints can be warranted and authorized for clients in some cases.
- Restraints are either physical or chemical, such as neuroleptic medication to calm the client.
- A client may voluntarily request a temporary timeout in cases in which the environment is disturbing or seems too stimulating. A timeout is different from prescribed seclusion since a timeout is by the request of the client.
- In general, the provider should prescribe seclusion and/or restraint for the shortest duration necessary, and only if less restrictive measures are not sufficient. They are for the physical protection of the client and/or the protection of other clients and staff. **Qs**
- Less restrictive measures
  - Verbal interventions such as telling the client to calm down
  - Diversion or redirection
  - Providing a calm, quiet environment
  - Offering a PRN medication (though technically a chemical restraint, medications are considered less restrictive than a mechanical restraint)

- The nurse should never use seclusion or restraint for
  - Convenience of the staff
  - Punishment of the client
  - Clients who are extremely physically or mentally unstable
  - Clients who cannot tolerate the decreased stimulation of a seclusion room
- When the nurse has tried all other less restrictive means to prevent a client from harming self or others, the following must occur in order to use seclusion or restraint.
  - The provider must prescribe the seclusion or restraint in writing.
  - Time limits for seclusion or restraints are based upon the age of the client.
    - Age 18 years and older: 4 hr
    - Age 9 to 17 years: 2 hr
    - Age 8 years and younger: 1 hr
  - If the need for seclusion or restraint continues the provider must reassess the client and rewrite the prescription, specifying the type of restraint, every 24 hr or the frequency of time specified by facility policy.
  - The facility protocol should identify the nursing responsibilities, including how often the client should be Q_{EBP}
    - Assessed (including for safety and physical needs), and the client's behavior documented
    - Offered food and fluid
    - Toileted
    - Monitored for vital signs
    - Monitored for pain
  - Complete documentation every 15 to 30 minutes (or according to facility policy) includes a description of the following.
    - Precipitating events and behavior of the client prior to seclusion or restraint
    - Alternative actions taken to avoid seclusion or restraint
    - The time treatment began
    - The client's current behavior, what foods or fluids were offered and taken, needs provided for, and vital signs
    - Medication administration
    - Time released from restraints
- The nurse can use seclusion or restraints without first obtaining a provider's written prescription if it is an emergency situation. If this emergency treatment is initiated, the nurse must obtain the written prescription within a specified period of time (usually 15 to 30 min).

TORT LAW IN THE MENTAL HEALTH SETTING

Although intentional torts can occur in any health care setting, they are particularly likely to occur in mental health settings due to the increased likelihood of violence and client behavior that can be challenging to facility staff. A tort is referred to as a civil wrong doing, in which monetary damages can potentially be awarded to the plaintiff (injured party) and collected from the defendant (responsible party).

EXAMPLES OF TORTS

False imprisonment: Confining a client to a specific area, such as a seclusion room, is false imprisonment if the reason for such confinement is for the convenience of the staff.

Assault: Making a threat to a client's person, such as approaching the client in a threatening manner with a syringe in hand, is considered assault.

Battery: Touching a client in a harmful or offensive way is considered battery. This would occur if the nurse threatening the client with a syringe actually grabbed the client and gave an injection.

DOCUMENTATION

It is vital to clearly and objectively document information related to violent or other unusual episodes. The nurse should document the following. Q_{QI}

Client behavior in a clear and objective manner

> Example: The client suddenly began to run down the hall with both hands in the air, screaming obscenities.

Staff response to disruptive, violent, or potentially harmful behavior, such as suicide threats or potential or actual harm to others, including timelines and the extent of response

> Example: The client states, "I'm going to pound (other client) into the ground." Client has picked up a chair and is standing 3 ft from other client with chair held over his head in both hands. Nurse calls for help. Client is immediately told by nurse, "Put down the chair, and back away from (the other person)." Other client moved away to safe area. Five other staff members respond to verbal call for help within 30 seconds and stood several yards from client. Client then put the chair down, quietly turned around, walked to his room, and sat on the bed.

Time the nurse notified the provider and any prescriptions received.

Application Exercises

1. A nurse in an emergency mental health facility is caring for a group of clients. The nurse should identify that which of the following clients requires a temporary emergency admission?

   A. A client who has schizophrenia with delusions of grandeur

   B. A client who has manifestations of depression and attempted suicide a year ago

   C. A client who has borderline personality disorder and assaulted a homeless man with a metal rod

   D. A client who has bipolar disorder and paces quickly around the room while talking to himself

2. A nurse decides to put a client who has a psychotic disorder in seclusion overnight because the unit is very short-staffed, and the client frequently fights with other clients. The nurse's actions are an example of which of the following torts?

   A. Invasion of privacy

   B. False imprisonment

   C. Assault

   D. Battery

3. A client tells a nurse, "Don't tell anyone, but I hid a sharp knife under my mattress in order to protect myself from my roommate, who is always yelling at me and threatening me." Which of the following actions should the nurse take?

   A. Keep the client's communication confidential, but talk to the client daily, using therapeutic communication to convince him to admit to hiding the knife.

   B. Keep the client's communication confidential, but watch the client and his roommate closely.

   C. Tell the client that this must be reported to the health care team because it concerns the health and safety of the client and others.

   D. Report the incident to the health care team, but do not inform the client of the intention to do so.

4. A nurse is caring for a client who is in mechanical restraints. Which of the following statements should the nurse include in the documentation? (Select all that apply.)

   A. "Client ate most of his breakfast."

   B. "Client was offered 8 oz of water every hr."

   C. "Client shouted obscenities at assistive personnel."

   D. "Client received chlorpromazine 15 mg by mouth at 1000."

   E. "Client acted out after lunch."

5. A nurse hears a newly licensed nurse discussing a client's hallucinations in the hallway with another nurse. Which of the following actions should the nurse take first?

   A. Notify the nurse manager.

   B. Tell the nurse to stop discussing the behavior.

   C. Provide an in-service program about confidentiality.

   D. Complete an incident report.

PRACTICE Active Learning Scenario

A nurse in a mental health facility is caring for an adult client who has bipolar disorder. The client becomes violent and begins throwing objects at other clients. After calling for assistance, what actions should the nurse take next? Use the ATI Active Learning Template: Basic Concept to complete this item.

NURSING INTERVENTIONS: Describe at least four nursing interventions with rationales.

Application Exercises Key

1.   A. The presence of delusions does not constitute a clear reason for a temporary emergency admission unless they present a danger for the client or others.

    B. Clinical findings of depression do not constitute a clear reason for a temporary emergency admission unless the client is currently at risk for suicide.

    C. **CORRECT:** A client who is a current danger to self or others is a candidate for a temporary emergency admission.

    D. A client who is pacing does not constitute a clear reason for a temporary emergency admission.

    Ⓝ *NCLEX® Connection: Psychosocial Integrity, Crisis Intervention*

2.   A. Invasion of privacy is the sharing or obtaining of the client's confidential information without the client's consent.

    B. **CORRECT:** A civil wrong that violates a client's civil rights is a tort. In this case, it is false imprisonment, which is the confining of a client to a specific area, such as a seclusion room, if the reason for such confinement is for the convenience of staff.

    C. Assault is making a threat to the client's person.

    D. Justice involves the fair and equal treatment of clients.

    Ⓝ *NCLEX® Connection: Safety and Infection Control, Accident/Error/ Injury Prevention*

3.   A. The nurse should use therapeutic communication with the client. However, based on the nature of the information, the nurse cannot keep the information confidential from everyone despite the client's request.

    B. Based on the nature of the information, the nurse cannot keep the information confidential from everyone despite the client's request.

    C. **CORRECT:** The information presented by the client is a serious safety issue that the nurse must report to the health care team. Using the ethical principle of veracity, the student tells the client truthfully what must be done regarding the issue.

    D. The nurse should inform the if the information will be reported to the health care team.

    Ⓝ *NCLEX® Connection: Management of Care, Ethical Practice*

4.   A. The nurse should document objective information regarding intake in the client's medical record.

    B. **CORRECT:** How much water was offered and how often it was offered is objective data that the nurse should document when caring for a client in mechanical restraints.

    C. **CORRECT:** A description of the client's verbal communication is objective data that the nurse should document when caring for a client in mechanical restraints.

    D. **CORRECT:** The dosage and time of medication administration is objective data that the nurse should document when caring for a client in mechanical restraints

    E. The nurse should document objective information regarding the client's behavior in the client's medical record.

    Ⓝ *NCLEX® Connection: Safety and Infection Control, Use of Restraints/Safety Devices*

5.   A. The nurse should notify the nurse manager if the client's right to privacy is violated. However, there is another action that the nurse should take first.

    B. **CORRECT:** The greatest risk to this client is an invasion of privacy through the sharing of confidential information in a public place. The first action the nurse should take is to tell the newly licensed nurse to stop discussing the client's hallucinations in a public location.

    C. The nurse should provide an in-service program for staff about confidentiality. However, there is another action that the nurse should take first.

    D. The nurse should complete an incident report about the violation of the client's right to privacy. However, there is another action that the nurse should take first.

    Ⓝ *NCLEX® Connection: Management of Care, Confidentiality/ Information Security*

PRACTICE Answer

Using the ATI Active Learning Template: Basic Concept

NURSING INTERVENTIONS

- Tell the client calmly to sit down. Verbal intervention is the least restrictive method when dealing with an aggressive client.
- Provide the client with a decreased-stimulation environment and attempt diversion or redirection. These interventions are less restrictive than seclusion or restraint and the nurse should attempt these interventions prior to more restrictive actions.
- Offer the client a PRN medication, such as diazepam. It can be necessary for the nurse to administer diazepam to calm the client and is considered less restrictive than mechanical restraints.
- Place the client in a monitored seclusion room. It can become necessary to place the client in seclusion if the client persists in the behavior after attempting less restrictive interventions.
- Obtain a prescription for mechanical restraints. Follow facility policy for the application of restraints and the monitoring and documentation required for the client's care.

Ⓝ *NCLEX® Connection: Psychosocial Integrity, Behavioral Interventions*

UNIT 1 FOUNDATIONS FOR MENTAL HEALTH NURSING

CHAPTER 3 *Effective Communication*

Communication is a complex process of sending, receiving, and comprehending messages between two or more people. It is a dynamic and ongoing process that creates a unique experience between the participants.

Communicating effectively is a skill that the nurse develops. Nurses use communication when providing care to establish relationships, demonstrate caring, obtain information, and assist with changing behaviors. Foundational to the nurse-client relationship is therapeutic communication.

BASIC COMMUNICATION

BASIC LEVELS OF COMMUNICATION Qpcc

Intrapersonal communication: Communication that occurs within an individual. Also identified as "self-talk." This occurs within one's self and is the internal discussion that takes place when an individual is thinking thoughts and not outwardly verbalizing them. In nursing, intrapersonal communication allows the nurse to perform a self-assessment of her values or beliefs prior to caring for a client whose diagnosis can trigger an emotional response.

Interpersonal communication: Communication that occurs one-on-one with another individual. In nursing, interpersonal communication is used when the nurse obtains a psychosocial history from a client or when listening to a client discuss his feelings.

Small-group communication: Communication that occurs between two or more people in a small group. In nursing, small-group communication allows the nurse to discuss a change in the client's behavior with the health care team or discuss concerns with clients during a group therapy session.

Public communication: Communication that occurs within large groups of people. In nursing, this commonly occurs during educational endeavors where the nurse is teaching a large group of individuals. For example, the nurse may teach about suicide prevention with high school students at a school assembly.

Transpersonal communication: Communication that addresses an individual's spiritual needs and provides interventions to meet those needs. In nursing, transpersonal communication is used when the nurse assists the client with meditation as a means of relaxation.

Verbal communication

Vocabulary
- These are the words that are used to communicate either a written or a spoken message.
- Limited vocabulary or speaking a language other than English can make it difficult for the nurse to communicate with the client. Use of medical jargon can decrease client understanding.

Denotative/connotative meaning
- When communicating, participants must share meanings.
- Words that have multiple meanings can cause miscommunication if they are interpreted differently.

Clarity/brevity
- The shortest, simplest communication is usually most effective.
- The client can have difficulty understanding communication that is long and complex.

Timing/relevance
- Knowing when to communicate allows the receiver to be more attentive to the message.
- Communicating with a client who is in pain or distracted will make it difficult for the nurse to convey the message.

Pacing
- The rate of speech can communicate a meaning to the receiver.
- Speaking rapidly can communicate the impression that the nurse is in a rush and does not have time for the client.

Intonation
- The tone of voice can communicate a variety of feelings.
- The nurse can communicate feelings, such as acceptance, judgment, and dislike through tone of voice.

Nonverbal communication

Nurses should be aware of how they communicate nonverbally. The nurse should assess the client's nonverbal communications for the meaning being conveyed, remembering that culture impacts interpretation.

Attention to the following behaviors is important, as it is compared to the verbal message being conveyed.
- Appearance
- Posture
- Gait
- Facial expressions
- Eye contact
- Gestures
- Sounds
- Territoriality
- Personal space
- Silence

THERAPEUTIC COMMUNICATION

Therapeutic communication is the purposeful use of communication to build and maintain helping relationships with clients, families, and significant others. Therapeutic communication is essential when caring for a client who has a mental health disorder because of the emotional as well as the physical effects of the disorder on the client. Qpcc

- The nurse uses interactive, purposeful communication skills to
  - Elicit and attend to the client's thoughts, feelings, concerns, and needs.
  - Express empathy and genuine concern for the client's and family's issues.
  - Obtain information and give feedback about the client's condition.
  - Intervene to promote functional behavior and effective interpersonal relationships.
  - Evaluate the client's progress toward goals and outcomes.
- Children and older adults frequently require altered techniques to enhance communication. Ⓖ
- Effective use of the nursing process depends on therapeutic communication between the nurse, the client, the client's family, and the interprofessional team.

CHARACTERISTICS
- Client centered: not social or reciprocal
- Purposeful, planned, and goal-directed

ESSENTIAL COMPONENTS

Time
- Plan for and allow adequate time to communicate.
- The nurse should be aware that clients who have certain mental health disorders such as major depressive disorder or schizophrenia can require a longer period of time to respond to questions.

Attending behaviors or active listening
- These are nonverbal means of conveying interest in another.
- Eye contact typically conveys interest and respect but varies by situation and culture.
- Body language and posture can demonstrate level of comfort and ease.
- Vocal quality enhances rapport and emphasizes particular topics or issues.
- Verbal tracking provides feedback by restating or summarizing a client's statements.

Caring attitude: Show concern and facilitate an emotional connection with the client and the client's family.

Honesty: Be open, direct, truthful, and sincere.

Trust: Demonstrate reliability without doubt or question.

Empathy: Convey an objective awareness and understanding of the feelings, emotions, and behaviors of others, including trying to envision what it must be like to be in the position of the client and the client's family.

Nonjudgmental attitude: This is a display of acceptance that will encourage open, honest communication.

NURSING PROCESS

ASSESSMENT
- Assess verbal and nonverbal communication needs.
- Identify any cultural considerations that can impact communication, such as the use of eye contact or perception of personal space or touch. Qpcc
- Consider the client's developmental level and how communication should be altered during the assessment phase.

CHILDREN
- Use simple, straightforward language.
- Be aware of own nonverbal messages, as children are sensitive to nonverbal communication.
- Enhance communication by being at the child's eye level.
- Incorporate play in interactions.
- Be aware of the child's level of development.

ADOLESCENTS
- Determine how the adolescent perceives the mental health diagnosis. Is the adolescent at risk for refusal of treatment due to a desire to be "normal"?
- Identify if the mental health diagnosis affects the client's relationship with her peers.

OLDER ADULT CLIENTS Ⓖ
- Recognize that the client might require amplification.
- Minimize distractions, and face the client when speaking.
- Allow plenty of time for the client to respond.
- When impaired communication is assessed, ask for input from caregivers or family to determine the extent of the deficits and how best to communicate.

PLANNING
- Minimize distractions.
- Provide for privacy.
- Identify mutually agreed-upon client outcomes.
- Set priorities according to the client's needs.
- Plan for adequate time for interventions.

IMPLEMENTATION
- Establish a trusting nurse-client relationship. The client feels more at ease during the implementation phase once a helping relationship is established.
- Provide empathetic responses and explanations to the client by using observations and providing hope, humor, and information.

EFFECTIVE COMMUNICATION SKILLS AND TECHNIQUES

Silence: Silence allows time for meaningful reflection.

Active listening: The nurse is able to hear, observe, and understand what the client communicates and to provide feedback.

Questions: Questions allow the nurse to obtain specific or additional information from the client.
- **Open-ended questions:** Facilitates spontaneous responses and interactive discussion.
- **Closed-ended questions:** Helpful if used sparingly during the initial interaction to obtain specific data. The nurse should avoid using repeated closed-ended questions which can block further communication.
- **Projective questions:** Uses "what if" or similar questions to assist clients in exploring feelings and to gain greater understanding of problems and possible solutions
- **Presupposition questions:** Explores the client's life goals or motivations by presenting a hypothetical situation in which the client no longer has the mental health disorder

Clarifying techniques: This technique is used to determine if the message received was accurate:
- **Restating:** Uses the client's exact words.
- **Reflecting:** Directs the focus back to the client in order for the client to examine his feelings.
- **Paraphrasing:** Restates the client's feelings and thoughts for the client to confirm what has been communicated.
- **Exploring:** Allows the nurse to gather more information regarding important topics mentioned by the client.

Offering general leads, broad opening statements: This encourages the client to determine where the communication can start and to continue talking.

Showing acceptance and recognition: This technique acknowledges the nurse's interest and nonjudgmental attitude.

Focusing: This technique helps the client to concentrate on what is important.

Giving information: This technique provides details that the client might need for decision making.

Presenting reality: This technique is used to help the client focus on what is actually happening and to dispel delusions, hallucinations, or faulty beliefs.

Summarizing: Summarizing emphasizes important points and reviews what has been discussed.

Offering self: Use of this technique demonstrates a willingness to spend time with the client. Indicates to the client that the nurse has genuine concern.

Touch: If appropriate, therapeutic touch communicates caring and can provide comfort to the client.

BARRIERS TO EFFECTIVE COMMUNICATION

- Asking irrelevant personal questions
- Offering personal opinions
- Giving advice
- Giving false reassurance
- Minimizing feelings
- Changing the topic
- Asking "why" questions
- Offering value judgments
- Excessive questioning
- Responding approvingly or disapprovingly

Application Exercises

1. A charge nurse is conducting a class on therapeutic communication to a group of newly licensed nurses. Which of the following aspects of communication should the nurse identify as a component of verbal communication?

    A. Personal space

    B. Posture

    C. Eye contact

    D. Intonation

2. A nurse in an acute mental health facility is communicating with a client. The client states, "I can't sleep. I stay up all night." The nurse responds, "You are having difficulty sleeping?" Which of the following therapeutic communication techniques is the nurse demonstrating?

    A. Offering general leads

    B. Summarizing

    C. Focusing

    D. Restating

3. A nurse is communicating with a client who was just admitted for treatment of a substance use disorder. Which of the following communication techniques should the nurse identify as a barrier to therapeutic communication?

    A. Offering advice

    B. Reflecting

    C. Listening attentively

    D. Giving information

4. A nurse caring for a client who has anorexia nervosa. Which of the following examples demonstrates the nurse's use of interpersonal communication?

    A. The nurse discusses the client's weight loss during a health care team meeting.

    B. The nurse examines her own personal feelings about clients who have anorexia nervosa.

    C. The nurse asks the client about her body image perception.

    D. The nurse presents an educational session about anorexia nervosa to a large group of adolescents.

5. A nurse is caring for the parents of a child who has demonstrated recent changes in behavior and mood. When the mother of the child asks the nurse for reassurance about her son's condition, which of the following responses should the nurse make?

    A. "I think your son is getting better. What have you noticed?"

    B. "I'm sure everything will be okay. It just takes time to heal."

    C. "I'm not sure what's wrong. Have you asked the doctor about your concerns?"

    D. "I understand you're concerned. Let's discuss what concerns you specifically."

PRACTICE Active Learning Scenario

A nurse in a mental health facility is preparing to conduct a class with older adult clients on grief and loss. Use the ATI Active Learning Template: Basic Concept to complete this item.

NURSING INTERVENTIONS: Describe at least four verbal or nonverbal communication interventions the nurse should employ when working with older adult clients.

Application Exercises Key

1. A. Personal space is a component of nonverbal communication.

    B. Posture is a component of nonverbal communication.

    C. Eye contact is a component of nonverbal communication.

    D. **CORRECT:** The nurse should identify intonation as a component of verbal communication. Intonation is the tone of one's voice and can communicate a variety of feelings.

    Ⓝ *NCLEX® Connection: Psychosocial Integrity, Therapeutic Communication*

2. A. Offering general leads allows the nurse to take the direction of the discussion.

    B. Summarizing enables the nurse to bring together important points of discussion to enhance understanding.

    C. Focusing concentrates the attention on one single point.

    D. **CORRECT:** Restating allows the nurse to repeat the main idea expressed.

    Ⓝ *NCLEX® Connection: Psychosocial Integrity, Therapeutic Communication*

3. A. **CORRECT:** Offering advice to a client is a barrier to therapeutic communication that the nurse should avoid using. Advice tends to interfere with the client's ability to make personal decisions and choices.

    B. The technique of reflection, directs the focus back to the client in order for the client to examine his feelings.

    C. The skill of active listening is an important therapeutic technique to help the nurse hear and understand the information and messages the client is trying to convey.

    D. Giving information informs the client of needed information to assist in the treatment planning process.

    Ⓝ *NCLEX® Connection: Psychosocial Integrity, Therapeutic Communication*

4. A. The nurse's discussion of client information with members of the healthcare team is an example of small-group communication.

    B. The nurse's self-assessment of feelings is an example of intrapersonal communication.

    C. **CORRECT:** The nurse's one-on-one communication with the client is an example of interpersonal communication.

    D. The nurse's educational presentation to a large group of adolescents is an example of public communication.

    Ⓝ *NCLEX® Connection: Psychosocial Integrity, Therapeutic Communication*

5. A. This nontherapeutic response interjects the nurse's opinion and can cause the parents to withhold their thoughts and feelings.

    B. This nontherapeutic response interjects the nurse's opinion and provides false reassurance which can cause the parents to withhold their thoughts and feelings.

    C. This nontherapeutic response avoids addressing the parent's concerns directly and indicates disinterest by the nurse for wanting to discuss the concerns with the parents.

    D. **CORRECT:** This therapeutic response reflects upon, and accepts, the parents' feelings, and it allows them to clarify what they are feeling.

    Ⓝ *NCLEX® Connection: Psychosocial Integrity, Therapeutic Communication*

PRACTICE Answer

Using the ATI Active Learning Template: Basic Concept

NURSING INTERVENTIONS
- Recognize that the client might require amplification.
- Minimize distractions, and face the client when speaking.
- Allow plenty of time for the client to respond.
- When impaired communication is assessed, ask for input from caregivers or family to determine the extent of the deficits and how best to communicate.
- Provide for privacy.

Ⓝ *NCLEX® Connection: Psychosocial Integrity, Grief and Loss*

CHAPTER 4 Stress and Defense Mechanisms

Stress can result from a change in one's environment that is threatening, causes challenges, or is perceived as damaging to that person's well-being. Stress causes anxiety. Dysfunctional behavior may occur when a defense mechanism is used as a response to anxiety.

Individuals may use defense mechanisms as a way to manage conflict in response to anxiety. Defense mechanisms are reversible, and the client can use them in either an adaptive or maladaptive manner. Adaptive use of defense mechanisms helps people to achieve their goals in acceptable ways. Defense mechanisms become maladaptive when they interfere with functioning, relationships, and orientation to reality. It is important that the defense mechanism used is appropriate to the situation, and that an individual uses a variety of defense mechanisms, rather than having the same reaction to every stressful situation.

Defense mechanisms

Altruism and sublimation are defense mechanisms that are always healthy. Other defense mechanisms can be used in a healthy manner. However, they can become maladaptive if used inappropriately or repetitively.

Altruism

Dealing with anxiety by reaching out to others

ADAPTIVE USE: A nurse who lost a family member in a fire is a volunteer firefighter.

MALADAPTIVE USE: n/a

Sublimation

Dealing with unacceptable feelings or impulses by unconsciously substituting acceptable forms of expression

ADAPTIVE USE: A person who has feelings of anger and hostility toward his work supervisor sublimates those feelings by working out vigorously at the gym during his lunch period.

MALADAPTIVE USE: n/a

Suppression

Voluntarily denying unpleasant thoughts and feelings

ADAPTIVE USE: A student puts off thinking about a fight she had with her friend so she can focus on a test.

MALADAPTIVE USE: A person who has lost his job states he will worry about paying his bills next week.

Repression

Unconsciously putting unacceptable ideas, thoughts, and emotions out of awareness

ADAPTIVE USE: A person preparing to give a speech unconsciously forgets about the time when he was young and kids laughed at him while on stage.

MALADAPTIVE USE: A person who has a fear of the dentist continually forgets to go to his dental appointments.

Regression

Sudden use of childlike or primitive behaviors that do not correlate with the person's current developmental level

ADAPTIVE USE: A young child temporarily wets the bed when she learns that her pet died.

MALADAPTIVE USE: A person who has a disagreement with a co-worker begins throwing things at her office.

Displacement

Shifting feelings related to an object, person, or situation to another less threatening object, person, or situation

ADAPTIVE USE: An adolescent angrily punches a punching bag after losing a game.

MALADAPTIVE USE: A person who is angry about losing his job destroys his child's favorite toy.

Reaction formation

Overcompensating or demonstrating the opposite behavior of what is felt

ADAPTIVE USE: A man who is trying to quit smoking repeatedly talks to adolescents about the dangers of nicotine.

MALADAPTIVE USE: A person who dislikes her neighbor tells others what a great neighbor she is.

Undoing

Performing an act to make up for prior behavior

ADAPTIVE USE: An adolescent completes his chores without being prompted after having an argument with his parent.

MALADAPTIVE USE: A man buys his wife flowers and gifts following an incident of domestic abuse.

Rationalization

Creating reasonable and acceptable explanations for unacceptable behavior

ADAPTIVE USE: An adolescent boy says, "she must already have a boyfriend" when rejected by a girl

MALADAPTIVE USE: A young adult explains he had to drive home from a party after drinking alcohol because he had to feed his dog.

Dissociation

Creating a temporary compartmentalization or lack of connection between the person's identity, memory, or how they perceive the environment

ADAPTIVE USE: A parent blocks out the distracting noise of her children in order to focus while driving in traffic.

MALADAPTIVE USE: A woman forgets who she is following a sexual assault.

Denial

Pretending the truth is not reality to manage the anxiety of acknowledging what is real

ADAPTIVE USE: A person initially says, "No, that can't be true" when told they have cancer.

MALADAPTIVE USE: A parent who is informed that his son was killed in combat tells everyone one month later that he is coming home for the holidays.

Compensation

Emphasizing strengths to make up for weaknesses

ADAPTIVE USE: An adolescent who is physically unable to play contact sports excels in academic competitions.

MALADAPTIVE USE: A person who is shy works at computer skills to avoid socialization.

Identification

Conscious or unconscious assumption of the characteristics of another individual or group

ADAPTIVE USE: A girl who has a chronic illness pretends to be a nurse for her dolls.

MALADAPTIVE USE: A child who observes his father be abusive toward his mother becomes a bully at school.

Intellectualization

Separation of emotions and logical facts when analyzing or coping with a situation or event

ADAPTIVE USE: A law enforcement officer blocks out the emotional aspect of a crime so he can objectively focus on the investigation.

MALADAPTIVE USE: A person who learns he has a terminal illness focuses on creating a will and financial matters rather than acknowledging his grief.

Conversion

Responding to stress through the unconscious development of physical manifestations not caused by a physical illness

ADAPTIVE USE: n/a

MALADAPTIVE USE: A person experiences deafness after his partner tells him she wants a divorce.

Splitting

Demonstrating an inability to reconcile negative and positive attributes of self or others

ADAPTIVE USE: n/a

MALADAPTIVE USE: A client tells a nurse that she is the only one who cares about her, yet the following day, the same client refuses to talk to the nurse.

Projection

Attributing one's unacceptable thoughts and feelings onto another who does not have them.

ADAPTIVE USE: n/a

MALADAPTIVE USE: A married woman who is attracted to another man accuses her husband of having an extramarital affair.

Anxiety

Anxiety is viewed on a continuum with increasing levels of anxiety leading to decreasing ability to function.

Normal

A healthy life force that is necessary for survival, normal anxiety motivates people to take action.

> For example, a potentially violent situation occurs on the mental health unit, and the nurse moves rapidly to defuse the situation. The anxiety experienced by the nurse during the situation helped him perform quickly and efficiently.

Acute (state)

This level of anxiety is precipitated by an imminent loss or change that threatens one's sense of security.

> For example, the sudden death of a loved one precipitates an acute state of anxiety.

Chronic (trait)

This level of anxiety is one that usually develops over time, often starting in childhood. The adult who experiences chronic anxiety might display that anxiety in physical manifestations, such as fatigue and frequent headaches.

ASSESSMENT

Assessment of a client's level of anxiety is basic to therapeutic intervention in any setting.

LEVELS OF ANXIETY

Mild

- Mild anxiety occurs in the normal experience of everyday living.
- It increases one's ability to perceive reality.
- There is an identifiable cause of the anxiety.
- Other characteristics include a vague feeling of mild discomfort, restlessness, irritability, impatience, and apprehension.
- The client can exhibit behaviors such as finger- or foot-tapping, fidgeting, or lip-chewing as mild tension-relieving behaviors.

Moderate

- Moderate anxiety occurs when mild anxiety escalates.
- Slightly reduced perception and processing of information occurs, and selective inattention can occur.
- Ability to think clearly is hampered, but learning and problem-solving can still occur.
- Other characteristics include concentration difficulties, tiredness, pacing, change in voice pitch, voice tremors, shakiness, and increased heart rate and respiratory rate.
- The client can report somatic manifestations including headaches, backache, urinary urgency and frequency, and insomnia.
- The client who has this type of anxiety usually benefits from the direction of others.

Severe

- Perceptual field is greatly reduced with distorted perceptions.
- Learning and problem-solving do not occur.
- Functioning is ineffective.
- Other characteristics include confusion, feelings of impending doom, hyperventilation, tachycardia, withdrawal, loud and rapid speech, and aimless activity.
- The client who has severe anxiety usually is not able to take direction from others.

Panic-level

- Panic-level anxiety is characterized by markedly disturbed behavior.
- The client is not able to process what is occurring in the environment and can lose touch with reality.
- The client experiences extreme fright and horror.
- The client experiences severe hyperactivity or flight.
- Immobility can occur.
- Other characteristics can include dysfunction in speech, dilated pupils, severe shakiness, severe withdrawal, inability to sleep, delusions, and hallucinations.

PATIENT-CENTERED CARE

Nursing interventions are implemented according to the level of anxiety that a client is experiencing.

NURSING INTERVENTIONS

Mild to moderate anxiety

Use active listening to demonstrate willingness to help, and use specific communication techniques (open-ended questions, giving broad openings, exploring, and seeking clarification).
THERAPEUTIC INTENT: Encourage the client to express feelings, develop trust, and identify the source of the anxiety.

Provide a calm presence, recognizing the client's distress.
THERAPEUTIC INTENT: Assists the client to focus and to begin to problem solve.

Evaluate past coping mechanisms.
THERAPEUTIC INTENT: Assists the client to identify adaptive and maladaptive coping mechanisms.

Explore alternatives to problem situations.
THERAPEUTIC INTENT: Offers options for problem-solving.

Encourage participation in activities, such as exercise that can temporarily relieve feelings of inner tension.
THERAPEUTIC INTENT: Provides an outlet for pent-up tension, promotes endorphin release, and improves mental well-being.

Severe to panic-level anxiety

Provide an environment that meets the physical and safety needs of the client. Remain with the client.
THERAPEUTIC INTENT: Minimizes risk to the client, who might be unaware of the need for basic things, such as fluids, food, and sleep. Qs

Provide a quiet environment with minimal stimulation.
THERAPEUTIC INTENT: Helps to prevent intensification of the current level of anxiety.

Use medications and restraint, but only after less restrictive interventions have failed to decrease anxiety to safer levels.
THERAPEUTIC INTENT: Medications and/or restraint might be necessary to prevent harm to the client, other clients, and providers.

Encourage gross motor activities, such as walking and other forms of exercise.
THERAPEUTIC INTENT: Provides an outlet for pent-up tension, promotes endorphin release, and improves mental well-being.

Set limits by using firm, short, and simple statements. Repetition may be necessary.
THERAPEUTIC INTENT: Can minimize risk to the client and providers. Clear, simple communication facilitates understanding.

Direct the client to acknowledge reality and focus on what is present in the environment.
THERAPEUTIC INTENT: Focusing on reality assists with reducing the client's anxiety level.

Application Exercises

1. A nurse is caring for a client who smokes and has lung cancer. The client reports, "I'm coughing because I have that cold that everyone has been getting." The nurse should identify that the client is using which of the following defense mechanisms?

   A. Reaction formation

   B. Denial

   C. Displacement

   D. Sublimation

2. A nurse is providing preoperative teaching for a client who was just informed that she requires emergency surgery. The client, has a respiratory rate 30/min, and says, "This is difficult to comprehend. I feel shaky and nervous." The nurse should identify that the client is experiencing which of the following levels of anxiety?

   A. Mild

   B. Moderate

   C. Severe

   D. Panic

3. A nurse is caring for a client who is experiencing moderate anxiety. Which of the following actions should the nurse take when trying to give necessary information to the client? (Select all that apply.)

   A. Reassure the client that everything will be okay.

   B. Discuss prior use of coping mechanisms with the client.

   C. Ignore the client's anxiety so that she will not be embarrassed.

   D. Demonstrate a calm manner while using simple and clear directions.

   E. Gather information from the client using closed-ended questions.

Application Exercises Key

1. A. This is not an example of reaction formation, which is overcompensating or demonstrating the opposite behavior of what is felt.

   B. **CORRECT:** This is an example of denial, which is pretending the truth is not reality to manage the anxiety of acknowledging what is real.

   C. This is not an example of displacement, which is shifting feelings related to an object, person, or situation to another less threatening object, person, or situation.

   D. This is not an example of sublimation, which is dealing with unacceptable feelings or impulses by unconsciously substituting acceptable forms of expression.

   Ⓝ *NCLEX® Connection: Psychosocial Integrity, Mental Health Concepts*

2. A. In mild anxiety, the client's ability to understand information may actually increase.

   B. **CORRECT:** Moderate anxiety decreases problem-solving and may hamper the client's ability to understand information. Vital signs may increase somewhat, and the client is visibly anxious.

   C. Severe anxiety causes restlessness, decreased perception, and an inability to take direction.

   D. During a panic attack, the person is completely distracted, unable to function, and may lose touch with reality.

   Ⓝ *NCLEX® Connection: Psychosocial Integrity, Behavioral Interventions*

3. A. Providing false reassurance is an example of nontherapeutic communication.

   B. **CORRECT:** Discussing the prior use of coping mechanisms assists the client in identifying ways of effectively coping with the current stressor.

   C. Recognizing the client's current level of anxiety assists the client to begin the process of problem solving.

   D. **CORRECT:** Providing a calm presence assists the client in feeling secure and promotes relaxation. Clients experiencing moderate levels of anxiety often benefit from the direction of others.

   E. Using open-ended questions for client communication encourages the client to express feelings and identify the source of the anxiety.

   Ⓝ *NCLEX® Connection: Psychosocial Integrity, Behavioral Interventions*

UNIT 1 FOUNDATIONS FOR MENTAL HEALTH NURSING

CHAPTER 5 *Creating and Maintaining a Therapeutic and Safe Environment*

Therapeutic encounters can occur in any nursing setting if a nurse is sensitive to a client's needs and uses effective communication skills.

The therapeutic nurse-client relationship is foundational to mental health nursing care.

The therapeutic nurse-client relationship differs from social and intimate relationships.

A therapeutic nurse-client relationship is:

- Purposeful and goal-directed.
- Well-defined with clear boundaries.
- Structured to meet the client's needs.
- Characterized by an interpersonal process that is safe, confidential, reliable, and consistent.

MILIEU THERAPY

Milieu therapy creates an environment that is supportive, therapeutic, and safe. (5.1)

- Milieu therapy began as an effort to provide an environment conducive to the treatment of children who have mental illness.
- Management of the milieu refers to the management of the total environment of the mental health unit in order to provide the least amount of stress, while promoting the greatest benefit for all the clients.
- The goal is that while the client is in this therapeutic environment, he will learn the tools necessary to cope adaptively, interact more effectively and appropriately, and strengthen relationship skills. The hope is that the client will use these tools in all other aspects of his life.
- The nurse, as manager of care, is responsible for structuring and/or implementing aspects of the therapeutic milieu within the mental health facility.
- One structure of the therapeutic milieu is regular community meetings, which include both the clients and the nursing staff.

THERAPEUTIC NURSE-CLIENT RELATIONSHIP

ROLES OF THE NURSE

- Consistently focus on the client's ideas, experiences, and feelings.
- Identify and explore the client's needs and problems. Qpcc
- Discuss problem-solving alternatives with the client.
- Help to develop the client's strengths and new coping skills.
- Encourage positive behavior change in the client.
- Assist the client to develop a sense of autonomy and self-reliance.
- Portray genuineness, empathy, and a positive regard toward the client. The nurse practices empathy by remaining nonjudgmental and attempting to understand the client's actions and feelings. This differs from sympathy, in which the nurse allows herself to feel the way the client does and is nontherapeutic.

5.1 Characteristics of the therapeutic milieu

Physical setting

Unit should be clean and orderly.

The setting should include comfortable furniture placed so that it promotes interaction, solitary spaces for reading and thinking alone, comfortable places conducive to meals, and quiet areas for sleeping.

Color scheme and overall design should be appropriate for the client's age.

Materials used for such features as floors should be attractive, easy to clean, and safe.

Traffic-flow considerations should be conducive to client and staff movement.

Health care team member responsibilities

Promote independence for self-care and individual growth in clients.

Treat clients as individuals.

Allow choices for clients within the daily routine and within individual treatment plans.

Apply rules of fair treatment for all clients.

Model good social behavior for clients, such as respect for the rights of others.

Work cooperatively as a team to provide care.

Maintain boundaries with clients.

Maintain a professional appearance and demeanor.

Promote safe and satisfying peer interactions among the clients.

Practice open communication techniques with health team members and clients.

Promote feelings of self-worth and hope for the future.

EMOTIONAL CLIMATE

Clients should feel safe from harm (self-harm, as well as harm from the disruptive behaviors of other clients).

Clients should feel cared for and accepted by the staff and others.

BENEFITS OF THE THERAPEUTIC RELATIONSHIP

Therapeutic relationships contribute to the well-being of those who have a mental illness, as well as other clients, although the treatment goals will be individualized. **(5.2)**

- These relationships take time to establish, but even time-limited therapeutic encounters can have positive outcomes.
- Therapeutic relationships have a positive impact on the success of treatment.
- **Supervision** by peers or the clinical team enhances the nurse's ability to examine her own thoughts and feelings, maintain boundaries, and continue to learn from nurse-client relationships.
- Factors that positively affect the development of the therapeutic relationship include:
  - NURSE FACTORS
    - Consistent approach to interaction
    - Adjustment of pace to client's needs
    - Attentive listening
    - Positive initial impressions
    - Comfort level during the relationship
    - Self-awareness of own thoughts and feelings
    - Consistent availability
  - CLIENT FACTORS
    - Trusting attitude
    - Willingness to talk
    - Active participation
    - Consistent availability

BOUNDARIES OF THE THERAPEUTIC RELATIONSHIP

Boundaries must be established in order to maintain a safe and professional nurse-client relationship.

- Blurred boundaries occur if the relationship begins to meet the needs of the nurse rather than those of the client, or if the relationship becomes social rather than therapeutic.
  - **Social relationship**: Primary purpose is for socialization or friendship with a focus on the mutual needs of the individuals involved in the relationship.
  - **Therapeutic relationship**: Primary purpose is to identify the client's problems or needs and then focus on assisting the client in meeting or resolving those issues.

5.2 Phases and tasks of a therapeutic relationships

Orientation

NURSE

Introduce self to the client and state purpose.

Set the contract: meeting time, place, frequency, duration, and date of termination.

Discuss confidentiality.

Build trust by establishing expectations and boundaries.

Set goals with the client.

Explore the client's ideas, issues, and needs.

Explore the meaning of testing behaviors.

Enforce limits on testing or other inappropriate behaviors.

CLIENT

Meet with the nurse.

Agree to the contract.

Understand the limits of confidentiality.

Understand the expectations and limits of the relationship.

Participate in setting goals.

Begin to explore own thoughts, experiences, and feelings.

Explore the meaning of own behaviors.

Working

NURSE

Maintain relationship according to the contract.

Perform ongoing assessment to plan and evaluate therapeutic measures.

Facilitate the client's expression of needs and issues.

Encourage the client to problem-solve.

Promote the client's self-esteem.

Foster positive behavioral change.

Explore and deal with resistance and other defense mechanisms.

Recognize transference and countertransference issues.

Reassess the client's problems and goals, and revise plans as necessary.

Support the client's adaptive alternatives and use of new coping skills.

Remind the client about the date of termination.

CLIENT

Explore problematic areas of life.

Reconsider usual coping behaviors.

Examine own world view and self-concept.

Describe major conflicts and various defenses.

Experience intense feelings and learn to cope with anxiety reactions.

Test new behaviors.

Begin to develop awareness of transference situations.

Try alternative solutions.

Termination

NURSE

Provide opportunity for the client to discuss thoughts and feelings about termination and loss.

Discuss the client's previous experience with separations and loss.

Elicit the client's feelings about the therapeutic work in the nurse-client relationship.

Summarize goals and achievements.

Review memories of work in the sessions.

Express own feelings about sessions to validate the experience with the client.

Discuss ways for the client to incorporate new healthy behaviors into life.

Maintain limits of final termination.

CLIENT

Discuss thoughts and feelings about termination.

Examine previous separation and loss experiences.

Explore the meaning of the therapeutic relationship.

Review goals and achievements.

Discuss plans to continue new behaviors.

Express any feelings of loss related to termination.

Make plans for the future.

Accept termination as final.

The nurse must work to maintain a consistent level of involvement with the client, to reflect on boundary issues frequently, and to maintain awareness of how behaviors can be perceived by others (clients, family members, other health team members).

- **Transference** occurs when the client views a member of the health care team as having characteristics of another person who has been significant to the client's personal life.
  - BEHAVIORS
    - Client expects exclusive services from the nurse (e.g. extra session time)
    - Client demonstrates jealousy of the nurse's time or attention
    - Client compares the nurse to a former authority figure
  - EXAMPLE: A client may see a nurse as being like his mother and thus may demonstrate some of the same behaviors with the nurse as he demonstrated with his mother.
  - NURSING IMPLICATIONS: A nurse should be aware that transference by a client is more likely to occur with a person in authority.
- **Countertransference** occurs when a health care team member displaces characteristics of people in her past onto a client.
  - BEHAVIORS
    - Nurse overly identifies with client
    - Nurse competes with client
    - Nurse argues with client
  - EXAMPLE: A nurse may feel defensive and angry with a client for no apparent reason if the client reminds her of a friend who often elicited those feelings.
  - NURSING IMPLICATIONS: A nurse should be aware that clients who induce very strong personal feelings may become objects of countertransference.

PHYSICAL SAFETY

- The nurses' station and other areas should be placed to allow for easy observation of clients by staff and access to staff by clients.
- Special safety features, such as bathroom bars and wheelchair accessibility for clients who are disabled, should be addressed.
- Set up the following provisions to prevent client self-harm or harm by others. Qs
  - No access to sharp or otherwise harmful objects
  - Restriction of client access to restricted or locked areas
  - Monitoring of visitors
  - Restriction of alcohol and illegal substance access or use
  - Restriction of sexual activity among clients
  - Deterrence of elopement from facility
  - Rapid de-escalation of disruptive and potentially violent behaviors through planned interventions by trained staff

- Seclusion rooms and restraints should be set up for safety and used only after all less-restrictive measures have been exhausted. When used, facility policies and procedures must be followed.
- Plan for safe access to recreational areas, occupational therapy, and meeting rooms.
- Teach fire, evacuation, and other safety rules to all staff.
  - Provide clear plans for keeping clients and staff safe in emergencies.
  - Maintain staff skills, such as cardiopulmonary resuscitation.
- Considerations of room assignments on a 24-hr care unit should include:
  - Personalities of each roommate.
  - The likelihood of nighttime disruptions for a roommate if one client has difficulty sleeping.
  - Mental health and medical diagnoses, such as how two clients who have severe paranoia might interact with each other.

ACTIVITIES WITHIN THE THERAPEUTIC MILIEU

Activities are structured and include time for the following:
- **Community meetings** on the mental health unit should enhance the emotional climate of the therapeutic milieu by promoting: QEBP
  - Interaction and communication between staff and clients.
  - Decision making skills of clients.
  - A feeling of self-worth among clients.
  - Discussions of common unit objectives, such as encouraging clients to meet treatment goals and plan for discharge.
  - Discussion of issues of concern to all members of the unit, including common problems, future activities, and the introduction of new clients to the unit.
  - Meetings may be structured so that they are client-led with decisions made by the group as a whole.
- **Individual therapy** is characterized by scheduled sessions with a mental health provider to address specific mental health concerns, such as depression.
- **Group therapy** is characterized by scheduled sessions for a group of clients to address common mental health issues, such as substance use disorder.
- **Psychoeducational groups** are based on clients' level of functioning and personal needs, such as adverse effects of medication.
- **Recreational activities** include games and community outings.
- **Unstructured, flexible time** includes opportunities for the nurse and other staff to observe clients as they interact spontaneously within the milieu.

Application Exercises

1. A nurse is talking with a client who is at risk for suicide following the death of his spouse. Which of the following statements should the nurse make?

   A. "I feel very sorry for the loneliness you must be experiencing."

   B. "Suicide is not the appropriate way to cope with loss."

   C. "Losing someone close to you must be very upsetting."

   D. "I know how difficult it is to lose a loved one."

2. A charge nurse is discussing the characteristics of a nurse-client relationship with a newly licensed nurse. Which of the following characteristics should the nurse include in the discussion? (Select all that apply.)

   A. The needs of both participants are met.

   B. An emotional commitment exists between the participants.

   C. It is goal-directed.

   D. Behavioral change is encouraged.

   E. A termination date is established.

3. A nurse is in the working phase of a therapeutic relationship with a client who has methamphetamine use disorder. Which of the following actions indicates transference behavior?

   A. The client asks the nurse whether she will go out to dinner with him.

   B. The client accuses the nurse of telling him what to do just like his ex-girlfriend.

   C. The client reminds the nurse of a friend who died from a substance overdose.

   D. The client becomes angry and threatens harm to himself.

4. A nurse is planning care for the termination phase of a nurse-client relationship. Which of the following actions should the nurse include in the plan of care?

   A. Discussing ways to use new behaviors

   B. Practicing new problem-solving skills

   C. Developing goals

   D. Establishing boundaries

5. A nurse is orienting a new client to a mental health unit. When explaining the unit's community meetings, which of the following statements should the nurse make?

   A. "You and a group of other clients will meet to discuss your treatment plans."

   B. "Community meetings have a specific agenda that is established by staff."

   C. "You and the other clients will meet with staff to discuss common problems."

   D. "Community meetings are an excellent opportunity to explore your personal mental health issues."

PRACTICE Active Learning Scenario

A charge nurse is discussing the therapeutic milieu during the orientation of a newly hired nurse. Use the ATI Active Learning Template: Basic Concept to complete this item.

UNDERLYING PRINCIPLES: Identify at least five responsibilities of the health care team to maintain a therapeutic milieu.

NURSING INTERVENTIONS: Identify at least four interventions to prevent client self-harm or harm by others.

Application Exercises Key

1. A. This statement focuses on the nurse's feelings and is sympathetic rather than empathetic.

   B. This statement implies judgment and is therefore not an empathetic or therapeutic response.

   C. **CORRECT:** This statement is an empathetic response that attempts to understand the client's feelings.

   D. This statement focuses on the nurse's experiences rather than the client's and is therefore not therapeutic.

   Ⓝ *NCLEX® Connection: Psychosocial Integrity, Therapeutic Communication*

2. A. A therapeutic nurse-client relationship focuses on the needs of the client.

   B. An emotional commitment between the participants is characteristic of an intimate or social relationship rather than one that is therapeutic.

   C. **CORRECT:** A therapeutic nurse-client relationship is goal-directed.

   D. **CORRECT:** A therapeutic nurse-client relationship encourages positive behavioral change.

   E. **CORRECT:** A therapeutic nurse-client relationship has an established termination date.

   Ⓝ *NCLEX® Connection: Psychosocial Integrity, Therapeutic Environment*

3. A. This indicates the need to discuss boundaries but does not indicate transference.

   B. **CORRECT:** When a client views the nurse as having characteristics of another person who has been significant to his personal life, such as his ex-girlfriend, this indicates transference.

   C. This indicates countertransference rather than transference.

   D. This indicates the need for safety intervention but does not indicate transference.

   Ⓝ *NCLEX® Connection: Psychosocial Integrity, Therapeutic Environment*

4. A. **CORRECT:** Discussing ways for the client to incorporate new healthy behaviors into life is an appropriate task for the termination phase.

   B. Practicing new problem-solving skills is an appropriate task for the working phase.

   C. Developing goals is an appropriate task for the orientation phase.

   D. Establishing boundaries is an appropriate task for the orientation phase.

   Ⓝ *NCLEX® Connection: Psychosocial Integrity, Behavioral Interventions*

5. A. Individual treatment plans are discussed during individual therapy rather than a community meeting.

   B. Community meetings may be structured so that they are client-led with decisions made by the group as a whole.

   C. **CORRECT:** Community meetings are an opportunity for clients to discuss common problems or issues affecting all members of the unit.

   D. Personal mental health issues are discussed during individual therapy rather than a community meeting.

   Ⓝ *NCLEX® Connection: Psychosocial Integrity, Therapeutic Environment*

PRACTICE Answer

Using ATI Active Learning Template: Basic Concept

UNDERLYING PRINCIPLES

- Promote independence for self-care and individual growth.
- Treat clients as individuals.
- Allow choices for clients within the daily routine and treatment plan.
- Apply rules of fair treatment for all clients.
- Model good social behavior.
- Work cooperatively as a team to provide care.
- Maintain boundaries with clients.
- Maintain a professional appearance and demeanor.
- Promote safe and satisfying peer interactions among clients.
- Practice open communication techniques with health team members and clients.
- Promote feelings of self-worth and hope for the future.

NURSING INTERVENTIONS

- Prevent access to sharp or harmful objects.
- Restrict client access to restricted or locked areas.
- Monitor visitors.
- Restrict alcohol and illegal substance access and use.
- Restrict sexual activity among clients.
- Deter elopement from facility.
- Provide rapid de-escalation of disruptive and potentially violent behaviors.
- Be aware of facility policies and procedures for seclusion or restraints.
- Provide safe access to recreational areas, therapy, and meeting rooms.

Ⓝ *NCLEX® Connection: Psychosocial Integrity, Therapeutic Environment*

UNIT 1   FOUNDATIONS FOR MENTAL HEALTH NURSING

CHAPTER 6   *Diverse Practice Settings*

Mental health nursing occurs in acute care and community settings, as well as in forensic nursing settings.

In all settings, nurses are advocates for clients who have mental illness. Referral of clients and their families to organizations and agencies that provide additional resources can provide significant support to individuals.

For example, the National Alliance on Mental Illness (NAMI), is a grassroots organization with the goals of improving the quality of life for persons with mental illness and providing research to better treat or eradicate mental illness. For more information, go to www.nami.org. Q℡

SETTINGS FOR MENTAL HEALTH CARE

ACUTE CARE

This setting provides intensive treatment and supervision in locked units for clients who have severe mental illness.
- Care in these facilities helps stabilize mental illness manifestations and promotes the clients' rapid return to the community.
- Staff is made up of an interprofessional team with management provided by nurses developing individualized plans that are client and family centered. Facilities might be privately owned or general hospitals, with payment provided by private funds or insurance. Q℡
- Facilities also might be state owned, with much of the funding provided for indigent clients. State-run facilities also often provide full-time acute care for forensic clients (those in a correctional setting) who have severe mental illness.
- Case management programs assist with client transition to a community setting after discharge from the acute care facility.

COMMUNITY

Primary care is provided in community-based settings, which include clinics, schools and day-care centers, partial hospitalization programs, substance treatment facilities, forensic settings, psychosocial rehabilitation programs, telephone crisis counseling centers, and home health care.
- Nurses working in community care programs help to stabilize or improve clients' mental functioning within a community. They also teach, support, and make referrals in order to promote positive social activities.
- Nursing interventions in community settings provide for primary treatment as well as primary, secondary, and tertiary prevention of mental illness.

FORENSIC NURSING

Forensic nursing is a combination of biophysical education and forensic science. The registered nurses use scientific investigation, collection of evidence, analysis, prevention, and treatment of trauma and/or death of perpetrators and victims of violence, abuse, and traumatic accidents.

HISTORY OF MENTAL HEALTH CARE IN THE UNITED STATES

- Most clients who have severe mental illness were treated solely in acute care facilities before the middle of the twentieth century.
- Congress passed a series of acts in 1946, 1955, and 1963 in response to the appalling condition of facilities for the mentally ill. This began a trend to deinstitutionalize mental health care.
- Clients who had lived in acute care mental health facilities for many years were discharged into the community at a time when community mental health facilities were often unprepared to deal with this influx.
- The concept of the case manager was introduced around 1970 to meet the individual needs of clients in a mental health setting.
- Managed care through health maintenance organizations (HMOs), preferred provider organizations (PPOs), and others began limiting hospital stays for clients in a general medical setting starting around 1980.
- Managed Behavioral Healthcare Organizations (MBHOs) later developed to coordinate care and limit stays in acute care facilities for clients needing mental health care.
- This began the trend to develop a continuum of acute care facilities and community mental health facilities to provide for all levels of behavioral health care needs.
- Complete and accurate documentation of client needs and progress by nurses and other health care professionals is needed to ensure quality care for each client. Q๑ı
- Factors that will affect the future of mental health care include the following:
  - An increase in the aging population
  - An increase in cultural diversity within the United States
  - The expansion of technology, which might provide new settings for client care, as well as new ways to treat mental illness more effectively

CLIENT CARE

ACUTE MENTAL HEALTH CARE SETTINGS

- Criteria to justify admission to an acute care facility include: Q_{PCC}
  - A clear risk of the client's danger to self or others
  - An inability to meet own basic needs
  - Failure to meet expected outcomes of community-based treatment
  - A dangerous decline in the mental health status of a client undergoing long-term treatment
  - A client having a medical need in addition to a mental illness
- Goals of acute mental health treatment include the following:
  - Prevention of the client harming self or others
  - Stabilizing mental health crises
  - Return of clients who are severally ill to some type of community care

Interprofessional team members

- Team members in acute care include nurses, mental health technicians (who perform duties similar to assistive personnel in other health care facilities), psychologists, psychiatrists, other general health care providers, social workers, counselors, occupational and other specialty therapists, and pharmacists. Q_{TC}
- The interprofessional team has the primary responsibility of planning and monitoring individualized treatment plans or clinical pathways of care, depending on the philosophy and policy of the facility.
- Plans for discharge to home or to a community facility begin from the time of admission and continue with the implementation of the initial treatment plan or clinical pathway.

Nursing role

Nurses in acute care mental health facilities use the nursing process and a holistic approach to provide care. Nursing roles include the following:

- Overall management of the unit, including client activities and therapeutic milieu
- Ensuring safe administration and monitoring of all client medications
- Implementation of individual client treatment plans, including client teaching
- Documentation of the nursing process for each client
- Managing crises as they arise

COMMUNITY HEALTH SETTINGS

- Nurses are mainly responsible for linking acute care facilities with community care facilities.
- Intensive outpatient programs promote community reintegration for clients.

Levels of prevention

Three levels of prevention are used by nurses when implementing community care interventions/teaching. Q_{TC}

Primary prevention promotes health and prevents mental health problems from occurring.

> A nurse teaches a community education program on stress reduction techniques.

Secondary prevention focuses on early detection of mental illness.

> A nurse screens older adults in the community for depression.

Tertiary prevention focuses on rehabilitation and prevention of further problems in clients who have previous diagnoses.

> A nurse leads a support group for clients who have completed a substance use disorder program.

Community-based mental health programs

Community-based mental health programs are a continuum of mental health agencies with varying treatment intensity levels to allow clients to remain safe in the least restrictive environment possible.

Partial hospitalization programs
- These programs provide intense short-term treatment for clients who are well enough to go home every night and who have a responsible person at home to provide support and a safe environment.
- Certain detoxification programs are a specialized form of partial hospitalization for clients who require medical supervision, stress management, substance use disorder counseling, and relapse prevention.

Assertive community treatment (ACT)
- This includes nontraditional case management and treatment by an interprofessional team for clients who have severe mental illness and are noncompliant with traditional treatment.
- ACT helps to reduce reoccurrences of hospitalizations and provides crisis intervention, assistance with independent living, and information regarding resources for necessary support services.

Community mental health centers
These facilities provide a variety of services for a wide range of community clients, including:
- Educational groups
- Medication dispensing programs
- Individual and family counseling programs

Psychosocial rehabilitation programs
These programs provide a structured range of programs for clients in a mental health setting, including:
- Residential services
- Day programs for older adults

Home care: Home care provides mental health assessment, interventions, and family support in the client's home. This is implemented most often for children, older adults, and clients who have medical conditions.

ROLES OF NURSES IN DIVERSE MENTAL HEALTH PRACTICE SETTINGS

REGISTERED NURSE

- Educational preparation: diploma, associate degree, or baccalaureate degree in nursing, with additional on-the-job training and continuing education in mental health care
- May work in either an acute care or community-based facility
- Functions within a facility using the nursing process to provide care and treatment, such as medication
- Manages care for a group of clients within a unit of the facility

ADVANCED PRACTICE NURSE

- Educational preparation: advanced nursing degree in behavioral health (master's degree, doctorate, nurse practitioner, or clinical nurse specialist)
- May work independently, often supervising individuals or groups in either an acute care or community-based setting
- May have prescription privileges and is able to independently recommend interventions
- May manage and administrate the care for an entire facility

Application Exercises

1. A nurse is caring for several clients who are attending community-based mental health programs. Which of the following clients should the nurse plan to visit first?
   - A. A client who recently burned her arm while using a hot iron at home
   - B. A client who requests that her antipsychotic medication be changed due to some new adverse effects
   - C. A client who says he is hearing a voice that tells him he is not worthy of living anymore
   - D. A client who tells the nurse he experienced manifestations of severe anxiety before and during a job interview

2. A community mental health nurse is planning care to address the issue of depression among older adult clients in the community. Which of the following interventions should the nurse plan as a method of tertiary prevention?
   - A. Educating clients on health promotion techniques to reduce the risk of depression
   - B. Performing screenings for depression at community health programs
   - C. Establishing rehabilitation programs to decrease the effects of depression
   - D. Providing support groups for clients at risk for depression

3. A nurse is working in a community mental health facility. Which of the following services does this type of program provide? (Select all that apply.)
   - A. Educational groups
   - B. Medication dispensing programs
   - C. Individual counseling programs
   - D. Detoxification programs
   - E. Family therapy

4. A nurse in an acute mental health facility is assisting with discharge planning for a client who has a severe mental illness and requires supervision much of the time. The client's wife works all day but is home by late afternoon. Which of the following strategies should the nurse suggest as appropriate follow-up care?
   - A. Receiving daily care from a home health aide
   - B. Having a weekly visit from a nurse case worker
   - C. Attending a partial hospitalization program
   - D. Visiting a community mental health center on a daily basis

5. A nurse is caring for a group of clients. Which of the following clients should a nurse consider for referral to an assertive community treatment (ACT) group?
   - A. A client in an acute care mental health facility who has fallen several times while running down the hallway
   - B. A client who lives at home and keeps "forgetting" to come in for his monthly antipsychotic injection for schizophrenia
   - C. A client in a day treatment program who says he is becoming more anxious during group therapy
   - D. A client in a weekly grief support group who says she still misses her deceased husband who has been dead for 3 months

Application Exercises Key

1. A. This client has needs that should be met, but there is another client whom the nurse should see first.

   B. This client has needs that should be met, but there is another client whom the nurse should see first.

   C. **CORRECT:** A client who hears a voice telling him he is not worthy is at greatest risk for self-harm, and the nurse should visit this client first.

   D. This client has needs that should be met, but there is another client whom the nurse should see first.

   Ⓝ *NCLEX® Connection: Management of Care, Establishing Priorities*

2. A. This intervention is an example of primary prevention.

   B. This intervention is an example of secondary prevention.

   C. **CORRECT:** Rehabilitation programs are an example of tertiary prevention. Tertiary prevention deals with prevention of further problems in clients already diagnosed with mental illness.

   D. This intervention is an example of primary prevention.

   Ⓝ *NCLEX® Connection: Psychosocial Integrity, Mental Health Concepts*

3. A. **CORRECT:** Educational groups are services provided in a community mental health facility.

   B. **CORRECT:** Medication dispensing programs are services provided in a community mental health facility.

   C. **CORRECT:** Individual counseling programs are services provided in a community mental health facility.

   D. Detoxification programs are services provided in a partial hospitalization program.

   E. **CORRECT:** Family therapy is a service provided in a community mental health facility.

   Ⓝ *NCLEX® Connection: Management of Care, Referrals*

4. A. Daily care provided by a home health aide will not provide adequate supervision for this client.

   B. Weekly visits from a case worker will not provide adequate care and supervision for this client.

   C. **CORRECT:** A partial hospitalization program can provide treatment during the day while allowing the client to spend nights at home, as long as a responsible family member is present.

   D. Daily visits to a community mental health center will not provide consistent supervision for this client.

   Ⓝ *NCLEX® Connection: Psychosocial Integrity, Mental Health Concepts*

5. A. A client in acute care who has been running and falling should be helped by the treatment team on her unit.

   B. **CORRECT:** An ACT group works with clients who are nonadherent with traditional therapy, such as the client in a home setting who keeps "forgetting" his injection.

   C. A client who has anxiety might be referred to his counselor or mental health provider.

   D. A client who is grieving for her husband who died 3 months ago is currently involved in an appropriate intervention.

   Ⓝ *NCLEX® Connection: Management of Care, Referrals*

PRACTICE Active Learning Scenario

A nurse is conducting an in-service education program regarding acute mental health treatment for a group of newly licensed nurses. What should the nurse include in this presentation? Use the ATI Active Learning Template: Basic Concept to complete this item.

RELATED CONTENT: Identify two criteria for admitting a client to a mental health facility.

UNDERLYING PRINCIPLES: Describe two concepts of mental health treatment.

NURSING INTERVENTIONS: Describe two interventions that apply to acute mental health care.

PRACTICE Answer

Using the ATI Active Learning Template: Basic Concept

RELATED CONTENT

- Clear risk of the client's danger to self and others.
- Failure to meet expected outcomes of community-based treatment.
- A dangerous decline in the mental health status of a client undergoing long-term treatment
- A client having a medical need in addition to a mental illness.

UNDERLYING PRINCIPLES

- Goals of acute mental health treatment:
  ○ Prevention of the client harming self or others
  ○ Stabilizing mental health crises
  ○ Return of clients who are severally ill to some type of community care
- Interprofessional team members in acute care include nurses, mental health technicians, psychologists, psychiatrists, other general health care providers, social workers, counselors, occupational and other specialty therapists, and pharmacists.

NURSING INTERVENTIONS

- Who: The interprofessional team member's primary responsibility is planning and monitoring individualized treatment plans or clinical pathways of care.
- When: Plans for discharge to home or to a community facility begin from the time of admission.
- How: Nursing roles include overall management of the unit, including client activities and therapeutic milieu.
- Ensuring safe administration and monitoring of client medications.
- Implementation of individual client treatment plans, including client teaching.
- Documentation of the nursing process for each client. Manage crises as they arise.

Ⓝ *NCLEX® Connection: Psychosocial Integrity, Mental Health Concepts*

When reviewing the following chapters, keep in mind the relevant topics and tasks of the NCLEX outline, in particular:

Client Needs: Psychosocial Integrity

BEHAVIORAL INTERVENTIONS: Participate in group sessions.

FAMILY DYNAMICS
Assess family dynamics to determine plan of care.

Assess parental techniques related to discipline.

Evaluate resources available to assist family functioning.

MENTAL HEALTH CONCEPTS: Apply knowledge of client psychopathology to mental health concepts applied in individual/group/family therapy.

STRESS MANAGEMENT
Assess stressors, including environmental, that affect client care.

Provide information to client on stress management techniques.

SUPPORT SYSTEMS: Encourage the client's involvement in the health care decision-making process.

Client Needs: Reduction of Risk Potential

POTENTIAL FOR COMPLICATIONS OF DIAGNOSTIC TESTS/TREATMENTS/PROCEDURES
Provide care for the client undergoing electroconvulsive therapy.

Use precautions to prevent injury and/or complications associated with a procedure or diagnosis.

UNIT 2   TRADITIONAL NONPHARMACOLOGICAL
            THERAPIES

CHAPTER 7 *Psychoanalysis,*
           Psychotherapy,
           and Behavioral
           Therapies

Psychoanalysis, psychotherapy, and behavioral therapies are approaches to addressing mental health issues using various methods and theoretical bases.

Nurses working in mental health settings need to be familiar with the methods that are part of these approaches and their application in practice.

PSYCHOANALYSIS

Classical psychoanalysis is a therapeutic process of assessing unconscious thoughts and feelings, and resolving conflict by talking to a psychoanalyst. Clients attend many sessions over the course of months to years.
- Due to the length of psychoanalytic therapy and health insurance constraints, classical psychoanalysis is unlikely to be the sole therapy of choice.
- Psychoanalysis was first developed by Sigmund Freud to resolve internal conflicts which, he contended, always occur from early childhood experiences.
- Past relationships are a common focus for therapy.

THERAPEUTIC TOOLS

Free association, which is the spontaneous, uncensored verbalization of whatever comes to a client's mind

Dream analysis and interpretation, believed by Freud to be urges and impulses of the unconscious mind that played out through the dreams of clients

Transference, which includes feelings that the client has developed toward the therapist in relation to similar feelings toward significant persons in the client's early childhood

Use of **defense mechanisms**

PSYCHOTHERAPY

Psychotherapy involves more verbal therapist-to-client interaction than classic psychoanalysis. The client and the therapist develop a trusting relationship to explore the client's problems.

Psychodynamic psychotherapy employs the same tools as psychoanalysis, but it focuses more on the client's present state, rather than his early life.

Interpersonal psychotherapy (IPT) assists clients in addressing specific problems. It can improve interpersonal relationships, communication, role-relationship, and bereavement.

Cognitive therapy is based on the cognitive model, which focuses on individual thoughts and behaviors to solve current problems. It treats depression, anxiety, eating disorders, and other issues that can improve by changing a client's attitude toward life experiences.

Behavioral therapy
- In protest of Freud's psychoanalytic theory, behavioral theorists such as Ivan Pavlov, John B. Watson, and B.F. Skinner felt that changing behavior was the key to treating problems such as anxiety or depressive disorders.
- Behavioral therapy is based on the theory that behavior is learned and has consequences. Abnormal behavior results from an attempt to avoid painful feelings. Changing abnormal or maladaptive behavior can occur without the need for insight into the underlying cause of the behavior.
- Behavioral therapies teach clients ways to decrease anxiety or avoidant behavior and give clients an opportunity to practice techniques. Behavioral therapy teaches activities to help the client reduce anxious and avoidant behavior like relaxation training and modeling.
- Behavioral therapy has been used successfully to treat clients who have phobias, substance use or addictive disorders, and other issues.

Cognitive-behavioral therapy uses both cognitive and behavioral approaches to assist a client with anxiety management.

Dialectical behavior therapy is a cognitive-behavioral therapy for clients who have a personality disorder and exhibit self-injurious behavior. This therapy focuses on gradual behavior changes and provides acceptance and validation for these clients.

USE OF COGNITIVE THERAPY

Cognitive reframing

Changing cognitive distortions can decrease anxiety. Cognitive reframing assists clients to identify negative thoughts that produce anxiety, examine the cause, and develop supportive ideas that replace negative self-talk. For example, a client who has a depressive disorder might say he is "a bad person" who has "never done anything good" in his life. Through therapy, this client can change his thinking to realize that he might have made some bad choices, but that he is not "a bad person."

Priority restructuring: Assists clients to identify what requires priority, such as devoting energy to pleasurable activities.

Journal keeping: Helps clients write down stressful thoughts and has a positive effect on well-being.

Assertiveness training: Teaches clients to express feelings, and solve problems in a nonaggressive manner.

Monitoring thoughts: Helps clients to be aware of negative thinking.

TYPES AND USES OF BEHAVIORAL THERAPY

Modeling

A therapist or others serve as role models for a client, who imitates this modeling to improve behavior.

USE IN MENTAL HEALTH NURSING: Modeling can occur in the acute care milieu to help clients improve interpersonal skills. The therapist demonstrates appropriate behavior in a stressful situation with the goal of having the client imitate the behavior.

Operant conditioning

The client receives positive rewards for positive behavior (positive reinforcement).

USE IN MENTAL HEALTH NURSING: As an example: a client receives tokens for good behavior, and he can exchange them for a privilege or other items.

Systematic desensitization

This therapy is the planned, progressive, or graduated exposure to anxiety-provoking stimuli in real-life situations, or by imagining events that cause anxiety. During exposure, the client uses relaxation techniques to suppress anxiety response.

USE IN MENTAL HEALTH NURSING: Systematic desensitization begins with the client mastering relaxation techniques. Then, the client is exposed to increasing levels of the anxiety-producing stimulus (either imagined or real) and uses relaxation to overcome anxiety. The client is then able to tolerate a greater and greater level of the stimulus until anxiety no longer interferes with functioning.

Aversion therapy

Pairing of a maladaptive behavior with a punishment or unpleasant stimuli to promote a change in the behavior.

USE IN MENTAL HEALTH NURSING: A therapist or treatment team can use unpleasant stimuli, such as bitter taste or mild electric shock, as punishment for behaviors such as alcohol use disorder, violence, self-mutilation, and thumb-sucking.

Meditation, guided imagery, diaphragmatic breathing, muscle relaxation, and biofeedback

This therapy uses various techniques to control pain, tension, and anxiety.

USE IN MENTAL HEALTH NURSING: A nurse can teach diaphragmatic breathing to a client having a panic attack, or to a female client in labor.

OTHER TECHNIQUES

Flooding: Exposing a client, while in the company of a therapist, to a great deal of an undesirable stimulus in an attempt to turn off the anxiety response

Response prevention: Preventing a client from performing a compulsive behavior with the intent that anxiety will diminish

Thought stopping: Teaching a client, when negative thoughts or compulsive behaviors arise, to say or shout, "stop," and substitute a positive thought. The goal over time is for the client to use the command silently.

Application Exercises

1. A nurse is teaching a client who has an anxiety disorder and is scheduled to begin classical psychoanalysis. Which of the following client statements indicates an understanding of this form of therapy?

   A. "Even if my anxiety improves, I will need to continue this therapy for 6 weeks."

   B. "The therapist will focus on my past relationships during our sessions."

   C. "Psychoanalysis will help me reduce my anxiety by changing my behaviors."

   D. "This therapy will address my conscious feelings about stressful experiences."

2. A nurse is discussing free association as a therapeutic tool with a client who has major depressive disorder. Which of the following client statements indicates understanding of this technique?

   A. "I will write down my dreams as soon as I wake up."

   B. "I may begin to associate my therapist with important people in my life."

   C. "I can learn to express myself in a nonaggressive manner."

   D. "I should say the first thing that comes to my mind."

3. A nurse is preparing to implement cognitive reframing techniques for a client who has an anxiety disorder. Which of the following techniques should the nurse include in the plan of care? (Select all that apply.)

   A. Priority restructuring

   B. Monitoring thoughts

   C. Diaphragmatic breathing

   D. Journal keeping

   E. Meditation

4. A nurse is caring for a client who has a new prescription for disulfiram for treatment of alcohol use disorder. The nurse informs the client that this medication can cause nausea and vomiting if he drinks alcohol. Which of the following types of treatment is this method an example?

   A. Aversion therapy

   B. Flooding

   C. Biofeedback

   D. Dialectical behavior therapy

5. A nurse is assisting with systematic desensitization for a client who has an extreme fear of elevators. Which of the following actions should the nurse implement with this form of therapy?

   A. Demonstrate riding in an elevator, and then ask the client to imitate the behavior.

   B. Advise the client to say "stop" out loud every time he begins to feel an anxiety response related to an elevator.

   C. Gradually expose the client to an elevator while practicing relaxation techniques.

   D. Stay with the client in an elevator until his anxiety response diminishes.

PRACTICE Active Learning Scenario

A nurse working in an acute mental health unit is caring for a client who has a personality disorder. The client refuses to attend group meetings and will not speak to other clients or attend unit activities. The client enjoys visiting with staff and requests daily to take a walk outside with a staff member. The provider prescribes behavioral therapy with operant conditioning. Use the ATI Active Learning Template: Therapeutic Procedure to complete this item.

DESCRIPTION OF PROCEDURE: Discuss behavioral therapy and operant conditioning.

OUTCOMES/EVALUATION: Identify an appropriate client outcome.

NURSING INTERVENTIONS: Identify an appropriate nursing action to implement operant conditioning with this client.

Application Exercises Key

1. A. Classical psychoanalysis is a therapeutic process that requires many sessions over months to years.

   B. **CORRECT:** Classical psychoanalysis places a common focus on past relationships to identify the cause of the anxiety disorder.

   C. Classical psychoanalysis focuses on identifying and resolving the cause of the anxiety rather than changing behavior.

   D. Classical psychoanalysis assesses unconscious, rather than conscious, thoughts and feelings.

   Ⓝ *NCLEX® Connection: Physiological Adaptation, Illness Management*

2. A. Dream analysis and interpretation are therapeutic tools. However, they are not an example of free association.

   B. Associating the therapist with significant persons in the client's life is an example of transference rather than free association.

   C. Learning to express feelings and solve problems in a nonaggressive manner is an example of assertiveness training, rather than free association.

   D. **CORRECT:** Free association is the spontaneous, uncensored verbalization of whatever comes to a client's mind.

   Ⓝ *NCLEX® Connection: Psychosocial Integrity, Therapeutic Communication*

3. A. **CORRECT:** Priority restructuring is a cognitive reframing technique.

   B. **CORRECT:** Monitoring thoughts is a cognitive reframing technique.

   C. Diaphragmatic breathing is a form of behavioral therapy rather than a cognitive reframing technique.

   D. **CORRECT:** Journal keeping is a cognitive reframing technique.

   E. Meditation is a form of behavioral therapy rather than a cognitive reframing technique.

   Ⓝ *NCLEX® Connection: Psychosocial Integrity, Behavioral Interventions*

4. A. **CORRECT:** Aversion therapy pairs a maladaptive behavior with unpleasant stimuli to promote a change in behavior.

   B. Flooding is planned exposure to an undesirable stimulus in an attempt to turn off the anxiety response.

   C. Biofeedback is a behavioral therapy to control pain, tension, and anxiety.

   D. Dialectical behavior therapy is a cognitive-behavioral therapy for clients who have a personality disorder and exhibit self-injurious behavior.

   Ⓝ *NCLEX® Connection: Psychosocial Integrity, Chemical and Other Dependencies/Substance Use Disorder*

5. A. Demonstration followed by client imitation of the behavior is an example of modeling.

   B. Teaching a client to say "stop" when anxiety occurs is an example of thought stopping.

   C. **CORRECT:** Systematic desensitization is the planned, progressive exposure to anxiety-provoking stimuli. During this exposure, relaxation techniques suppress the anxiety response.

   D. Exposing the client to a great deal of an undesirable stimulus in an attempt to turn off the anxiety response is an example of flooding.

   Ⓝ *NCLEX® Connection: Psychosocial Integrity, Behavioral Interventions*

PRACTICE Answer

Using the ATI Active Learning Template: Therapeutic Procedure

DESCRIPTION OF PROCEDURE
- Behavioral therapy is based on the theory that behavior is learned and has consequences. These therapies teach clients ways to decrease anxiety or avoidant behavior and give clients an opportunity to practice techniques.
- Operant conditioning provides the client with positive rewards for positive behavior.

OUTCOMES/EVALUATION
- The client will attend group meetings.
- The client will attend unit activities.
- The client will appropriately socialize with other clients on the unit.

NURSING INTERVENTIONS
- The nurse will use tokens, or something similar, to reward the client for a positive change in behavior. The client can use these tokens for larger rewards, such as a walk outside with a staff member.
- The nurse will provide positive feedback and encouragement for a positive change in behavior.

Ⓝ *NCLEX® Connection: Psychosocial Integrity, Behavioral Interventions*

UNIT 2 TRADITIONAL NONPHARMACOLOGICAL THERAPIES

CHAPTER 8 *Group and Family Therapy*

Therapy is an intensive treatment that involves open therapeutic communication with participants who are willing to take part in therapy. Although individual therapy is an important treatment for mental illness, group and family therapies are also a part of the treatment plan for many clients in a mental health setting.

Family composition has become more complex through the years, departing from the traditional nuclear household of mother, father, and children. Disciplining children is an important aspect of family life. Discipline techniques can be healthy or unhealthy.

Leaders guide group and family therapy, and they may employ various leadership styles. Democratic leadership supports group interaction and decision making to solve problems. Laissez-faire leadership progresses without any attempt by the leader to control the direction. In autocratic leadership, the leader completely controls the direction and structure of the group without allowing group interaction or decision making to solve problems.

Examples of group therapy include stress management, substance use disorders, medication education, understanding mental illness, and dual diagnosis groups.

Group therapy

Group process is the verbal and nonverbal communication that occurs during group sessions, including how the work progresses.

Group norm is the way the group behaves during sessions, and, over time, it provides structure for the group. For example, a group norm could be that members raise their hand to be recognized by the leader before they speak. Another norm could be that all members sit in the same places for each session.

Hidden agenda: Some group members (or the leader) might have goals different from the stated group goals that may disrupt group processes. For example, three members might try to embarrass another member whom they dislike.

A **subgroup** is a small number of people within a larger group who function separately from the group.

Groups can be open (new members join as old members leave) or closed (no new members join after formation of the group).

A **homogeneous group** is one in which all members share a certain chosen characteristic, such as diagnosis or gender. Membership of heterogeneous groups is not based on a shared chosen personal characteristic. An example of a heterogeneous group is all clients on a unit, including a mixture of men and women who have a wide range of diagnoses.

8.1 Focus and goals for individual, family, and group therapies

Individual	*Family*	*Group*
FOCUS	**FOCUS**	**FOCUS**
Client needs and problems	Family needs and problems within family dynamics	Helping individuals develop more functional and satisfying relations within a group setting
The therapeutic relationship	Improving family functioning	
GOALS	**GOALS**	**GOALS**
Make more positive individual decisions.	Learn effective ways for dealing with mental illness within the family.	Goals vary depending on type of group, but clients generally:
Make productive life decisions.	Improve understanding among family members.	Discover that members share some common feelings, experiences, and thoughts.
Develop a strong sense of self.	Maximize positive interaction among family members.	Experience positive behavior changes as a result of group interaction and feedback.

COMPONENTS OF THERAPY SESSIONS

- Use of open and clear communication
- Cohesiveness and guidelines for the therapy session
- Direction toward a particular goal
- Opportunities for development of interpersonal skills; resolution of personal and family issues; and development of appropriate, satisfying relationships.
- Encouragement of the client to maximize positive interactions, feel empowered to make decisions, and strengthen feelings of self-worth
- Communication regarding respect among all members
- Support, as well as education regarding things such as available community resources for support

GROUP THERAPY GOALS

- Sharing common feelings and concerns
- Sharing stories and experiences
- Diminishing feelings of isolation
- Creating a community of healing and restoration
- Providing a more cost-effective environment than that of individual therapy

AGE GROUPS IN GROUP THERAPY

Children: In the form of play while talking about a common experience

Adolescent: Especially valuable, as this age group typically has strong peer relationships Qᴘᴄᴄ

Older adult: Helps with socialization and sharing of memories

PHASES OF GROUP DEVELOPMENT

Orientation phase

PRIMARY FOCUS: Define the purpose and goals of the group.

RESPONSIBILITIES
- The group leader sets a tone of respect, trust, and confidentiality among members.
- Members get to know each other and the group leader.
- There is a discussion about termination.

Working phase

PRIMARY FOCUS: Promote problem-solving skills to facilitate behavioral changes. Power and control issues may dominate in this phase.

RESPONSIBILITIES
- The group leader uses therapeutic communication to encourage group work toward meeting goals.
- Members take informal roles within the group, which may interfere with, or favor, group progress toward goals.

Termination phase

PRIMARY FOCUS: This marks the end of group sessions.

RESPONSIBILITIES
- Group members discuss termination issues.
- The leader summarizes work of the group and individual contributions.
- Members of a group can take on any of a number of roles.

ROLES

Maintenance roles: Members who take on these roles tend to help maintain the purpose and process of the group. For example, the harmonizer attempts to prevent conflict in the group.

Task roles: Members take on various tasks within the group process. An example is the recorder, who takes notes and records what occurs during each session.

Individual roles: These roles tend to prevent teamwork, because individuals take on roles to promote their own agenda. Examples include the dominator, who tries to control other members, and the recognition seeker, who boasts about personal achievements.

GROUP CHARACTERISTICS

Can vary depending on the health care setting.

Acute mental health setting: Members can vary on a daily basis, and the focus of the group is on relief. Unit activities will directly impact the group, and the leader must provide a higher level of structure.

Outpatient setting: Members are often consistent, the focus of the group is on growth, external influences are limited, and the leader can allow members an opportunity in determining the group's direction.

Families and family therapy

TYPES OF FAMILIES

Nuclear families: Include children who reside with married parents

Single-parent families: Include children who live with a single adult that can be related or nonrelated to the children

Adoptive families: Include children who live with parents who have adopted them

Blended families: Include children who live with one biological or adoptive parent and an nonrelated stepparent who are married

Cohabitating families: Include children who live with one biological parent and a nonrelated adult who are cohabitating

Extended families: Include children living with one biological or adoptive parent and a related adult who is not their parent (e.g., grandparent, aunt, uncle)

Other families: Include children living with related or nonrelated adults who are neither biological nor adoptive parents (e.g., grandparents, adult siblings, foster parents)

> Family is the first system to which a person is attached.

- Families go through various developmental stages. The roles the family members fulfill change throughout the stages. For instance, when adults become parents they care for and model behavior for their children. As children mature, they rely on their parents less. Later on, the parents may have to depend on their children to meet their needs.
- Families can have healthy or dysfunctional characteristics in one or more areas of functioning.

AREAS OF FUNCTIONING

Communication

HEALTHY FAMILIES: There are clear, understandable messages between family members, and each member is encouraged to express individual feelings and thoughts.

DYSFUNCTIONAL FAMILIES
One or more members use unhealthy patterns, such as
- **Blaming:** Members blame others to shift focus away from their own inadequacies.
- **Manipulating:** Members use dishonesty to support their own agendas.
- **Placating:** One member takes responsibility for problems to keep peace at all costs.
- **Distracting:** A member inserts irrelevant information during attempts at problem solving.
- **Generalizing:** Members use overall descriptions such as "always" and "never" in describing family encounters.

Management

HEALTHY FAMILIES: Adults of a family agree on important issues, such as rule making, finances, and plans for the future.

DYSFUNCTIONAL FAMILIES: Management may be chaotic, with a child making management decisions at times.

Boundaries

HEALTHY FAMILIES: Boundaries are distinguishable between family roles. Clear boundaries define roles of each member and are understood by all. Each family member is able to function appropriately.

DYSFUNCTIONAL FAMILIES
- **Enmeshed boundaries:** Thoughts, roles, and feelings blend so much that individual roles are unclear.
- **Rigid boundaries:** Rules and roles are completely inflexible. These families tend to have members that isolate themselves.

Socialization

HEALTHY FAMILIES: All members interact, plan, and adopt healthy ways of coping. Children learn to function as family members, as well as members of society. Members are able to change as the family grows and matures.

DYSFUNCTIONAL FAMILIES: Children do not learn healthy socialization skills within the family and have difficulty adapting to socialization roles of society.

Emotional/supportive

HEALTHY FAMILIES: Emotional needs of family members are met most of the time, and members have concerns about each other. Conflict and anger do not dominate.

DYSFUNCTIONAL FAMILIES: Negative emotions predominate most of time. Members are isolated and afraid and do not show concern for each other.

OTHER CONCEPTS RELATED TO FAMILY DYSFUNCTION

Scapegoating: A member of the family with little power is blamed for problems within the family. For example, one child who has not completed his chores may be blamed for the entire family not being able to go on an outing.

Triangulation: A third party is drawn into the relationship with two members whose relationship is unstable. For example, one parent may develop an alliance with a child, leaving the other parent relatively uninvolved with both.

Multigenerational issues: These are emotional issues or themes within a family that continue for at least three generations, such as a pattern of substance use or addictive behavior, dysfunctional grief patterns, triangulation patterns, divorce.

DISCIPLINE

Family behavior that can be healthy or dysfunctional is the action of disciplining. Setting limits on children's behavior protects their safety and provides them with security. Disciplining should be consistent, timely, and age appropriate. Parents should administer discipline in private, when they are calm. Caregivers should be in unison on when and how to discipline

TYPES OF DISCIPLINE Qs

Reasoning: A healthy style of disciplining that is appropriate for older children, wherein the parent explains why a particular behavior is unacceptable. Younger children cannot cognitively understand the concepts involved.

Scolding: Reasoning can often lead to scolding, which can be an unhealthy form of disciplining as the parent sends the message that the child is bad, rather than the behavior being bad.

Behavior modification: Based on positive and negative reinforcement, the parent rewards good behavior with verbal praise and a small gift (stars and stickers for younger children, tokens to be redeemed later for older children). Negative reinforcement takes the form of ignoring. To be a valid technique, the parent must be consistent in its use.

Consequences: Children undergo outcomes for misbehavior. Consequences can be a natural occurrence (missing a treat by not showing up on time), logical (not being able to go outside to play until toys are picked up) or unrelated (having privileges taken away or being placed in time-out).

Corporal or physical punishment: Short-term solution based on the premise that pain caused from spanking will deter misbehavior. The technique has a negative impact in that it promotes violence as an acceptable behavior, poses a risk of hurting the child, and must become more severe over time as children get used to being spanked.

FAMILY THERAPY

A family is defined as a group with reciprocal relationships in which members are committed to each other. Examples of a family vary widely and are often nontraditional, such as a family made up of a child living with her grown brother and his wife. Areas of functioning for families include management, boundaries, communication, emotional support, and socialization. Dysfunction can occur in any one or more areas.

- In family therapy, the focus is on the family as a system, rather than on each person as an individual.
- Family assessments include focused interviews and use of various family assessment tools.
- Nurses work with families to provide teaching. For example, an RN might instruct a family on medication administration, or ways to help a family member manage his mental health disorder. Qpcc
- Nurses also work to mobilize family resources, to improve communication, and to strengthen the family's ability to cope with the illness of one member.

Application Exercises

1. A nurse wants to use democratic leadership with a group whose purpose is to learn appropriate conflict resolution techniques. The nurse is correct in implementing this form of group leadership when she demonstrates which of the following actions?

   A. Observes group techniques without interfering with the group process

   B. Discusses a technique and then directs members to practice the technique

   C. Asks for group suggestions of techniques and then supports discussion

   D. Suggests techniques and asks group members to reflect on their use

2. A nurse is planning group therapy for clients dealing with bereavement. Which of the following activities should the nurse include in the initial phase? (Select all that apply.)

   A. Encourage the group to work toward goals.

   B. Define the purpose of the group.

   C. Discuss termination of the group.

   D. Identify informal roles of members within the group.

   E. Establish an expectation of confidentiality within the group.

3. A nurse working on an acute mental health unit forms a group to focus on self-management of medications. At each of the meetings, two of the members use the opportunity to discuss their common interest in gambling on sports. This is an example of which of the following concepts?

   A. Triangulation

   B. Group process

   C. Subgroup

   D. Hidden agenda

4. A nurse is conducting a family therapy session. The adolescent son tells the nurse that he plans ways to make his sister look bad so his parents will think he's the better sibling, which he believes will give him more privileges. The nurse should identify this dysfunctional behavior as which of the following?

   A. Placation

   B. Manipulation

   C. Blaming

   D. Distraction

5. A nurse is working with an established group and identifies various member roles. Which of the following should the nurse identify as an individual role?

   A. A member who praises input from other members

   B. A member who follows the direction of other members

   C. A member who brags about accomplishments

   D. A member who evaluates the group's performance toward a standard

---

PRACTICE Active Learning Scenario

A nurse is creating a plan of care for a family that is planning to begin therapy to improve the emotional and supportive aspect of the family unit. Use the ATI Active Learning Template: Basic Concept to complete this item.

RELATED CONTENT: Identify the definition of a family.

UNDERLYING PRINCIPLES: Discuss the focus of family therapy.

NURSING INTERVENTIONS
- Identify at least two outcomes for emotional/supportive functioning.
- Identify at least two interventions to assist the family during therapy.

Application Exercises Key

1. A. Laissez-faire leadership allows the group process to progress without any attempt by the leader to control the direction of the group.

   B. Autocratic leadership controls the direction of the group.

   C. **CORRECT:** Democratic leadership supports group interaction and decision making to solve problems.

   D. Autocratic leadership controls the direction of the group.

   (N) *NCLEX® Connection: Management of Care, Collaboration with Interdisciplinary Team*

2. A. During the working phase, the group works toward goals.

   B. **CORRECT:** During the initial phase, the nurse should identify the purpose of the group.

   C. **CORRECT:** During the initial phase, the nurse should discuss termination of the group.

   D. During the working phase, the nurse should identify informal roles that other members in the group often assume.

   E. **CORRECT:** During the initial phase, the nurse should set the tone of the group, including an expectation of confidentiality.

   (N) *NCLEX® Connection: Psychosocial Integrity, Grief and Loss*

3. A. Triangulation is when a third party is drawn into a relationship with two members whose relationship is unstable.

   B. Group process is the verbal and nonverbal communication that occurs within the group during group sessions.

   C. A subgroup is a small number of people within a larger group who function separately from that group.

   D. **CORRECT:** A hidden agenda is when some group members have a different goal than the stated group goals. The hidden agenda is often disruptive to the effective functioning of the group.

   (N) *NCLEX® Connection: Psychosocial Integrity, Mental Health Concepts*

4. A. Placation is the dysfunctional behavior of taking responsibility for problems to keep peace among family members.

   B. **CORRECT:** Manipulation is the dysfunctional behavior of using dishonesty to support an individual agenda.

   C. Blaming is the dysfunctional behavior of blaming others to shift focus away from the individual's own inadequacies.

   D. Distraction is the dysfunctional behavior of inserting irrelevant information during attempts at problem solving.

   (N) *NCLEX® Connection: Psychosocial Integrity, Family Dynamics*

5. A. An individual who praises the input of others is acting in a maintenance role.

   B. An individual who is a follower is acting in a maintenance role.

   C. **CORRECT:** An individual who brags about accomplishments is acting in an individual role that does not promote the progression of the group toward meeting goals.

   D. An individual who evaluates the group's performance is acting in a task role.

   (N) *NCLEX® Connection: Psychosocial Integrity, Behavioral Intervention*

PRACTICE Answer

Using the ATI Active Learning Template: Basic Concept

RELATED CONTENT: A family is defined as a group with reciprocal relationships in which members are committed to each other.

UNDERLYING PRINCIPLES
- Family needs and problems within family dynamics
- Improve family functioning

NURSING INTERVENTIONS
- Outcomes
  - Family members will have emotional needs met the majority of the time.
  - Family members will show concern for each other.
  - Family members will maintain a positive emotional atmosphere rather than one of conflict and anger.
- Interventions
  - Teach the family effective ways to deal with emotional needs of family members.
  - Assist the family to improve understanding among family members.
  - Promote positive interaction among family members.
  - Identify common feelings, experiences, and thoughts among family members.

(N) *NCLEX® Connection: Psychosocial Integrity, Family Dynamics*

UNIT 2 TRADITIONAL NONPHARMACOLOGICAL
THERAPIES

CHAPTER 9 *Stress Management*

Stress is the body's nonspecific response to any demand made upon it. Stressors are physical or psychological factors that produce stress. Any stressor, whether it is perceived as "good" or "bad," produces a biological response in the body. Individuals need the presence of some stressors to provide interest and purpose to life; however, too much stress or too many stressors can cause distress. Anxiety and anger are damaging stressors that cause distress.

General adaptation syndrome (GAS) is the body's response to an increased demand. The first stage is the initial adaptive response, also known as the "fight or flight" mechanism. If stress is prolonged, maladaptive responses can occur.

Stress management is a client's ability to experience appropriate emotions and cope with stress. The client who manages stress in a healthy manner is flexible and uses a variety of coping techniques or mechanisms. Responses to stress and anxiety are affected by factors such as age, gender, culture, life experiences, and lifestyle. The effects of stressors are cumulative. For example, the death of a family member can cause a high amount of stress. If the client experiencing that stress is also experiencing other stressful events at the same time, this could cause illness due to the cumulative effect of those stressors. A client's ability to use successful stress management techniques can improve stress-related medical conditions and improve functioning.

ASSESSMENT

Protective factors increasing a client's resilience, or ability to resist the effects of stress, include the following.
- Physical health
- Strong sense of self
- Religious or spiritual beliefs
- Optimism
- Hobbies and other outside interests
- Satisfying interpersonal relationships
- Strong social support systems
- Humor

EXPECTED FINDINGS

ACUTE STRESS (FIGHT OR FLIGHT)
- Apprehension
- Unhappiness or sorrow
- Decreased appetite
- Increased respiratory rate, heart rate, cardiac output, blood pressure
- Increased metabolism and glucose use
- Depressed immune system

PROLONGED STRESS (MALADAPTIVE RESPONSE)
- Chronic anxiety or panic attacks
- Depression, chronic pain, sleep disturbances
- Weight gain or loss
- Increased risk for myocardial infarction, stroke
- Poor diabetes control, hypertension, fatigue, irritability, decreased ability to concentrate
- Increased risk for infection

STANDARDIZED SCREENING TOOLS

Life-changing events questionnaires, such as the Holmes and Rahe stress scale to measure Life Change Units, and Lazarus's Cognitive Appraisal. Q**EBP**

PATIENT-CENTERED CARE

NURSING CARE

Most nursing care involves teaching stress-reduction strategies to clients.

Cognitive techniques

Cognitive reframing
- The client is helped to look at irrational cognitions (thoughts) in a more realistic light and to restructure those thoughts in a more positive way.
- As an example, a client may think he is "a terrible father to my daughter." A health professional, using therapeutic communication techniques, could help the client reframe that thought into a positive thought, such as, "I've made some bad mistakes as a parent, but I've learned from them and have improved my parenting skills."

Behavioral techniques

RELAXATION TECHNIQUES

- Meditation includes formal meditation techniques, as well as prayer for those who believe in a higher power.
- **Guided imagery:** The client is guided through a series of images to promote relaxation. Images vary depending on the individual. For example, one client might imagine walking on a beach, while another client might imagine himself in a position of success.
- **Breathing exercises** are used to decrease rapid breathing and promote relaxation.
- **Progressive muscle relaxation:** A person trained in this method can help a client attain complete relaxation within a few minutes.
- **Physical exercise** (yoga, walking, biking) causes release of endorphins that lower anxiety, promote relaxation, and have antidepressant effects.
- Use nursing judgment to determine the appropriateness of relaxation techniques for clients who are experiencing acute manifestations of a psychotic disorder. Qs

Journal writing

- Journaling has been shown to allow for a therapeutic release of stress.
- This activity can help the client identify stressors and make specific plans to decrease stressors.

Priority restructuring

- The client learns to prioritize differently to reduce the number of stressors affecting her.
- For example, a person who is under stress due to feeling overworked might delegate some tasks to others rather than doing them all herself.

Biofeedback

A nurse or other health professional trained in this method uses a sensitive mechanical device to assist the client to gain voluntary control of such autonomic functions as heart rate and blood pressure.

Mindfulness

- The client is encouraged to be mindful of his surroundings using all of his senses, such as the relaxing warmth of sunlight or the sound of a breeze blowing through the trees.
- The client learns to restructure negative thoughts and interpretations into positive ones. For example, instead of saying, "It's so frustrating that the elevator isn't working," the client restructures the thought into, "Using the stairs is a great opportunity to burn off some extra calories."

Assertiveness training

- The client learns to communicate in a more assertive manner in order to decrease psychological stressors.
- For example, one technique teaches the client to assert his feelings by describing a situation or behavior that causes stress, stating his feelings about the behavior or situation, and then making a change. The client states, "When you keep telling me what to do, I feel angry and frustrated. I need to try making some of my own decisions."

Other individual stress-reduction techniques

- The nurse should assist each client in identifying individual strategies that improve her ability to cope with stress. Qpcc
- Examples include individual hobbies, such as fishing or scrapbooking, music therapy, and pet therapy.

Application Exercises

1. A nurse is preparing to provide an educational seminar on stress to other nursing staff. Which of the following information should the nurse include in the discussion?

   A. Excessive stressors cause the client to experience distress.

   B. The body's initial adaptive response to stress is denial.

   C. Absence of stressors results in homeostasis.

   D. Negative, rather than positive, stressors produce a biological response.

2. A nurse is discussing acute vs. prolonged stress with a client. Which of the following effects should the nurse identify as an acute stress response? (Select all that apply.)

   A. Chronic pain

   B. Depressed immune system

   C. Increased blood pressure

   D. Panic attacks

   E. Unhappiness

3. A nurse is teaching a client about stress-reduction techniques. Which of the following client statements indicates understanding of the teaching?

   A. "Cognitive reframing will help me change my irrational thoughts to something positive."

   B. "Progressive muscle relaxation uses a mechanical device to help me gain control over my pulse rate."

   C. "Biofeedback causes my body to release endorphins so that I feel less stress and anxiety."

   D. "Mindfulness allows me to prioritize the stressors that I have in my life so that I have less anxiety."

4. A client says she is experiencing increased stress because her significant other is "pressuring me and my kids to go live with him. I love him, but I'm not ready to do that." Which of the following recommendations should the nurse make to promote a change in the client's situation?

   A. Learn to practice mindfulness.

   B. Use assertiveness techniques.

   C. Exercise regularly.

   D. Rely on the support of a close friend.

5. A nurse is caring for a client who states, "I'm so stressed at work because of my coworker. He expects me to finish his work because he's too lazy!" When discussing effective communication, which of the following statements by the client to his coworker indicates client understanding?

   A. "You really should complete your own work. I don't think it's right to expect me to complete your responsibilities."

   B. "Why do you expect me to finish your work? You must realize that I have my own responsibilities."

   C. "It is not fair to expect me to complete your work. If you continue, then I will report your behavior to our supervisor."

   D. "When I have to pick up extra work, I feel very overwhelmed. I need to focus on my own responsibilities."

PRACTICE Active Learning Scenario

A nurse is leading a peer group discussion about general adaptation syndrome (GAS). Use the ATI Active Learning Template: Basic Concept and the Fundamentals Review Module to complete this item.

RELATED CONTENT: Define GAS.

UNDERLYING PRINCIPLES: Discuss the three stages of GAS.

Application Exercises Key

1. A. **CORRECT:** Distress is the result of excessive or damaging stressors, such as anxiety or anger.

   B. Denial is part of the grief process. The body's initial adaptive response to stress is known as the fight-or-flight mechanism.

   C. Individuals need the presence of some stressors to provide interest and purpose to life.

   D. Both positive and negative stressors produce a biological response in the body.

   Ⓝ *NCLEX® Connection: Psychosocial Integrity, Mental Health Concepts*

2. A. Chronic pain indicates a prolonged or maladaptive stress response.

   B. **CORRECT:** A depressed immune system is an indicator of acute stress.

   C. **CORRECT:** Increased blood pressure is an indicator of acute stress.

   D. Panic attacks indicate a prolonged or maladaptive stress response.

   E. **CORRECT:** Unhappiness is an indicator of acute stress.

   Ⓝ *NCLEX® Connection: Psychosocial Integrity, Stress Management*

3. A. **CORRECT:** Cognitive reframing helps the client look at irrational cognitions (thoughts) in a more realistic light and to restructure those thoughts in a more positive way.

   B. Biofeedback, rather than progressive muscle training, uses a mechanical device to promote voluntary control over autonomic functions.

   C. Physical exercise, rather than biofeedback, causes a release of endorphins that lower anxiety and reduce stress.

   D. Priority restructuring, rather than mindfulness, teaches the client to prioritize differently to reduce the number of stressors.

   Ⓝ *NCLEX® Connection: Psychosocial Integrity, Stress Management*

4. A. Mindfulness is appropriate to decrease the client's stress. However, it does not promote a change in the client's situation.

   B. **CORRECT:** Assertive communication allows the client to assert her feelings and then make a change in the situation.

   C. Regular exercise is appropriate to decrease the client's stress. However, it does not promote a change in the client's situation.

   D. Social support is appropriate to decrease the client's stress. However, it does not promote a change in the client's situation.

   Ⓝ *NCLEX® Connection: Psychosocial Integrity, Stress Management*

5. A. This statement is an example of disapproving/disagreeing, which can prompt a defensive reaction and is therefore nontherapeutic.

   B. This statement uses a "why" question, which implies criticism and can prompt a defensive reaction and is therefore nontherapeutic.

   C. This statement is aggressive and threatening, which can prompt a defensive reaction and is therefore nontherapeutic.

   D. **CORRECT:** This response demonstrates assertive communication, which allows the client to state his feelings about the behavior and then promote a change.

   Ⓝ *NCLEX® Connection: Psychosocial Integrity, Therapeutic Communication*

PRACTICE Answer

Using ATI Active Learning Template: Basic Concept

RELATED CONTENT: GAS is the body's response to an increased demand created by stressors.

UNDERLYING PRINCIPLES

- Stage 1: Alarm Reaction: The alarm reaction is the body's initial adaptive response to a stressor. Also known as the fight-or-flight mechanism, body functions are heightened to respond to stressors. Indicators of the alarm reaction include elevated blood pressure and heart rate, heightened mental alertness, and increased secretion of epinephrine and norepinephrine.
- Stage 2: Resistance Stage: During the resistance stage, body functions normalize while responding to the stressor. The body attempts to cope with the stressor.
- Stage 3: Exhaustion Stage: If the client reaches the exhaustion stage, body functions are no longer able to maintain an adaptive response to the stressor.

Ⓝ *NCLEX® Connection: Psychosocial Integrity, Stress Management*

UNIT 2   TRADITIONAL NONPHARMACOLOGICAL
THERAPIES

CHAPTER 10   *Brain Stimulation Therapies*

Brain stimulation therapies offer a nonpharmacological treatment for clients who have certain mental health disorders. Brain stimulation therapies include electroconvulsive therapy (ECT), transcranial magnetic stimulation (TMS), and vagus nerve stimulation (VNS).

Electroconvulsive therapy

ECT uses electrical current to induce brief seizure activity while the client is anesthetized. The exact mechanism of ECT is still unknown. One theory suggests that the seizure activity produced by ECT may enhance the effects of neurotransmitters (serotonin, dopamine, and norepinephrine) in the brain.

INDICATIONS

POTENTIAL DIAGNOSES

Major depressive disorder

- Clients whose manifestations are not responsive to pharmacological treatment
- Clients for whom the risks of other treatments outweigh the risks of ECT, such as a client who is in her first trimester of pregnancy
- Clients who are suicidal or homicidal and for whom there is a need for rapid therapeutic response Q**EBP**
- Clients who are experiencing psychotic manifestations

Schizophrenia spectrum disorders

- Clients who have schizophrenia with catatonic manifestations
- Clients who have schizoaffective disorder
- Clients who are pregnant and have a schizophrenia spectrum disorder, therefore having an increased risk for adverse effects from medication therapy

Acute manic episodes

- Clients who have bipolar disorder with rapid cycling (four or more episodes of acute mania within 1 year)
- Clients who are unresponsive to treatment with lithium and antipsychotic medications

CONTRAINDICATIONS

There are no absolute contraindications. However, the nurse should assess for medical conditions that place clients at higher risk of adverse effects. These conditions include the following.

- **Cardiovascular disorders:** Recent myocardial infarction, hypertension, heart failure, cardiac arrhythmias. ECT increases the stress on the heart due to seizure activity that occurs during the treatment.
- **Cerebrovascular disorders:** History of stroke, brain tumor, subdural hematoma. ECT increases intracranial pressure and blood flow through the brain during treatment.

Mental health conditions for which ECT has not been found useful include the following.
- Substance use disorders
- Personality disorders
- Dysphoric disorder

CONSIDERATIONS

PROCEDURAL CARE

- The typical course of ECT treatment is two to three times a week for a total of six to 12 treatments.
- The provider obtains informed consent. If ECT is involuntary, the provider may obtain consent from next of kin or a court order.
- MEDICATION MANAGEMENT
  - Thirty minutes prior to the beginning of the procedure, an IM injection of atropine sulfate or glycopyrrolate is administered to decrease secretions that could cause aspiration and to counteract any vagal stimulation effects, such as bradycardia. Q**s**
  - At the time of the procedure, an anesthesia provider administers a short-acting anesthetic, such as methohexital or propofol, via IV bolus.
  - A muscle relaxant, such as succinylcholine, is then administered to paralyze the client's muscles during the seizure activity, which decreases the risk for injury.

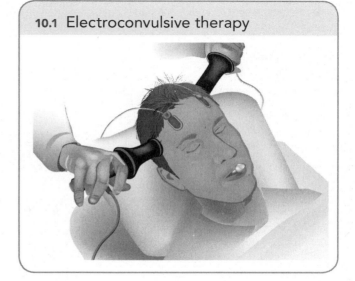

10.1 Electroconvulsive therapy

- Severe hypertension should be controlled because a short period of hypertension occurs immediately after the ECT procedure.
- Any cardiac conditions, such as dysrhythmias or hypertension, should be monitored and treated before the procedure.
- The nurse monitors vital signs and mental status before and after the ECT procedure.
- The nurse assesses the client's and family's understanding and knowledge of the procedure and provides teaching as necessary. Many clients and family have misconceptions about ECT due to media portrayals of the procedure. Due to the use of anesthesia and muscle relaxants, the tonic–clonic seizure activity associated with the procedure in the past is no longer an effect of the treatment.
- An IV line is inserted and maintained until full recovery.
- Electrodes are applied to the scalp for electroencephalogram (EEG) monitoring.
- The client receives 100% oxygen during and after ECT until the return of spontaneous respirations.
- Ongoing cardiac monitoring is provided, including blood pressure, electrocardiogram (ECG), and oxygen saturation.
- Clients are expected to become alert about 15 min following ECT.

COMPLICATIONS

Memory loss and confusion

Short-term memory loss, confusion, and disorientation occurs immediately following the procedure may persist for several hours. Memory loss can persist for several weeks. Whether ECT causes permanent memory loss is controversial, but most clients fully recover from any memory deficits.

NURSING ACTIONS
- Provide frequent orientation.
- Provide a safe environment to prevent injury. Qs
- Assist the client with personal hygiene as needed.

Reactions to anesthesia

NURSING ACTIONS: Provide continuous monitoring during the procedure and in the immediate recovery phase.

Cardiovascular changes

NURSING ACTIONS: Monitor vital signs and cardiac rhythm regularly per protocol.

Headache, muscle soreness, and nausea

Can occur during and following the immediate recovery period

NURSING ACTIONS
- Observe the client to determine the degree of discomfort.
- Administer antiemetic and analgesic medications as needed.

Relapse of depression

NURSING ACTIONS: Advise the client that ECT is not a permanent cure. Weekly or monthly maintenance ECT can decrease the incidence of relapse.

Transcranial magnetic stimulation

TMS is a noninvasive therapy that uses magnetic pulsations to stimulate the cerebral cortex of the brain.

INDICATIONS

TMS is approved by the United States Food and Drug Administration (FDA) for the treatment of major depressive disorder for clients who are not responsive to pharmacological treatment.

CONSIDERATIONS

Educate the client about TMS.
- TMS is commonly prescribed daily for a period of 4 to 6 weeks.
- TMS can be performed as an outpatient procedure.
- The TMS procedure lasts 30 to 40 min.
- A noninvasive electromagnet is placed on the client's scalp, allowing the magnetic pulsations to pass through.
- The client is alert during the procedure.
- Clients might feel a tapping or knocking sensation in the head, scalp skin contraction, and tightening of the jaw muscles during the procedure.

COMPLICATIONS

- Common adverse effects include mild discomfort or a tingling sensation at the site of the electromagnet and headaches.
- Monitor for lightheadedness after the procedure.
- Seizures are a rare but potential complication.
- TMS is not associated with systemic adverse effects or neurologic deficits.

Vagus nerve stimulation

- VNS provides electrical stimulation through the vagus nerve to the brain through a device that is surgically implanted under the skin on the client's chest.
- VNS is believed to result in an increased level of neurotransmitters.

INDICATIONS

- Depression that is resistant to pharmacological treatment and/or ECT. The treatment is approved by the FDA.
- Current research studies are determining the effectiveness for VNS in clients who have anxiety disorders, obesity, and pain.

CONSIDERATIONS

- Educate the client about VNS.
  - VNS is commonly performed as an outpatient surgical procedure.
  - The VNS device delivers around-the-clock programmed pulsations, usually every 5 minutes for a duration of 30 seconds.
  - Therapeutic antidepressant effects usually take several weeks to achieve.
  - The client can turn off the VNS device at any time by placing a special external magnet over the site of the implant.
- Assist the provider in obtaining informed consent.

COMPLICATIONS

- Voice changes due to the proximity of the implanted lead on the vagus nerve to the larynx and pharynx.
- Other potential adverse effects include hoarseness, throat or neck pain, dysphagia. These commonly improve with time.
- Dyspnea, especially with physical exertion, is possible. Therefore, the client might want to turn off the VNS during exercise or when periods of prolonged speaking are required. Qs

---

PRACTICE Active Learning Scenario

A nurse is preparing to assist in providing electroconvulsive therapy (ECT) treatment for a client. Use the ATI Active Learning Template: Therapeutic Procedure to complete this item.

DESCRIPTION OF PROCEDURE

NURSING INTERVENTIONS (PRE, INTRA, POST)
- Identify two preprocedure medication management actions.
- Identify at least two intraprocedure actions.

Application Exercises

1. A nurse is providing teaching for a client who is scheduled to receive ECT for the treatment of major depressive disorder. Which of the following client statements indicates understanding of the teaching?

   A. "It is common to treat depression with ECT before trying medications."

   B. "I can have my depression cured if I receive a series of ECT treatments."

   C. "I should receive ECT once a week for 6 weeks."

   D. "I will receive a muscle relaxant to protect me from injury during ECT."

2. A charge nurse is discussing TMS with a newly licensed nurse. Which of the following statements by the newly licensed nurse indicates an understanding of the teaching?

   A. "TMS is indicated for clients who have schizophrenia spectrum disorders."

   B. "I will provide postanesthesia care following TMS."

   C. "TMS treatments usually last 5 to 10 minutes."

   D. "I will schedule the client for daily TMS treatments for the first several weeks."

3. A nurse is assessing a client immediately following an ECT procedure. Which of the following findings should the nurse expect? (Select all that apply.)

   A. Hypotension

   B. Paralytic ileus

   C. Memory loss

   D. Nausea

   E. Confusion

4. A nurse is leading a peer group discussion about the indications for ECT. Which of the following indications should the nurse include in the discussion?

   A. Borderline personality disorder

   B. Acute withdrawal related to a substance use disorder

   C. Bipolar disorder with rapid cycling

   D. Dysphoric disorder

5. A nurse is planning care for a client following surgical implantation of a VNS device. The nurse should plan to monitor for which of the following adverse effects? (Select all that apply.)

   A. Voice changes

   B. Seizure activity

   C. Disorientation

   D. Dysphagia

   E. Neck pain

Application Exercises Key

1. A. ECT is indicated for clients who have major depressive disorder and who are not responsive to pharmacological treatment.

   B. ECT does not cure depression. However, it can reduce the incidence and severity of relapse.

   C. The typical course of ECT treatment is two to three times a week for a total of six to 12 treatments.

   D. **CORRECT:** A muscle relaxant, such as succinylcholine, is administered to reduce the risk for injury during induced seizure activity.

   Ⓝ *NCLEX® Connection: Reduction of Risk Potential, Potential for Complications of Diagnostic Tests/Treatments/Procedures*

2. A. TMS is indicated for the treatment of major depressive disorder that is not responsive to pharmacological treatment. ECT is indicated for the treatment of schizophrenia spectrum disorders.

   B. Postanesthesia care is not necessary after TMS because the client does not receive anesthesia and is alert during the procedure.

   C. The TMS procedure lasts 30 to 40 min.

   D. **CORRECT:** TMS is commonly prescribed daily for a period of 4 to 6 weeks.

   Ⓝ *NCLEX® Connection: Physiological Adaptation, Illness Management*

3. A. Immediately following ECT, the client's blood pressure is expected to be elevated.

   B. Paralytic ileus is not an expected finding of ECT.

   C. **CORRECT:** Transient short-term memory loss is an expected finding immediately following ECT.

   D. **CORRECT:** Nausea is an expected finding immediately following ECT.

   E. **CORRECT:** Confusion is an expected finding immediately following ECT.

   Ⓝ *NCLEX® Connection: Reduction of Risk Potential, Potential for Complications of Diagnostic Tests/Treatments/Procedures*

4. A. ECT has not been found to be effective for the treatment of personality disorders.

   B. ECT has not been found to be effective for the treatment of substance use disorders.

   C. **CORRECT:** ECT is indicated for the treatment of bipolar disorder with rapid cycling.

   D. ECT has not been found effective for the treatment of dysphoric disorder.

   Ⓝ *NCLEX® Connection: Physiological Adaptation, Illness Management*

5. A. **CORRECT:** Voice changes are a common adverse effect of VNS due to the proximity of the implanted lead on the vagus nerve to the larynx and pharynx.

   B. Seizure activity is associated with ECT rather than VNS.

   C. Disorientation is associated with ECT rather than VNS.

   D. **CORRECT:** Dysphagia is a potential adverse effect of VNS. However, this usually subsides with time.

   E. **CORRECT:** Neck pain is a potential adverse effect of VNS. However, this usually subsides with time.

   Ⓝ *NCLEX® Connection: Reduction of Risk Potential, Potential for Complications of Diagnostic Tests/Treatments/Procedures*

PRACTICE Answer

Using ATI Active Learning Template: Therapeutic Procedure

DESCRIPTION OF PROCEDURE: ECT is a nonpharmacologic brain stimulation therapy for the treatment of mental health disorders, especially major depressive disorder. ECT induces seizure activity, which is thought to enhance the effects of neurotransmitters in the brain.

NURSING ACTIONS (PRE, INTRA, POST)

- Preprocedure medication management actions
  - Administer atropine sulfate or glycopyrrolate 30 min prior to ECT.
  - Establish IV access prior to ECT.
  - Inform the client that the anesthesia provider will administer a short-acting anesthetic, such as methohexital or propofol, via IV bolus.
  - Inform the client that a muscle relaxant, sch as succinylcholine, is administered to paralyze the client's muscles during the seizure activity, which decreases the risk for injury.
- Intraprocedure actions
  - Apply electrodes to the scalp for EEG monitoring.
  - Apply cardiac electrodes for ECG monitoring.
  - Assist with the administration of 100% oxygen during and after ECT until the return of spontaneous respirations.
  - Monitor vital signs.

Ⓝ *NCLEX® Connection: Reduction of Risk Potential, Potential for Complications of Diagnostic Tests/Treatments/Procedures*

When reviewing the following chapters, keep in mind the relevant topics and tasks of the NCLEX outline, in particular:

Client Needs: Psychosocial Integrity

CRISIS INTERVENTION: Identify the client in crisis.

BEHAVIORAL INTERVENTIONS
Assist the client to develop and use strategies to decrease anxiety.

Assess the client's appearance, mood and psychomotor behavior and identify/respond to inappropriate/abnormal behavior.

CHEMICAL AND OTHER DEPENDENCIES/SUBSTANCE USE DISORDER: Assess client for drug-alcohol dependencies, withdrawal, or toxicities and intervene as appropriate.

MENTAL HEALTH CONCEPTS
Recognize signs and symptoms of acute and chronic mental illness.

Assess client for alterations in mood, judgment, cognition and reasoning.

Provide care and education for acute and chronic psychosocial health issues.

THERAPEUTIC COMMUNICATION: Encourage the client to verbalize feelings.

SENSORY/PERCEPTUAL ALTERATIONS: Provide care for a client experiencing visual, auditory or cognitive distortions.

Client Needs: Safety and Infection Control

ACCIDENT/ERROR/INJURY PREVENTION
Identify factors that influence accident/injury prevention.

Protect client from injury.

Client Needs: Health Promotion and Maintenance

DEVELOPMENTAL STAGES AND TRANSITIONS:
Compare client development to expected age/ developmental stage and report and deviations.

HEALTH PROMOTION/DISEASE PREVENTION:
Identify risk factors for disease/illness.

Client Needs: Reduction of Risk Potential

SYSTEM SPECIFIC ASSESSMENTS
Assess the client for abnormal neurological status.

Recognize trends and changes in client condition
and intervene as appropriate.

Perform a risk assessment.

Client Needs: Physiological Adaptation

ALTERATIONS IN BODY SYSTEMS: Evaluate
achievement of client treatment goals.

PATHOPHYSIOLOGY: Identify pathophysiology
related to an acute or chronic condition.

Client Needs: Pharmacological and Parenteral Therapies

**ADVERSE EFFECTS/CONTRAINDICATIONS/
SIDE EFFECTS/INTERACTIONS:** Assess the client for
actual or potential adverse effects of medications.

EXPECTED ACTIONS/OUTCOMES: Evaluate
client response to medication.

UNIT 3   PSYCHOBIOLOGIC DISORDERS

CHAPTER 11 *Anxiety Disorders*

Normal anxiety is a healthy response to stress that is essential for survival. Elevated or persistent anxiety can result in anxiety disorders causing behavior changes and impairment in functioning. Anxiety disorders tend to be persistent and are often disabling.

Anxiety levels can be mild (restlessness, increased motivation, irritability), moderate (agitation, muscle tightness), severe (inability to function, ritualistic behavior, unresponsive), or panic (distorted perception, loss of rational thought, immobility).

TYPES OF DISORDERS

ANXIETY DISORDERS

Anxiety disorders recognized and defined by the DSM-5 include the following:

Separation anxiety disorder: The client experiences excessive fear or anxiety when separated from an individual to which the client is emotionally attached.

Specific phobias: The client experiences an irrational fear of a certain object or situation. Specific clinical names are used to refer to specific phobias (monophobia = phobia of being alone; zoophobia = phobia of animals; acrophobia = phobia of heights).

Agoraphobia: The client experiences an extreme fear of certain places (such as the outdoors or being on a bridge) where the client feels vulnerable or unsafe.

Social anxiety disorder (social phobia): The client experiences excessive fear of social or performance situations.

Panic disorder: The client experiences recurrent panic attacks.

Generalized anxiety disorder (GAD): The client exhibits uncontrollable, excessive worry for at least 6 months.

OBSESSIVE COMPULSIVE DISORDERS

Obsessive-compulsive and related disorders are not actual anxiety disorders but have similar effects and include the following:

Obsessive compulsive disorder (OCD): The client has intrusive thoughts of unrealistic obsessions and tries to control these thoughts with compulsive behaviors (e.g., repetitive cleaning of a particular object or washing of hands).

Hoarding disorder: The client has difficulty parting with possessions, resulting in extreme stress and functional impairments.

Body dysmorphic disorder: The client has a preoccupation with perceived flaws or defects in physical appearance.

ASSESSMENT

RISK FACTORS

- Most anxiety disorders are more likely to occur in women. Obsessive-compulsive and related disorders also affect women more than men with the exception of hoarding disorder which has a higher prevalence rate among men. Anxiety and obsessive-compulsive disorders have a genetic and neurobiological link.
- Clients can experience anxiety due to an acute medical condition, such as hyperthyroidism or pulmonary embolism. It is important to assess the manifestations of anxiety in a medical facility to rule out a physical cause. QEBP
- Adverse effects of many medications can mimic anxiety disorders.
- Substance-induced anxiety is related to current use of a chemical substance or to withdrawal effects from a substance, such as alcohol.

EXPECTED FINDINGS

Separation anxiety disorder

- The client exhibits excessive levels of anxiety and concern when separated from someone to whom they have an emotional attachment, fearing that something tragic will occur resulting in permanent separation.
- The client's anxiety disrupts the ability to participate in routine daily activities.
- Physical manifestations of anxiety develop during the separation or in anticipation of the separation and include headaches, nausea and vomiting, and sleep disturbances.

Specific phobias

- The client reports a fear of specific objects, such as spiders, snakes, or strangers.
- The client reports a fear of specific experiences, such as flying, being in the dark, riding in an elevator, or being in an enclosed space.
- The client might experience anxiety manifestations just by thinking of the feared object or situation and might attempt to decrease the anxiety through the use of alcohol or other substances.

Agoraphobia

- The client avoids certain places or situations that cause anxiety. This avoidance might disrupt the client's ability to maintain employment or participate in routine activities of daily life.
- The client's fear and manifestations of anxiety are out of proportion with the actual danger of the place or situation.

Social phobia

- The client reports difficulty performing or speaking in front of others or participating in social situations due to an excessive fear of embarrassment or poor performance.
- The client might report physical manifestations (actual or factitious) in an attempt to avoid the social situation or need to perform.

Panic disorder

- Panic attacks typically last 15 to 30 min.
- Four or more of the following manifestations are present during a panic attack:
  - Palpitations
  - Shortness of breath
  - Choking or smothering sensation
  - Chest pain
  - Nausea
  - Feelings of depersonalization
  - Fear of dying or insanity
  - Chills or hot flashes
- The client might experience behavior changes and/or persistent worries about when the next attack will occur.

Generalized anxiety disorder

- The client exhibits uncontrollable, excessive worry for more than 6 months.
- GAD causes significant impairment in one or more areas of functioning, such as work-related duties.
- Manifestations of GAD include the following:
  - Restlessness
  - Muscle tension
  - Avoidance of stressful activities or events
  - Increased time and effort required to prepare for stressful activities or events
  - Procrastination in decision making
  - Seeks repeated reassurance

Obsessive-compulsive disorders

OCD: The client attempts to suppress persistent thoughts or urges that cause anxiety through compulsive or obsessive behaviors, such as repetitive handwashing. Obsessions or compulsions are time-consuming and result in impaired social and occupational functioning.

Hoarding disorder: The client has an obsessive desire to save items regardless of value and experiences extreme stress with thoughts of discarding or getting rid of items. The client's hoarding behavior results in social and occupational impairment and often leads to an unsafe living environment.

Body dysmorphic disorder: The client attempts to conceal a perceived physical flaw and practices repetitive behaviors, such as mirror checking or comparison to others, in response to the anxiety experienced over the perception. The client might have social and occupational impairment in response to the perceived physical defects or flaws.

STANDARDIZED SCREENING TOOLS

- Hamilton Rating Scale for Anxiety QEBP
- Fear Questionnaire (phobias)
- Panic Disorder Severity Scale
- Yale-Brown Obsessive Compulsive Scale
- Hoarding Scale Self-Report

PATIENT-CENTERED CARE

NURSING CARE

- Provide a structured interview to keep the client focused on the present.
- Assess for comorbid condition of substance use disorder.
- Provide safety and comfort to the client during the crisis period of these disorders, as clients in severe- to panic-level anxiety are unable to problem solve and focus. Clients experiencing panic-level anxiety benefit from a calm, quiet environment.
- Remain with the client during the worst of the anxiety to provide reassurance.
- Perform a suicide risk assessment. Qs
- Provide a safe environment for other clients and staff.
- Provide milieu therapy that employs the following:
  - A structured environment for physical safety and predictability
  - Monitoring for, and protection from, self-harm or suicide
  - Daily activities that encourage the client to share and be cooperative
  - Use of therapeutic communication skills, such as open-ended questions, to help the client express feelings of anxiety, and to validate and acknowledge those feelings
  - Client participation in decision making regarding care
- Use relaxation techniques with the client as needed for relief of pain, muscle tension, and feelings of anxiety.
- Instill hope for positive outcomes (but avoid false reassurance).
- Enhance client self-esteem by encouraging positive statements and discussing past achievements.
- Assist the client to identify defense mechanisms that interfere with recovery.
- Postpone health teaching until after acute anxiety subsides. Clients experiencing a panic attack or severe anxiety are unable to concentrate or learn.

MEDICATIONS

SSRI antidepressants, such as sertraline or paroxetine, are the first line of treatment for anxiety and obsessive-compulsive disorders.

SNRI antidepressants, such as venlafaxine or duloxetine, are effective in the treatment of anxiety disorders.

Antianxiety medications are helpful in treating the manifestations of anxiety disorders. **Benzodiazepines**, such as diazepam, are indicated for short-term use. **Buspirone** is effective in managing anxiety and can be taken for long-term treatment of anxiety.

Other medications that can be used to treat anxiety disorders include **beta blockers** and **antihistamines** to decrease anxiety. **Anticonvulsants** are used as mood stabilizers for the client who is experiencing anxiety.

THERAPEUTIC PROCEDURES

Cognitive behavioral therapy

The anxiety response can be decreased by changing cognitive distortions. This therapy uses cognitive reframing to help the client identify negative thoughts that produce anxiety, examine the cause, and develop supportive ideas that replace negative self-talk. Ⓠ**EBP**

Behavioral therapies

Behavioral therapies teach clients ways to decrease anxiety or avoidant behavior and allow an opportunity to practice techniques.

Relaxation training is used to control pain, tension, and anxiety. Refer to the chapter on *Stress Management*, which covers relaxation training techniques.

Modeling allows a client to see a demonstration of appropriate behavior in a stressful situation. The goal of therapy is that the client will imitate the behavior.

Systematic desensitization begins with mastering of relaxation techniques. Then, a client is exposed to increasing levels of an anxiety-producing stimulus (either imagined or real) and uses relaxation to overcome the resulting anxiety. The goal of therapy is that the client is able to tolerate a greater and greater level of the stimulus until anxiety no longer interferes with functioning. This form of therapy is especially effective for clients who have phobias.

Flooding involves exposing the client to a great deal of an undesirable stimulus in an attempt to turn off the anxiety response. This therapy is useful for clients who have phobias.

Response prevention focuses on preventing the client from performing a compulsive behavior with the intent that anxiety will diminish.

Thought stopping teaches a client to say "stop" when negative thoughts or compulsive behaviors arise, and substitute a positive thought. The goal of therapy is that with time, the client uses the command silently.

CLIENT EDUCATION

- Educate the client regarding identification of manifestations of anxiety.
- Instruct the client to notify the provider of worsening effects and to not adjust medication dosages. Warn the client against stopping or increasing medication without consulting the provider.
- Assist the client to evaluate coping mechanisms that work and do not work for controlling the anxiety, and assist the client to learn new methods. Use of alternative stress relief and coping mechanisms might increase medication effectiveness and decrease the need for medication in most cases. Ⓠ**PCC**

Application Exercises

1. A nurse observes a client who has OCD repeatedly applying, removing, and then reapplying makeup. The nurse identifies that repetitive behavior in a client who has OCD is due to which of the following underlying reasons?

   A. Narcissistic behavior
   B. Fear of rejection from staff
   C. Attempt to reduce anxiety
   D. Adverse effect of antidepressant medication

2. A nurse is caring for a client who is experiencing a panic attack. Which of the following actions should the nurse take?

   A. Discuss new relaxation techniques.
   B. Show the client how to change his behavior.
   C. Distract the client with a television show.
   D. Stay with the client and remain quiet.

3. A nurse is assessing a client who has generalized anxiety disorder. Which of the following findings should the nurse expect? (Select all that apply.)

   A. Excessive worry for 6 months
   B. Impulsive decision making
   C. Delayed reflexes
   D. Restlessness
   E. Need for reassurance

4. A nurse is planning care for a client who has body dysmorphic disorder. Which of the following actions should the nurse plan to take first?

   A. Assessing the client's risk for self-harm
   B. Instilling hope for positive outcomes
   C. Encouraging the client to participate in group therapy sessions
   D. Encouraging the client to participate in treatment decisions

5. A nurse is caring for a client who has acute stress disorder and is experiencing severe anxiety. Which of the following statements actions should the nurse make?

   A. "Tell me about how you are feeling right now."
   B. "You should focus on the positive things in your life to decrease your anxiety."
   C. "Why do you believe you are experiencing this anxiety?"
   D. "Let's discuss the medications your provider is prescribing to decrease your anxiety."

PRACTICE Active Learning Scenario

A nurse working in a mental health clinic is teaching a client who has a specific phobia of riding on an elevator about the use of systematic desensitization as a form of behavioral therapy. Use the ATI Active Learning Template: Therapeutic Procedure to complete this item.

DESCRIPTION OF PROCEDURE

INDICATIONS: Describe one.

OUTCOMES/EVALUATION: Identify at least two client outcomes.

Application Exercises Key

1. A. Clients who have OCD demonstrate repetitive behavior but not out of narcissism, which might be associated with personality disorders.

   B. Clients who have OCD demonstrate repetitive behavior but not out of fear of rejection, which might be associated with social phobia anxiety disorder.

   C. **CORRECT:** Clients who have OCD demonstrate repetitive behavior in an attempt to suppress persistent thoughts or urges that cause anxiety.

   D. Clients who have OCD might take an antidepressant to help control repetitive behavior.

   Ⓝ *NCLEX® Connection: Psychosocial Integrity, Mental Health Concepts*

2. A. During a panic attack, the client is unable to concentrate on learning new information.

   B. During a panic attack, the client is unable to concentrate on learning new information.

   C. During a panic attack, the nurse should avoid further stimuli that can increase the client's level of anxiety.

   D. **CORRECT:** During a panic attack, the nurse should quietly remain with the client. This promotes safety and reassurance without additional stimuli.

   Ⓝ *NCLEX® Connection: Psychosocial Integrity, Behavioral Interventions*

3. A. **CORRECT:** Generalized anxiety disorder is characterized by uncontrollable, excessive worry for more than 3 months.

   B. Generalized anxiety disorder is characterized by procrastination in decision making.

   C. Generalized anxiety disorder is characterized by muscle tension.

   D. **CORRECT:** Generalized anxiety disorder is characterized by restlessness.

   E. **CORRECT:** Generalized anxiety disorder is characterized by the need for repeated reassurance.

   Ⓝ *NCLEX® Connection: Psychosocial Integrity, Mental Health Concepts*

4. A. **CORRECT:** The greatest risk to a client who has an anxiety or obsessive-compulsive disorder is self-harm or suicide. Therefore, the first action the nurse should plan to take is to assess the client's risk for self-harm to ensure that the client is provided with a safe environment.

   B. The nurse should instill hope for positive outcomes, without providing false reassurance, as part of milieu therapy; however, there is another action that the nurse should take first.

   C. The nurse should encourage the client to participate in group therapy to assist the client in order to address social impairments that result from the disorder; however, there is another action that the nurse should take first.

   D. The nurse should encourage the client to participate in treatment decisions as part of milieu therapy; however, there is another action that the nurse should take first.

   Ⓝ *NCLEX® Connection: Physiological Adaptation, Pathophysiology*

5. A. **CORRECT:** Asking an open-ended question is therapeutic and assists the client in identifying anxiety.

   B. Offering advice is nontherapeutic and can hinder further communication.

   C. Asking the client a "why" question is nontherapeutic and can promote a defensive client response.

   D. Postpone health teaching until after acute anxiety subsides. Clients experiencing severe anxiety are unable to concentrate or learn.

   Ⓝ *NCLEX® Connection: Psychosocial Integrity, Stress Management*

PRACTICE Answer

Using the ATI Active Learning Template: Therapeutic Procedure

DESCRIPTION OF PROCEDURE: Systematic desensitization is a behavioral therapy that exposes clients to increasing levels of an anxiety-producing stimulus.

INDICATIONS: Systematic desensitization is indicated for the treatment of anxiety disorders associated with an anxiety-producing stimulus.

OUTCOMES/EVALUATION
- The client will demonstrate effective relaxation techniques to overcome anxiety.
- The client's level of functioning will not be impaired by the phobia.
- The client will verbalize decreased feelings of anxiety when encountering the stimulus.

Ⓝ *NCLEX® Connection: Psychosocial Integrity, Stress Management*

UNIT 3   PSYCHOBIOLOGIC DISORDERS

CHAPTER 12 *Trauma- and Stressor-Related Disorders*

Clients can develop a trauma- or stressor-related disorder following exposure to a traumatic event, such as military combat, or to an extreme stressor, such as the unexpected death of a family member. It is important that nurses have an understanding of how to effectively assess and care for clients experiencing this type of disorder.

SPECIFIC DISORDERS

Acute stress disorder (ASD): Exposure to traumatic events causes anxiety, detachment and other manifestations about the event for at least 3 days but for not more than 1 month following the event.

Posttraumatic stress disorder (PTSD): Exposure to traumatic events causes anxiety, detachment, and other manifestations about the event for longer than 1 month following the event. Manifestations can last for years.

Adjustment disorder: A stressor triggers a reaction causing changes in mood and/or dysfunction in performing usual activities. The stressor and effects are less severe than with ASD or PTSD.

Dissociative disorders
- **Depersonalization/derealization disorder:** This disorder is characterized by a temporary change in awareness displaying depersonalization, derealization, or both. Depersonalization is the feeling that a person is observing one's own personality or body from a distance. Derealization is the feeling that outside events are unreal or part of a dream, or that objects appear larger or smaller than they should.
- **Dissociative amnesia:** Inability to recall personal information regarding stressful events for a period of time
- **Dissociative fugue:** A type of dissociative amnesia in which the client travels to a new area and is unable to remember one's own identity and at least some of one's past. Can last weeks to months and usually follows a traumatic event.
- **Dissociative identity disorder:** Client displays more than one distinct personality, with a stressful event precipitating the change from one personality to another.

HEALTH PROMOTION AND DISEASE PREVENTION

The nurse should monitor for and recognize child physical and sexual abuse, which can lead to ASD or PTSD, and report suspected cases to the proper authorities promptly to prevent severe trauma reactions from occurring.

The nurse should recognize occupations that have a high incidence of PTSD, such as participation in military combat. Clients should receive support and treatment before severe trauma reactions occur.

PTSD PREVENTION

Health promotion measures to prevent PTSD during and after a traumatic incident, such as a mass casualty incident involving police, paramedics, health care staff and others Q̣EBP
- During the incident, be aware of need for breaks, rest, adequate water, and nutrition.
- Provide emotional support for those involved in the incident.
- Encourage staff to support each other.
- Debrief with others following the incident.
- Encourage expression of feelings by all involved.
- Use offered counseling resources.

ASSESSMENT

RISK FACTORS

ASD, PTSD, and adjustment disorder

- Exposure to a traumatic event or experience, such as a motor vehicle crash, rape, physical abuse. For adjustment disorder, the event or experience can be less severe, such as a breakup of a relationship or loss of employment.
- Exposure to trauma experienced during a natural disaster, such as a fire, storm, or a man-made experience, such as terrorism
- Exposure or repeated re-exposure to trauma in an occupational setting, such as in military combat, or as experienced by medical personnel or law enforcement officers, can precipitate a trauma- and stressor-related disorder.
- Living through a traumatic event experienced by a family member or close friend, such as an airplane crash or homicide
- The client who has PTSD is also at risk for other disorders, including dissociative disorders, anxiety, depression, and substance use disorders

ASD and PTSD

- Characteristics about the trauma, such as duration of the experience, the amount of personal threat associated with the trauma and whether it occurs far from home or in familiar surroundings
- Characteristics about the individual, such as past coping mechanisms, personality, and pre-existing mental disorders
- Characteristics about the treatment environment following the trauma, such as client social supports, societal attitudes about the situation, and cultural influences

Adjustment disorder

- Pattern of life-long difficulty accepting change
- Learned pattern of difficulty with social skills or coping strategies which, when a stressor occurs, can trigger a stress response out of proportion to the stressor

Dissociative disorders

- Traumatic life event
- Childhood abuse or trauma

EXPECTED FINDINGS

ASD and PTSD

- Intrusive findings (presence of memories, flashbacks, dreams about the traumatic event)
- Memories of the event recur involuntarily and are distressing to the client
- Flashbacks (dissociative reactions where the client feels the traumatic event is recurring in the present), such as a military veteran feeling that he is reliving a combat situation after hearing a harmless loud noise
- Night-time dreams related to the traumatic event
- Avoidance of people, places, events, or situations that bring back reminders of the traumatic event
- Trying to avoid thinking of the event

MOOD AND COGNITIVE ALTERATIONS
- Anxiety or depressive disorders
- Anger, irritability frequently present
- Decreased interest in current activities
- Guilt, negative self-beliefs, and cognitive distortions, such as, "I am responsible for everything bad that happens."
- Detachment from others, including friends and family members
- Inability to experience positive emotional experiences, such as love and tenderness
- Dissociative manifestations, such as amnesia, derealization, or depersonalization

BEHAVIORAL MANIFESTATIONS
- Aggression, irritability, and angry responses toward others
- Hypervigilance with heightened startle responses
- Inability to focus and concentrate on work or other activities
- Sleep disturbances, such as insomnia
- Destructive behavior, such as suicidal thoughts or thoughts of harming others Qs

Adjustment disorder

- Depression
- Anxiety
- Changes in behavior, such as arguing with others or driving erratically

Dissociative disorders

Depersonalization/derealization disorder: Reports of feeling detached from one's body or feeling disconnected from his environment.

Dissociative amnesia: Lack of memory that can range from name or date of birth to the client's entire lifetime.

Dissociative identity disorder: Client displays two or more separate personalities. Each personality can be very distinct and different from the other.

DIAGNOSTIC PROCEDURES

ASD, PTSD, and adjustment disorder Qᴇʙᴘ

- Screening tools, such as the Primary Care PTSD Screen and the PTSD Checklist
- Screening tests for anxiety and depression
- Asking about suicidal ideation
- Mental status examination

Dissociative disorders

- Physical assessment, electroencephalogram, and x-ray studies to rule out physical trauma (traumatic brain injury, epilepsy)
- Screening to rule out substance use
- Mental status examination and nursing history

NURSING ACTIONS
- Assess recent and remote memory for gaps or contradictions.
- Check for family and occupational difficulties.
- Ask about occurrence of stressful events.
- Assess for depression, mood shifts, and anxiety.
- Use screening tools, such as the Dissociative Disorders Interview Schedule, Somatoform Dissociation Questionnaire and the Dissociative Experience Scale.

PATIENT-CENTERED CARE

NURSING CARE

ASD, PTSD, and adjustment disorder

- Establish a therapeutic relationship, and encourage the client to share feelings. Qᴘᴄᴄ
- Provide a safe, nonthreatening, routine environment.
- Assess clients for suicidal ideation, and take precautions as needed.
- Use multiple strategies to decrease anxiety, such as music therapy, guided imagery, massage, relaxation therapy, and breathing techniques.

Dissociative disorders

- During dissociative periods, help the client make decisions to lower stress.
- When the client shows readiness, encourage independence and decision making.
- Instruct clients in strategies to reduce anxiety.
- Use grounding techniques, such as having the client clap hands or touch an object.
- Allow clients to verbalize negative feelings and to progress at their own pace.
- Avoid giving the client too much information about past events to prevent increased stress.

MEDICATIONS

ASD and PTSD

- Antidepressants can decrease depression and relieve anxiety in ASD or PTSD.
  - Fluoxetine, a selective serotonin reuptake inhibitor
  - Venlafaxine, a serotonin norepinephrine reuptake inhibitor
  - Mirtazapine, a norepinephrine and serotonin specific antidepressant
  - Amitriptyline, a tricyclic antidepressant
- Prazosin, a centrally-acting alpha agonist, can decrease manifestations of hypervigilance and insomnia.
- Propranolol, a beta-adrenergic blocker, decreases elevated vital signs and manifestations of anxiety, panic, hypervigilance, and insomnia.

Adjustment disorder and dissociative disorders

Medications might not be prescribed for adjustment disorder or the dissociative disorders unless specific findings of depression or anxiety require treatment.

THERAPEUTIC PROCEDURES

Cognitive-behavioral therapy (cognitive restructuring): The client is helped to change appraisal of events and change negative thoughts.

Prolonged exposure therapy: Combines the use of relaxation techniques with exposure to the traumatic situation. The exposure can either be imagined through the use of repeated discussion of the traumatic event or practiced in real-world situations (in vivo) in which the client is exposed to the traumatic situation within safe limits. The repeated exposure eventually results in a decreased anxiety response.

Psychodynamic psychotherapy: Getting in touch with conscious and unconscious thought processes.

Eye movement desensitization and reprocessing (EMDR)
- A therapy using rapid eye movements during desensitization techniques in a multi-phase process by a trained therapist.
- Contraindicated for clients who have active suicidal ideation, psychosis, severe dissociative disorders, detached retina or glaucoma, or severe substance use disorder. Q EBP

Group or family therapy can include support groups or formal therapy.

Crisis intervention immediately following a traumatic incident.

Somatic therapy for dissociative disorders: Psychotherapy works over time to increase awareness of the present and decrease dissociation episodes.

Hypnotherapy can be used for dissociative disorders.

Biofeedback/neurofeedback helps the client learn how to increase awareness and gain control of reactions to a trigger.

INTERPROFESSIONAL CARE

- Refer clients to social workers/case managers for coordination of community care.
- Collaborate with psychotherapists to ensure coordination of care.

CLIENT EDUCATION

- Teach relaxation techniques and other anxiety-reducing strategies.
- Teach the client and family about causes and manifestations of the disorder.
- Instruct the client to avoid caffeine and alcohol.
- Teach grounding techniques for clients who have dissociative disorders. The client is taught to observe and experience physical objects or situations and to keep a written journal.

Application Exercises

1. A nurse working on an acute mental health unit is caring for a client who has posttraumatic stress disorder (PTSD). Which of the following findings should the nurse expect? (Select all that apply.)
   - A. Difficulty concentrating on tasks
   - B. Obsessive need to talk about the traumatic event
   - C. Negative self-image
   - D. Recurring nightmares
   - E. Diminished reflexes

2. A nurse is involved in a serious and prolonged mass casualty incident in the emergency department. Which of the following strategies should the nurse use to help prevent developing a trauma-related disorder? (Select all that apply)
   - A. Avoid thinking about the incident when it is over.
   - B. Take breaks during the incident for food and water.
   - C. Debrief with others following the incident.
   - D. Hold emotions in check in the days following the incident.
   - E. Take advantage of offered counseling.

3. A nurse is collecting an admission history for a client who has acute stress disorder (ASD). Which of the following information should the nurse expect to collect?
   - A. The client remembers many details about the traumatic incident.
   - B. The client expresses heightened elation about what is happening.
   - C. The client states he first noticed manifestations of the disorder 6 weeks after the traumatic incident occurred.
   - D. The client expresses a sense of unreality about the traumatic incident.

4. A nurse is caring for a client who has derealization disorder. Which of the following findings should the nurse identify as an indication of derealization?
   - A. The client explains that her body seems to be floating above the ground.
   - B. The client has the idea that someone is trying to kill her and steal her money.
   - C. The client states that the furniture in the room seems to be small and far away.
   - D. The client cannot recall anything that happened during the past 2 weeks.

5. A nurse in an acute mental health facility is planning care for a client who has dissociative fugue. Which of the following interventions should the nurse add to the plan of care?
   - A. Teach the client to recognize how stress brings on a personality change in the client.
   - B. Repeatedly present the client with information about past events.
   - C. Make decisions for the client regarding routine daily activities.
   - D. Work with the client on grounding techniques.

PRACTICE Active Learning Scenario

A nurse is caring for a client who has post traumatic stress disorder (PTSD) following several months in a military combat situation. Use the Active Learning Template: System Disorder to complete this item.

ALTERATION IN HEALTH (DIAGNOSIS): Differentiate PTSD from acute stress disorder (ASD).

EXPECTED FINDINGS: List three subjective and three objective manifestations of PTSD.

NURSING CARE: List three nursing actions for a client who has PTSD.

THERAPEUTIC PROCEDURES: Describe two therapeutic techniques used to treat a client who has PTSD.

Application Exercises Key

1. A. **CORRECT:** Manifestations of PTSD include the inability to concentrate on or complete tasks.

   B. A client who has PTSD is reluctant to talk about the traumatic event that triggered the disorder.

   C. **CORRECT:** Manifestations of PTSD include feeling guilty and having a negative self-image.

   D. **CORRECT:** Manifestations of PTSD include recurring nightmares or flashbacks.

   E. A client who has PTSD has an increased startle reflex and hypervigilance.

   Ⓝ *NCLEX® Connection: Psychosocial Integrity, Mental Health Concepts*

2. A. Thinking and talking about a traumatic incident can help prevent development of a trauma-related disorder.

   B. **CORRECT:** Taking breaks and remembering to drink water and eat nutritious foods while working during a traumatic incident can help prevent development of a trauma-related disorder.

   C. **CORRECT:** Debriefing with others following a traumatic incident can help prevent development of a trauma-related disorder.

   D. Displaying emotions following a traumatic incident can help prevent development of a trauma-related disorder.

   E. **CORRECT:** Taking advantage of counseling offered by an employer or others can help prevent development of a trauma-related disorder.

   Ⓝ *NCLEX® Connection: Psychosocial Integrity, Crisis Intervention*

3. A. The client who has ASD tends to be unable to remember details about the incident and can block the entire incident from memory.

   B. The client who has ASD reacts to what is happening with negative emotions such as anger, guilt, depression, and anxiety. Elation is an emotion that can occur in clients who have mania.

   C. Manifestations of ASD occur immediately to a few days following the event.

   D. **CORRECT:** The client who has ASD often expresses dissociative manifestations regarding the event, which includes a sense of unreality.

   Ⓝ *NCLEX® Connection: Psychosocial Integrity, Mental Health Concepts*

4. A. Feeling that one's body is floating above the ground is an example of depersonalization, in which the person seems to observe her own body from a distance.

   B. Having the idea that others are trying to hurt or kill her is an example of a paranoid delusion.

   C. **CORRECT:** Stating that one's surroundings are far away or unreal in some way is an example of derealization.

   D. Being unable to recall any events from the past 2 weeks is an example of amnesia.

   Ⓝ *NCLEX® Connection: Psychosocial Integrity, Mental Health Concepts*

5. A. The client who has dissociative identity disorder displays multiple personalities, while the client who has dissociative fugue has amnesia regarding her identity and past.

   B. The nurse should avoid flooding the client with information about past events, which can increase the client's level of anxiety.

   C. The nurse should encourage the client to make decisions regarding routine daily activities in order to promote improved self-esteem and decrease the client's feelings of powerlessness.

   D. **CORRECT:** Grounding techniques, such as stomping the feet, clapping the hands, or touching physical objects, are useful for clients who have a dissociative disorder and are experiencing manifestations of derealization.

   Ⓝ *NCLEX® Connection: Psychosocial Integrity, Mental Health Concepts*

PRACTICE Answer

Using the ATI Active Learning Template: System Disorder

ALTERATION IN HEALTH (DIAGNOSIS)
- Both disorders follow a traumatic incident or multiple experiences that the client perceives as traumatic.
- ASD manifestations occur soon after the incident but subside within 1 month of the trauma.
- PTSD findings can be delayed for weeks or months after the trauma has subsided and continue for months or years, often causing severe social and occupational implications.

EXPECTED FINDINGS
- Subjective manifestations: Client describes dreams and/or flashbacks of the traumatic event; client states he has insomnia; client verbalizes guilt and self-blame.
- Objective manifestations: Hyperactive startle reflexes; manifestations of anxiety, such as tachycardia, hyperventilation; inability to focus in order to complete a simple task.

NURSING CARE
- Monitor for suicidal ideation, and take precautions if it occurs.
- Provide a safe, routine environment for the client.
- Teach strategies to decrease anxiety, such as breathing techniques or music therapy.
- Encourage the client to share feelings.
- Use therapeutic communication techniques to assist a client who has cognitive distortions.

THERAPEUTIC PROCEDURES:
Therapeutic techniques for a client who has PTSD include eye movement desensitization and reprocessing (EMDR), group and family therapy, and cognitive behavioral therapy.

Ⓝ *NCLEX® Connection: Psychosocial Integrity, Mental Health Concepts*

UNIT 3 PSYCHOBIOLOGIC DISORDERS

CHAPTER 13 *Depressive Disorders*

Depression is a mood (affective) disorder that is a widespread issue, ranking high among causes of disability.

A client who has depression has a potential risk for suicide, especially if he has a family or personal history of suicide attempts, comorbid anxiety disorder or panic attacks, comorbid substance use disorder or psychosis, poor self-esteem, a lack of social support, or a chronic medical condition.

COMMON COMORBIDITIES

Anxiety disorders: These disorders are comorbid in approximately 70% of clients who have a depressive disorder. This combination makes a client's prognosis poorer, with a higher risk for suicide and disability.

Psychotic disorders, such as schizophrenia

Substance use disorders: Clients often use substances in an attempt to relieve manifestations of depression or self-treat mental health disorders.

Eating disorders

Personality disorders

DEPRESSIVE DISORDERS RECOGNIZED BY THE DSM-5

Major depressive disorder (MDD): A single episode or recurrent episodes of unipolar depression (not associated with mood swings from major depression to mania) resulting in a significant change in a client's normal functioning (social, occupational, self-care) accompanied by at least five of the following specific clinical findings, which must occur almost every day for a minimum of 2 weeks, and last most of the day.
- Depressed mood
- Difficulty sleeping or excessive sleeping
- Indecisiveness
- Decreased ability to concentrate
- Suicidal ideation
- Increase or decrease in motor activity
- Inability to feel pleasure
- Increase or decrease in weight of more than 5% of total body weight over 1 month

A bereavement exclusion was previously used when a client experienced clinical findings of depression within the first 2 months after a significant loss. Now, however, a client can be diagnosed with depression during this time so that needed treatment will not be delayed.

- MDD can be further diagnosed in the DSM-5 with a more specific classification (specifier), including the following.
  - **Psychotic features:** The presence of auditory hallucinations (e.g., voices telling the client she is sinful) or the presence of delusions (e.g., client thinking that she has a fatal disease)
  - **Postpartum onset:** A depressive episode that begins within 4 weeks of childbirth (known as postpartum depression) and can include delusions, which can put the newborn infant at high risk of being harmed by the mother

Seasonal affective disorder (SAD): A form of depression that occurs seasonally, usually during the winter, when there is less daylight. Light therapy is the first-line treatment for SAD.

Dysthymic disorder: A milder form of depression that usually has an early onset, such as in childhood or adolescence, and lasts at least 2 years for adults (1 year for children). Dysthymic disorder contains at least three clinical findings of depression and can, later in life, become major depressive disorder.

Premenstrual dysphoric disorder (PMDD): A depressive disorder associated with the luteal phase of the menstrual cycle. Primary manifestations include emotional lability and persistent or severe anger and irritability. Other manifestations include a lack of energy, overeating, and difficulty concentrating.

Substance-induced depressive disorder: Clinical findings of depression that are associated with the use of, or withdrawal from, drugs and alcohol.

CLIENT CARE

Care of a client who has MDD will mirror the phase of the disease that the client is experiencing. Q**pcc**

Acute phase: Severe clinical findings of depression
- Treatment is generally 6 to 12 weeks in duration.
- Potential need for hospitalization.
- Reduction of depressive manifestations is the goal of treatment.
- Assess suicide risk, and implement safety precautions or one-to-one observation as needed.

Continuation phase: Increased ability to function
- Treatment is generally 4 to 9 months in duration.
- Relapse prevention through education, medication therapy, and psychotherapy is the goal of treatment.

Maintenance phase: Remission of manifestations
- This phase can last for years.
- Prevention of future depressive episodes is the goal of treatment.

ASSESSMENT

RISK FACTORS

- **Family history and a previous personal history of depression** are the most significant risk factors.
- Depressive disorders are twice as common in **females between the ages of 15 and 40** than in males.
- Depression is very common among **clients over age 65**, but the disorder is more difficult to recognize in the older adult client and can go untreated. It is important to differentiate between early dementia and depression. Some clinical findings of depression that can look like dementia are memory loss, confusion, and behavioral problems such as social isolation or agitation. Clients can seek health care for somatic problems that are manifestations of untreated depression. ©
- **Neurotransmitter deficiencies**, such as a serotonin deficiency (affects mood, sexual behavior, sleep cycles, hunger, and pain perception) or a norepinephrine deficiency (affects attention and behavior), can be risk factors for depression. Imbalances of the neurotransmitters norepinephrine, dopamine, acetylcholine, GABA, and possibly glutamate can play a role in the occurrence of depression.

OTHER RISK FACTORS
- Stressful life events
- Presence of a medical illness
- A woman's postpartum period
- Poor social support network
- Comorbid substance use disorder
- Being unmarried
- Trauma occurring early in life

> Depressive disorders occur throughout all groups of people.

> Depression can be the primary disorder or a response to another physical or mental health disorder.

EXPECTED FINDINGS

- Anergia (lack of energy)
- Anhedonia (lack of pleasure in normal activities)
- Anxiety
- Reports of sluggishness (most common), or feeling unable to relax and sit still
- Vegetative findings, which include a change in eating patterns (usually anorexia in MDD; increased intake in dysthymia and PMDD), change in bowel habits (usually constipation), sleep disturbances, and decreased interest in sexual activity
- Somatic reports, such as fatigue, gastrointestinal changes, pain

PHYSICAL ASSESSMENT FINDINGS
- The client most often looks sad with blunted affect.
- The client exhibits poor grooming and lack of hygiene.
- Psychomotor retardation (slowed physical movement, slumped posture) is more common, but psychomotor agitation (restlessness, pacing, finger tapping) can also occur.
- The client becomes socially isolated, showing little or no effort to interact.
- Slowed speech, decreased verbalization, delayed response: The client might seem too tired to speak and can sigh often.

STANDARDIZED SCREENING TOOLS

- Hamilton Depression Scale
- Beck Depression Inventory
- Geriatric Depression Scale (short form) ©
- Zung Self-Rating Depression Scale
- Patient Health Questionnaire-9 (PHQ-9)

PATIENT-CENTERED CARE

NURSING CARE

Milieu therapy

Suicide risk: Assess the client's risk for suicide, and implement appropriate safety precautions.

Self-care: Monitor the client's ability to perform activities of daily living, and encourage independence as much as possible.

Communication: Relate therapeutically to the client who is unable or unwilling to communicate.
- Make time to be with the client, even if he does not speak.
- Make observations rather than asking direct questions, which can cause anxiety in the client. For example, the nurse might say, "I noticed that you attended the unit group meeting today," rather than asking, "Did you enjoy the group meeting?" Give directions in simple, concrete sentences because a client who has depression can have difficulty focusing on and comprehending long sentences. Q EBP
- Give the client sufficient time to respond when holding a conversation due to a possible delayed response time.

Maintenance of a safe environment

Counseling: This can include individual counseling to assist with the following.
- Problem-solving
- Increasing coping abilities
- Changing negative thinking to positive
- Increasing self-esteem
- Assertiveness training
- Using available community resources

MEDICATIONS

CLIENT TEACHING FOR ALL ANTIDEPRESSANTS

- Do not discontinue medication suddenly. Qs
- Therapeutic effects are not immediate, and it can take several weeks or more to reach full therapeutic benefits.
- Avoid hazardous activities, such as driving or operating heavy equipment/machinery, due to the potential adverse effect of sedation.
- Notify the provider of any thoughts of suicide.
- Avoid alcohol while taking an antidepressant.

Selective serotonin reuptake inhibitors (SSRIs)

Citalopram
Fluoxetine
Sertraline
Leading treatment for depression

CLIENT EDUCATION

- Advise the client that adverse effects can include nausea, headache, and central nervous system stimulation (agitation, insomnia, anxiety).
- Instruct the client that sexual dysfunction can occur and to notify provider if effects are intolerable.
- Advise the client to observe for manifestations of serotonin syndrome. If any occur, instruct the client to withhold the medication and notify the provider.
- Instruct the client to avoid the concurrent use of St. John's wort, which can increase the risk of serotonin syndrome.
- Instruct the client to follow a healthy diet and exercise regimen because weight gain can occur with long-term use.

Tricyclic antidepressants

Amitriptyline

CLIENT EDUCATION

- Advise the client to change positions slowly to minimize dizziness from orthostatic hypotension.
- To minimize anticholinergic effects, advise the client to chew sugarless gum, eat foods high in fiber, and increase fluid intake to 2 to 3 L/day from food and beverage sources.

Monoamine oxidase inhibitors

Phenelzine

CLIENT EDUCATION

- Due to the risk for hypertensive crisis, advise the client to avoid foods with tyramine (ripe avocados or figs, fermented or smoked meats, liver, dried or cured fish, most cheeses, some beer and wine, and protein dietary supplements).
- Due to the risk of medication interactions, instruct the client to avoid all medications, including over-the-counter, without first discussing them with the provider.

Atypical antidepressants

Bupropion

CLIENT EDUCATION

- Advise the client to observe for headache, dry mouth, GI distress, constipation, increased heart rate, nausea, restlessness, or insomnia, and to notify the provider if they become intolerable.
- Monitor the client's food intake and weight due to appetite suppression.
- Avoid administering to clients at risk for seizures.

Serotonin norepinephrine reuptake inhibitors

Venlafaxine
Duloxetine

CLIENT EDUCATION

- Adverse effects include nausea, insomnia, weight gain, diaphoresis, and sexual dysfunction.
- Caution in administering to clients who have a history of hypertension.

ALTERNATIVE OR COMPLEMENTARY THERAPIES

St. John's wort

A plant product (*Hypericum perforatum*), not regulated by the U.S. Food and Drug Administration, is taken by some individuals to relieve manifestations of mild depression.

NURSING CONSIDERATIONS

- Adverse effects include photosensitivity, skin rash, rapid heart rate, gastrointestinal distress, and abdominal pain.
- St. John's wort can increase or reduce levels of some medications if taken concurrently. The client should inform the provider if taking St. John's wort.

> **!** Medication interactions: Potentially fatal serotonin syndrome can result if St. John's wort is taken with SSRIs or other types of antidepressants. Foods containing tyramine should be avoided.

Light therapy

- First-line treatment for SAD, light therapy inhibits nocturnal secretion of melatonin.
- Exposure of the face to 10,000-lux light box 30 min/day, once or in two divided doses

THERAPEUTIC PROCEDURES

Electroconvulsive therapy

Can be useful for some clients who have a depressive disorder and are unresponsive to other treatments.

NURSING ACTIONS: A specially trained nurse is responsible for monitoring the client before and after this therapy.

Transcranial magnetic stimulation

Uses electromagnetic stimulation of the brain; it is indicated for depressive disorders that are resistant to other forms of treatment.

Vagus nerve stimulation

Uses an implanted device that stimulates the vagus nerve. It can be used for clients who have depression that is resistant to antidepressant medications.

INTERPROFESSIONAL CARE

Psychotherapy by a trained therapist can include individual cognitive-behavioral therapy (CBT), interpersonal therapy (IPT), group therapy, and family therapy.
- CBT assists the client to identify and change negative behavior and thought patterns.
- IPT encourages the client to focus on personal relationships that contribute to the depressive disorder.

CLIENT EDUCATION

Continuation phase followed by maintenance phase
- Review manifestations of depression with the client and family members in order to identify relapse.
- Reinforce intended effects and potential adverse effects of medication.
- Explain the benefits of adherence to therapy.
- Thirty minutes of exercise daily for 3 to 5 days each week improves clinical findings of depression and can help to prevent relapse. Even shorter intervals of exercise are helpful. Exercise should be regarded as an adjunct to other therapies for the client who has major depressive disorder. Q**EBP**

Application Exercises

1. A nurse working in an acute mental health facility is caring for a 35-year-old female client who has manifestations of depression. The client lives at home with her partner and two young children. She currently smokes and has a history of chronic asthma. Which of the following factors put the client at risk for depression? (Select all that apply.)

   A. Age

   B. Gender

   C. History of chronic asthma

   D. Smoking

   E. Being married

2. A nurse working on an acute mental health unit is admitting a client who has major depressive disorder and comorbid anxiety disorder. Which of the following actions is the nurse's priority?

   A. Placing the client on one-to-one observation

   B. Assisting the client to perform ADLs

   C. Encouraging the client to participate in counseling

   D. Teaching the client about medication adverse effects

3. A nurse working in an outpatient clinic is providing teaching to a client who has a new diagnosis of premenstrual dysphoric disorder (PMDD). Which of the following statements by the client indicates understanding of the teaching?

   A. "I can expect my problems with PMDD to be worst when I'm menstruating."

   B. "I will use light therapy 30 minutes a day to prevent further recurrences of PMDD."

   C. "I am aware that my PMDD causes me to have rapid mood swings."

   D. "I should increase my caloric intake with a nutritional supplement when my PMDD is active."

4. A charge nurse is discussing the care of a client who has major depressive disorder (MDD) with a newly licensed nurse. Which of the following statements by the newly licensed nurse indicates an understanding of the teaching?

   A. "Care during the continuation phase focuses on treating continued manifestations of MDD."

   B. "The treatment of MDD during the maintenance phase lasts for 6 to 12 weeks."

   C. "The client is at greatest risk for suicide during the first weeks of an MDD episode."

   D. "Medication and psychotherapy are most effective during the acute phase of MDD."

5. A nurse is interviewing a 25-year-old client who has a new diagnosis of dysthymic disorder. Which of the following findings should the nurse expect?

   A. Wide fluctuations in mood

   B. Report of a minimum of five clinical findings of depression

   C. Presence of manifestations for at least 2 years

   D. Inflated sense of self-esteem

PRACTICE Active Learning Scenario

A nurse working in an acute mental health facility is performing an admission assessment for a client who has major depressive disorder (MDD). Use the ATI Active Learning Template: System Disorder to complete this item.

ALTERATION IN HEALTH (DIAGNOSIS)

EXPECTED FINDINGS: Identify at least four expected findings.

NURSING CARE: Describe an appropriate communication technique to relate therapeutically with this client.

Application Exercises Key

1. A. **CORRECT:** Depressive disorders are more prevalent in adults between the ages of 15 and 40.

   B. **CORRECT:** Depressive disorders are twice as common in women than men.

   C. **CORRECT:** Depressive disorders are more common in clients who have a chronic medical illness.

   D. **CORRECT:** Depressive disorders are more common in clients who have a substance use disorder, such as nicotine use disorder.

   E. Depressive disorders are more common in unmarried clients.

   Ⓝ *NCLEX® Connection: Health Promotion and Maintenance, Health Promotion/Disease Prevention*

2. A. **CORRECT:** The greatest risk for a client who has MDD and comorbid anxiety is injury due to self-harm. The highest priority intervention is placing the client on one-to-one observation.

   B. The client who has MDD can require assistance with ADLs. However, this does not address the greatest risk to the client and is therefore not the priority intervention.

   C. The nurse should encourage the client who has MDD to participate in counseling. However, this does not address the greatest risk to the client and is therefore not the priority intervention.

   D. The nurse should teach the client who has MDD about medication adverse effects. However, this does not address the greatest risk to the client and is therefore not the priority intervention.

   Ⓝ *NCLEX® Connection: Psychosocial Integrity, Mental Health Concepts*

3. A. Clinical findings of PMDD are present during the luteal phase of the menstrual cycle just prior to menses.

   B. Light therapy is a first-line treatment for seasonal affective disorder.

   C. **CORRECT:** A clinical finding of PMDD is emotional lability. The client can experience rapid changes in mood.

   D. PMDD increases the client's risk for weight gain due to overeating. It is not appropriate to increase caloric intake.

   Ⓝ *NCLEX® Connection: Psychosocial Integrity, Mental Health Concepts*

4. A. The focus of the continuation phase is relapse prevention. Treatment of manifestations occurs during the acute phase of MDD.

   B. The maintenance phase of treatment for MDD can lasts for 1 year or more.

   C. **CORRECT:** The client is at greatest risk for suicide during the acute phase of MDD.

   D. Medication therapy and psychotherapy are used during the continuation phase to prevent relapse of MDD.

   Ⓝ *NCLEX® Connection: Psychosocial Integrity, Mental Health Concepts*

5. A. Wide fluctuations in mood are associated with bipolar disorder.

   B. MDD contains a minimum of five clinical findings of depression.

   C. **CORRECT:** Manifestations of dysthymic disorder last for at least 2 years in adults.

   D. A decreased, rather than inflated, sense of self-esteem is associated with dysthymic disorder.

   Ⓝ *NCLEX® Connection: Psychosocial Integrity, Mental Health Concepts*

PRACTICE Answer

Using the ATI Active Learning Template: System Disorder

ALTERATION IN HEALTH (DIAGNOSIS): MDD is a single episode or recurrent episodes of unipolar depression resulting in a significant change in a client's normal functioning (social, occupational, self-care) accompanied by at least five clinical findings of MDD, which must occur almost every day for a minimum of 2 weeks, and last most of the day.

EXPECTED FINDINGS
- Depressed mood
- Difficulty sleeping or excessive sleeping
- Indecisiveness
- Decreased ability to concentrate
- Suicidal ideation
- Increase or decrease in motor activity
- Inability to feel pleasure (anhedonia)
- Increase or decrease in weight of more than 5% of total body weight over 1 month

NURSING CARE
- Make time to be with the client even if he doesn't speak.
- Communicate with observations rather than asking direct questions.
- Give directions in simple, concrete sentences.
- Allow the client sufficient time to verbally respond.

Ⓝ *NCLEX® Connection: Psychosocial Integrity, Behavioral Interventions*

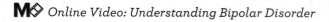
UNIT 3   PSYCHOBIOLOGIC DISORDERS

CHAPTER 14 *Bipolar Disorders*

Bipolar disorders are mood disorders with recurrent episodes of depression and mania.

Bipolar disorders usually emerge in early adulthood, but early-onset bipolar disorder can be diagnosed in pediatric clients. Because manifestations can mimic expected findings of attention deficit hyperactivity disorder (ADHD), it is more difficult to assess and diagnose bipolar disorders in children than in other client age groups.

Periods of normal functioning alternate with periods of illness, though some clients are not able to maintain full occupational and social functioning. Clients can exhibit psychotic, paranoid, and/or bizarre behavior during periods of mania.

CLIENT CARE

Care of a client who has bipolar disorder will mirror the phase of the disease that the client is experiencing.

Acute phase: Acute mania
- Hospitalization can be required.
- Reduction of mania and client safety are the goals of treatment.
- Risk of harm to self or others is determined.
- One-to-one supervision can be indicated for client safety. Qs

Continuation phase: Remission of manifestations
- Treatment is generally 4 to 9 months in duration.
- Relapse prevention through education, medication adherence, and psychotherapy is the goal of treatment.

Maintenance phase: Increased ability to function
- Treatment generally continues throughout the client's lifetime.
- Prevention of future manic episodes is the goal of treatment.

BEHAVIORS SHOWN WITH BIPOLAR DISORDERS

Mania: An abnormally elevated mood, which can also be described as expansive or irritable; usually requires hospitalization. Manic episodes last at least 1 week. (See the **ASSESSMENT** section in this chapter for specific findings.)

Hypomania: A less severe episode of mania that lasts at least 4 days accompanied by three or more manifestations of mania. Hospitalization is not required, and the client who has hypomania is less impaired. Hypomania can progress to mania.

Rapid cycling: Four or more episodes of hypomania or acute mania within 1 year.

TYPES OF BIPOLAR DISORDERS

Bipolar I disorder: The client has at least one episode of mania alternating with major depression.

Bipolar II disorder: The client has one or more hypomanic episodes alternating with major depressive episodes.

Cyclothymic disorder: The client has at least 2 years of repeated hypomanic manifestations that do not meet the criteria for hypomanic episodes alternating with minor depressive episodes.

COMORBIDITIES

- Substance use disorder
- Anxiety disorders
- Borderline personality disorder
- Oppositional defiant disorder
- Social phobia and specific phobias
- Seasonal affective disorder

ASSESSMENT

RISK FACTORS

Genetics: e.g., having an immediate family member who has a bipolar disorder

Psychological: e.g., stressful events or major life changes

Physiological: e.g., neurobiological and neuroendocrine disorders

Substance use disorder: e.g., alcohol or cocaine use disorder

RELAPSE

- Use of substances (alcohol, cocaine, caffeine) can lead to an episode of mania.
- Sleep disturbances can come before, be associated with, or be brought on by an episode of mania.
- Psychological stressors can trigger an episode of mania.

EXPECTED FINDINGS

MANIC CHARACTERISTICS
- Labile mood with euphoria
- Agitation and irritability
- Restlessness
- Dislike of interference and intolerance of criticism
- Increase in talking and activity
- Flight of ideas: rapid, continuous speech with sudden and frequent topic change
- Grandiose view of self and abilities (grandiosity)
- Impulsivity: spending money, giving away money or possessions
- Demanding and manipulative behavior
- Distractibility and decreased attention span
- Poor judgment
- Attention-seeking behavior: flashy dress and makeup, inappropriate behavior
- Impairment in social and occupational functioning
- Decreased sleep
- Neglect of ADLs, including nutrition and hydration
- Possible presence of delusions and hallucinations
- Denial of illness

DEPRESSIVE CHARACTERISTICS
- Flat, blunted, labile affect
- Tearfulness, crying
- Lack of energy
- Anhedonia: loss of pleasure and lack of interest in activities, hobbies, sexual activity
- Physical reports of discomfort/pain
- Difficulty concentrating, focusing, problem-solving
- Self-destructive behavior, including suicidal ideation
- Decrease in personal hygiene
- Loss or increase in appetite and/or sleep, disturbed sleep
- Psychomotor retardation or agitation

STANDARDIZED SCREENING TOOL

Mood Disorders Questionnaire: A standardized tool that places mood progression on a continuum from hypomania (euphoria) to acute mania (extreme irritability and hyperactivity) to delirious mania (completely out of touch with reality). Q**EBP**

PATIENT-CENTERED CARE

NURSING CARE

The care of the client is based on the phase of bipolar disorder that the client is experiencing. Nursing care is provided throughout this process.

Acute manic episode

Focus is on safety and maintaining physical health. Q**s**

THERAPEUTIC MILIEU (within acute care mental health facility)
- Provide a safe environment during the acute phase.
- Assess the client regularly for suicidal thoughts, intentions, and escalating behavior.
- Decrease stimulation without isolating the client if possible. Be aware of noise, music, television, and other clients, all of which can lead to an escalation of the client's behavior. In certain cases, seclusion might be the only way to safely decrease stimulation for the client.
- Follow agency protocols for providing client protection (restraints, seclusion, one-to-one observation) if a threat of self-injury or injury to others exists.
- Implement frequent rest periods.
- Provide outlets for physical activity. Do not involve the client in activities that last a long time or that require a high level of concentration and/or detailed instructions.
- Protect client from poor judgment and impulsive behavior, such as giving money away and sexual indiscretions.

MAINTENANCE OF SELF-CARE NEEDS
- Monitoring sleep, fluid intake, and nutrition.
- Providing portable, nutritious food because the client might not be able to sit down to eat.
- Supervising choice of clothes.
- Giving step-by-step reminders for hygiene and dress.

COMMUNICATION
- Use a calm, matter-of-fact, specific approach.
- Give concise explanations.
- Provide for consistency with expectations and limit-setting.
- Avoid power struggles, and do not react personally to the client's comments.
- Listen to and act on legitimate client grievances.
- Reinforce nonmanipulative behaviors.
- Use therapeutic communication techniques

MEDICATIONS

Mood stabilizers
- Lithium carbonate
- Anticonvulsants that act as mood stabilizers, including valproate, lamotrigine, carbamazepine

Antianxiety medications: e.g., lorazepam, clonazepam

Second-generation antipsychotic medications: including aripiprazole, clozapine, ziprasidone

Antidepressants: e.g., the SSRI fluoxetine, used to manage a major depressive episode

THERAPEUTIC PROCEDURES

Electroconvulsive therapy (ECT): Can be used to subdue extreme manic behavior, especially when pharmacological therapy, such as lithium, has not worked. Clients who are suicidal or those who have rapid cycling can also benefit from ECT.

CLIENT EDUCATION

- Case management to provide follow-up for the client the family Qᴛᴄ
- Group, family, and individual psychotherapy, such as cognitive-behavior therapy, to improve problem-solving and interpersonal skills

HEALTH TEACHING

- The chronicity of the disorder requiring long-term pharmacological and psychological support
- Benefits of psychotherapy and support groups to prevent relapse
- Indications of impending relapse and ways to manage the crisis
- Precipitating factors of relapse (e.g., sleep disturbance, use of alcohol, or caffeine)
- Importance of maintaining a regular sleep, meal, and activity pattern
- Medication administration and adherence

COMPLICATIONS

Physical exhaustion and possible death: A client in a true manic state usually will not stop moving, and does not eat, drink, or sleep. This can become a medical emergency.

NURSING ACTIONS

- Prevent client self-harm.
- Decrease client's physical activity.
- Ensure adequate fluid and food intake.
- Promote an adequate amount of sleep each night.
- Assist the client with self-care needs.
- Manage medication appropriately.

PRACTICE Active Learning Scenario

A nurse in an acute mental health facility is caring for a client who is experiencing acute mania. Use the ATI Active Learning Template: System Disorder to complete this item to include the following.

ALTERATION IN HEALTH (DIAGNOSIS)

EXPECTED FINDINGS: Identify four expected findings.

NURSING CARE: Identify two nursing actions.

CLIENT EDUCATION: Identify two client outcomes.

Application Exercises

1. A nurse is planning care for a client who has bipolar disorder and is experiencing a manic episode. Which of the following interventions should the nurse include in the plan of care? (Select all that apply.)
   - A. Provide flexible client behavior expectations.
   - B. Offer concise explanations.
   - C. Establish consistent limits.
   - D. Disregard client complaints.
   - E. Use a firm approach with communication.

2. A nurse is teaching a newly licensed nurse about the use of electroconvulsive therapy (ECT) for the treatment of bipolar disorder. Which of the following statements by the newly licensed nurse indicates understanding?
   - A. "ECT is the recommended initial treatment for bipolar disorder."
   - B. "ECT is contraindicated for clients who have suicidal ideation."
   - C. "ECT is effective for clients who are experiencing severe mania."
   - D. "ECT is prescribed to prevent relapse of bipolar disorder."

3. A nurse in an acute mental health facility is caring for a client who has bipolar disorder. Which of the following is the priority nursing action?
   - A. Set consistent limits for expected client behavior.
   - B. Administer prescribed medications as scheduled.
   - C. Provide the client with step-by-step instructions during hygiene activities.
   - D. Monitor the client for escalating behavior.

4. A nurse is caring for a client who has bipolar disorder. The client states, "I am very rich, and I feel I must give my money to you." Which of the following responses should the nurse make?
   - A. "Why do you think you feel the need to give money away?"
   - B. "I am here to provide care and cannot accept this from you."
   - C. "I can request that your case manager discuss appropriate charity options with you."
   - D. "You should know that giving away your money is inappropriate."

5. A nurse is discussing relapse prevention with a client who has bipolar disorder. Which of the following information should the nurse include in the teaching? (Select all that apply.)
   - A. Use caffeine in moderation to prevent relapse.
   - B. Difficulty sleeping can indicate a relapse.
   - C. Begin taking your medications as soon as a relapse begins.
   - D. Participating in psychotherapy can help prevent a relapse.
   - E. Anhedonia is a clinical manifestation of a depressive relapse.

Application Exercises Key

1. A. The nurse should establish consistent client behavior expectations to decrease the risk for client manipulation.

   B. **CORRECT:** Offering concise explanations improves the client's ability to focus and comprehend the information.

   C. **CORRECT:** Establishing consistent limits decreases the risk for client manipulation.

   D. The nurse should respond to valid client complaints to foster a trusting nurse-client relationship.

   E. **CORRECT:** Using a firm approach with client communication promotes structure and minimizes inappropriate client behaviors.

   Ⓝ *NCLEX® Connection: Psychosocial Integrity, Behavioral Interventions*

2. A. Pharmacological intervention is the recommended initial treatment for bipolar disorder.

   B. ECT is effective for clients who have bipolar disorder and suicidal ideation.

   C. **CORRECT:** ECT is appropriate for the treatment of severe mania associated with bipolar disorder.

   D. ECT is prescribed for clients experiencing an acute episode of bipolar disorder rather than for the prevention of relapse.

   Ⓝ *NCLEX® Connection: Reduction of Risk Potential, Potential for Complications of Diagnostic Tests/Treatments/Procedures*

3. A. The nurse should set consistent limits for expected client behavior. However, this does not address the client's priority need for safety and is therefore not the priority action.

   B. The nurse should administer prescribed medications as scheduled. However, this does not address the client's priority need for safety and is therefore not the priority action.

   C. The nurse should provide the client with step-by-step instructions during hygiene activities. However, this does not address the client's priority need for safety and is therefore not the priority action.

   D. **CORRECT:** Monitoring for escalating behavior addresses the client's priority need for safety and is therefore the priority nursing action.

   Ⓝ *NCLEX® Connection: Psychosocial Integrity, Mental Health Concepts*

4. A. Asking a "why" question is a nontherapeutic form of communication and can promote a defensive client response.

   B. **CORRECT:** This statement is matter-of-fact and concise and is a therapeutic response to a client who has bipolar disorder.

   C. This statement does not recognize the possibility of poor judgment, which is associated with bipolar disorder.

   D. This statement offers disapproval and can be interpreted by the client as aggressive, which can promote a defensive client response.

   Ⓝ *NCLEX® Connection: Psychosocial Integrity, Therapeutic Communication*

5. A. The client who has bipolar disorder should avoid the use of caffeine because it can precipitate a relapse.

   B. **CORRECT:** The client should be alert for sleep disturbances, which can indicate a relapse.

   C. The client who has bipolar disorder should take prescribed medications to prevent and minimize a relapse.

   D. **CORRECT:** The client who has bipolar disorder can participate in psychotherapy to help prevent a relapse.

   E. **CORRECT:** The client who has bipolar disorder should be aware of manifestations, including anhedonia, which is a depressive characteristic that can indicate a relapse.

   Ⓝ *NCLEX® Connection: Physiological Adaptation, Illness Management*

PRACTICE Answer

Using the ATI Active Learning Template: System Disorder

ALTERATION IN HEALTH (DIAGNOSIS): An abnormally elevated mood, which can also be described as expansive or irritable; usually requires hospitalization

EXPECTED FINDINGS
- Agitation and irritability
- Intolerance of interference or criticism
- Increase in talking and activity
- Flight of ideas
- Grandiosity
- Impulsivity
- Demanding and manipulative behavior
- Distractibility
- Poor judgment
- Attention-seeking behavior
- Impairment in social and occupational functioning
- Decreased sleep
- Neglect of ADLs
- Possible delusions and hallucinations
- Denial of illness

NURSING CARE
- Focus on safety as the priority of care.
- Maintain client's physical health and self-care needs.
- Provide a safe environment.
- Assess for suicidal thoughts, intentions, and escalating behavior.
- Decrease stimulation.
- Provide client protection with restraints, seclusion, or one-to-one observation if necessary.
- Implement frequent rest periods.
- Provide appropriate outlets for physical activity.
- Use calm and concise communication.

CLIENT EDUCATION: Client outcomes
- The client will refrain from self-harm.
- The client will sleep 6 to 8 hr each night.
- The client will maintain adequate fluid and food intake.
- The client will use appropriate communication skills to meet needs.
- The client will participate in self-care.

Ⓝ *NCLEX® Connection: Psychosocial Integrity, Crisis Intervention*

UNIT 3   PSYCHOBIOLOGIC DISORDERS

CHAPTER 15 *Psychotic Disorders*

Schizophrenia spectrum and other psychotic disorders affect thinking, behavior, emotions, and the ability to perceive reality. Schizophrenia probably results from a combination of genetic, neurobiological, and nongenetic (injury at birth, viral infection, and nutritional) factors.

The typical age at onset is late teens and early 20s, but schizophrenia has occurred in young children and can begin in later adulthood. Psychotic disorders become problematic when manifestations interfere with interpersonal relationships, self-care, and ability to work.

TYPES OF DISORDERS

The various types of psychotic disorders recognized and defined by the DSM–5 include the following.

Schizophrenia: The client has psychotic thinking or behavior present for at least 6 months. Areas of functioning, including school or work, self-care, and interpersonal relationships, are significantly impaired.

Schizotypal personality disorder: The client has impairments of personality (self and interpersonal) functioning. However, impairment is not as severe as with schizophrenia.

Delusional disorder: The client experiences delusional thinking for at least 1 month. Self or interpersonal functioning is not markedly impaired.

Brief psychotic disorder: The client has psychotic manifestations that last 1 day to 1 month in duration.

Schizophreniform disorder: The client has manifestations similar to schizophrenia, but the duration is 1 to 6 months, and social/occupational dysfunction might not be present.

Schizoaffective disorder: The client's disorder meets the criteria for both schizophrenia and depressive or bipolar disorder.

Substance-induced psychotic disorder: The client experiences psychosis due to substance intoxication or withdrawal. However, the psychotic manifestations are more severe than typically expected.

Psychotic or catatonic disorder not otherwise specified: The client exhibits psychotic features such as impaired reality testing or bizarre behavior (psychotic) or a significant change in motor activity behavior (catatonic) but does not meet criteria for diagnosis with another specific psychotic disorder.

ASSESSMENT

EXPECTED FINDINGS

Characteristic dimensions of psychotic disorders

POSITIVE SYMPTOMS: Manifestation of things that are not normally present. These are the most easily identified manifestations.
- Hallucinations
- Delusions
- Alterations in speech
- Bizarre behavior, such as walking backward constantly

NEGATIVE SYMPTOMS: Absence of things that are normally present. These manifestations are more difficult to treat successfully than positive symptoms.
- **Affect:** Usually blunted (narrow range of expression) or flat (facial expression never changes)
- **Alogia:** Poverty of thought or speech. The client might sit with a visitor but only mumble or respond vaguely to questions.
- **Anergia:** Lack of energy
- **Anhedonia:** Lack of pleasure or joy. The client is indifferent to things that often make others happy, such as looking at beautiful scenery.
- **Avolition:** Lack of motivation in activities and hygiene. For example, the client completes an assigned task, such as making his bed, but is unable to start the next common chore without prompting.

COGNITIVE SYMPTOMS: Problems with thinking make it very difficult for the client to live independently.
- Disordered thinking
- Inability to make decisions
- Poor problem-solving ability
- Difficulty concentrating to perform tasks
- Memory deficits
- Long-term memory
- Working memory, such as inability to follow directions to find an address

AFFECTIVE SYMPTOMS: Manifestations involving emotions
- Hopelessness
- Suicidal ideation

Alterations in thought (delusions)

Alterations in thought are false fixed beliefs that cannot be corrected by reasoning and are usually bizarre. These include the following.
- **Ideas of reference:** Misconstrues trivial events and attaches personal significance to them, such as believing that others, who are discussing the next meal, are talking about him
- **Persecution:** Feels singled out for harm by others (e.g., being hunted down by the FBI)
- **Grandeur:** Believes that she is all powerful and important, like a god
- **Somatic delusions:** Believes that his body is changing in an unusual way, such as growing a third arm
- **Jealousy:** Believes that her partner is sexually involved with another individual even though there is not any factual basis for this belief

- **Being controlled:** Believes that a force outside his body is controlling him
- **Thought broadcasting:** Believes that her thoughts are heard by others
- **Thought insertion:** Believes that others' thoughts are being inserted into his mind
- **Thought withdrawal:** Believes that her thoughts have been removed from her mind by an outside agency
- **Religiosity:** Is obsessed with religious beliefs
- **Magical thinking:** Believes his actions or thoughts are able to control a situation or affect others, such as wearing a certain hat makes him invisible to others

Alterations in speech

The following examples can occur.
- **Flight of ideas:** Associative looseness. The client might say sentence after sentence, but each sentence can relate to a different topic, and the listener is unable to follow the client's thoughts.
- **Neologisms:** Made-up words that have meaning only to the client, such as, "I tranged and flittled."
- **Echolalia:** The client repeats the words spoken to him.
- **Clang association:** Meaningless rhyming of words, often forceful, such as, "Oh fox, box, and lox."
- **Word salad:** Words jumbled together with little meaning or significance to the listener, such as, "Hip hooray, the flip is cast and wide-sprinting in the forest."

Alterations in perception

Hallucinations are sensory perceptions that do not have any apparent external stimulus. Examples include:
- **Auditory:** Hearing voices or sounds
  - **Command:** The voice instructs the client to perform an action, such as to hurt self or others. Qs
- **Visual:** Seeing persons or things
- **Olfactory:** Smelling odors
- **Gustatory:** Experiencing tastes
- **Tactile:** Feeling bodily sensations

Personal boundary difficulties

Disenfranchisement with one's own body, identity, and perceptions. This includes the following.
- **Depersonalization:** Nonspecific feeling that a person has lost her identity. Self is different or unreal.
- **Derealization:** Perception that the environment has changed (e.g., the client believes that objects in her environment are shrinking).

Alterations in behavior

- **Extreme agitation**, including pacing and rocking
- **Stereotyped behaviors:** Motor patterns that had meaning to client (sweeping the floor) but now are mechanical and lack purpose
- **Automatic obedience:** Responding in a robot-like manner
- **Waxy flexibility:** Maintaining a specific position for an extended period of time
- **Stupor:** Motionless for long periods of time, coma-like
- **Negativism:** Doing the opposite of what is requested
- **Echopraxia:** Purposeful imitation of movements made by others

STANDARDIZED SCREENING TOOLS

Abnormal Involuntary Movement Scale (AIMS): This tool is used to monitor involuntary movements and tardive dyskinesia in clients who take antipsychotic medication. QEBP

World Health Organization Disability Assessment Schedule (WHODAS): This scale helps to determine the client's level of global functioning.

PATIENT-CENTERED CARE

NURSING CARE

- Milieu therapy is used for clients who have a psychotic disorder both in acute mental health facilities and in community facilities, such as residential crisis centers, halfway houses, and day treatment programs.
  - Provide a structured, safe environment (milieu) for the client in order to decrease anxiety and to distract the client from constant thinking about hallucinations.
  - **Program of assertive community treatment (PACT):** Intensive case management and interprofessional team approach to assist clients with community-living needs. QTC
- Promote therapeutic communication to lower anxiety, decrease defensive patterns, and encourage participation in the milieu.
- Establish a trusting relationship with the client.
- Encourage the development of social skills and friendships.
- Encourage participation in group work and psychoeducation.
- Use appropriate communication to address hallucinations and delusions.
  - Ask the client directly about hallucinations. The nurse should not argue or agree with the client's view of the situation, but can offer a comment, such as, "I don't hear anything, but you seem to be feeling frightened."
  - Do not argue with a client's delusions, but focus on the client's feelings and possibly offer reasonable explanations, such as, "I can't imagine that the President of the United States would have a reason to kill a citizen, but it must be frightening for you to believe that."
  - Assess the client for paranoid delusions, which can increase the risk for violence against others.
  - If the client is experiencing command hallucinations, provide for safety due to the increased risk for harm to self or others. Qs
  - Attempt to focus conversations on reality-based subjects.
  - Identify symptom triggers, such as loud noises (can trigger auditory hallucinations in certain clients) and situations that seem to trigger conversations about the client's delusions.
  - Be genuine and empathetic in all dealings with the client.
- Assess discharge needs, such as ability to perform activities of daily living (ADLs).
- Promote self-care by modeling and teaching self-care activities within the mental health facility.

- Relate wellness to the elements of symptom management.
- Collaborate with the client to use symptom management techniques to cope with depressive symptoms and anxiety. Symptom management techniques include such strategies as using music to distract from "voices," attending activities, walking, talking to a trusted person when hallucinations are most bothersome, and interacting with an auditory or visual hallucination by telling it to stop or go away. Qᴘᴄᴄ
- Encourage medication compliance.
- Provide teaching regarding medications.
- Whenever possible, incorporate family in all aspects of care.

MEDICATIONS

First-generation/conventional antipsychotics

Used to treat mainly positive psychotic symptoms
- Haloperidol
- Loxapine
- Chlorpromazine
- Fluphenazine

NURSING CONSIDERATIONS
- To minimize anticholinergic effects, advise the client to chew sugarless gum, eat foods high in fiber, and to eat and drink 2 to 3 L of fluid a day from food and beverage sources.
- Instruct the client about indications of postural hypotension (e.g., lightheadedness, dizziness). If these occur, advise the client to sit or lie down. Minimize orthostatic hypotension by getting up slowly from a lying or sitting position.

Second-generation/atypical antipsychotics

Current medications of choice for psychotic disorders, and they generally treat both positive and negative symptoms.
- Risperidone
- Olanzapine
- Quetiapine
- Ziprasidone
- Clozapine

NURSING CONSIDERATIONS
- To minimize weight gain, advise the client to follow a healthy, low-calorie diet, engage in regular exercise, and monitor weight. Qᴇʙᴘ
- Adverse effects of agitation, dizziness, sedation, and sleep disruption can occur. Instruct the client to report these manifestations because the provider might need to change the medication.
- Inform the client of the need for blood tests to monitor for agranulocytosis.

Third-generation antipsychotics

Used to treat both positive and negative symptoms while improving cognitive function.
- Aripiprazole

NURSING CONSIDERATIONS
- Decreased risk of EPSs or tardive dyskinesia
- Lower risk for weight gain and anticholinergic effects

Antidepressants

Used to treat the depression seen in many clients who have a psychotic disorder.
- Paroxetine

NURSING CONSIDERATIONS
- Used temporarily to treat depression associated with psychotic disorders.
- Monitor the client for suicidal ideation because this medication can increase thoughts of self-harm, especially when first taking it. Qₛ
- Notify the provider of any adverse effects, such as deepened depression.
- Advise the client to avoid abrupt cessation of this medication to avoid a withdrawal effect.

Mood stabilizing agents and benzodiazepines

Used to treat the anxiety often found in clients who have psychotic disorders, as well as some of the positive and negative symptoms.
- Valproate
- Lamotrigine
- Lorazepam

NURSING CONSIDERATIONS
- Inform the client of sedative effects.
- Use these medications with caution in older adult clients.

CLIENT EDUCATION

- Case management to provide follow up for the client and family. Qᴛᴄ
- Group, family, and individual psychoeducation to improve problem-solving and interpersonal skills.
- Social skills training focuses on teaching social and ADL skills.

HEALTH TEACHING REGARDING THE FOLLOWING
- Understanding of the disorder
- Need for self-care to prevent relapse
- Medication effects, adverse effects, and importance of compliance
- Importance of attending support groups
- Abstinence from the use of alcohol and/or other substances
- Keeping a log or journal of feelings and changes in behavior to help monitor medication effectiveness

Application Exercises

1. A nurse is caring for a client who has substance-induced psychotic disorder and is experiencing auditory hallucinations. The client states, "The voices won't leave me alone!" Which of the following statements should the nurse make? (Select all that apply.)

   A. "When did you start hearing the voices?"

   B. "The voices are not real, or else we would both hear them."

   C. "It must be scary to hear voices."

   D. "Are the voices telling you to hurt yourself?"

   E. "Why are the voices talking to only you?"

2. A nurse is completing an admission assessment for a client who has schizophrenia. Which of the following findings should the nurse document as positive symptoms? (Select all that apply.)

   A. Auditory hallucination

   B. Lack of motivation

   C. Use of clang associations

   D. Delusion of persecution

   E. Constantly waving arms

   F. Flat affect

3. A nurse is caring for a client who has schizoaffective disorder. Which of the following statements indicates the client is experiencing depersonalization?

   A. "I am a superhero and am immortal."

   B. "I am no one, and everyone is me."

   C. "I feel monsters pinching me all over."

   D. "I know that you are stealing my thoughts."

4. A nurse is caring for a client on an acute mental health unit. The client reports hearing voices that are telling her to "kill your doctor." Which of the following actions should the nurse take first?

   A. Use therapeutic communication to discuss the hallucination with the client.

   B. Initiate one-to-one observation of the client.

   C. Focus the client on reality.

   D. Notify the provider of the client's statement.

5. A nurse is speaking with a client who has schizophrenia when he suddenly seems to stop focusing on the nurse's questions and begins looking at the ceiling and talking to himself. Which of the following actions should the nurse take?

   A. Stop the interview at this point, and resume later when the client is better able to concentrate.

   B. Ask the client, "Are you seeing something on the ceiling?"

   C. Tell the client, "You seem to be looking at something on the ceiling. I see something there, too."

   D. Continue the interview without comment on the client's behavior.

PRACTICE Active Learning Scenario

A nurse is caring for a client who has schizophrenia and is reviewing discharge instructions which include a new prescription for risperidone. Use the ATI Active Learning Template: Medication to complete the following.

THERAPEUTIC USES

CLIENT EDUCATION: Describe at least three teaching points.

Application Exercises Key

1. A. **CORRECT:** The nurse should ask the client directly about the hallucination.

   B. The nurse should not argue with the client's view of the situation.

   C. **CORRECT:** The nurse should focus on the client's feelings rather than agreeing with the client's hallucination.

   D. **CORRECT:** The nurse should assess for command hallucinations and the client's risk for injury to self or others.

   E. The nurse should avoid asking a "why" question, which is nontherapeutic and can promote a defensive client response.

   Ⓝ *NCLEX® Connection: Psychosocial Integrity, Support Systems*

2. A. **CORRECT:** Hallucinations are an example of a positive symptom.

   B. Lack of motivation, or avolition, is an example of a negative symptom.

   C. **CORRECT:** Alterations in speech are an example of a positive symptom.

   D. **CORRECT:** Delusions are an example of a positive symptom.

   E. **CORRECT:** Bizarre motor movements are an example of a positive symptom.

   F. Flat affect is an example of a negative symptom.

   Ⓝ *NCLEX® Connection: Psychosocial Integrity, Mental Health Concepts*

3. A. This comment indicates the client is experiencing delusions of grandeur.

   B. **CORRECT:** This comment indicates the client is experiencing a loss of identity or depersonalization.

   C. This comment indicates the client is experiencing a tactile hallucination.

   D. This comment indicates the client is experiencing thought withdrawal.

   Ⓝ *NCLEX® Connection: Psychosocial Integrity, Mental Health Concepts*

4. A. The nurse should use therapeutic communication to discuss the client's hallucination. However, there is another action the nurse should take first.

   B. **CORRECT:** A client who is experiencing a command hallucination is at risk for injury to self or others. Safety is the priority, and initiating one-to-one observation is the first action the nurse should take.

   C. The nurse should attempt to focus the client on reality. However, there is another action the nurse should take first.

   D. The nurse should notify the provider of the client's hallucination. However, there is another action the nurse should take first.

   Ⓝ *NCLEX® Connection: Reduction of Risk Potential, Potential for Complications of Diagnostic Tests/Treatments/Procedures*

5. A. The nurse should address the client's current needs related to the possible hallucination rather than stop the interview.

   B. **CORRECT:** The nurse should ask the client directly about the hallucination to identify client needs and assess for a potential risk for injury.

   C. The nurse should avoid agreeing with the client, which can promote psychotic thinking.

   D. The nurse should address the client's current needs related to the possible hallucination rather than ignoring the change in behavior.

   Ⓝ *NCLEX® Connection: Psychosocial Integrity, Mental Health Concepts*

PRACTICE Answer

Using the ATI Active Learning Template: Medication

THERAPEUTIC USE:
Risperidone is an second-generation/atypical antipsychotic medication used to treat positive and negative symptoms of schizophrenia.

CLIENT EDUCATION
- Advise the client to follow a healthy, low-calorie diet.
- Recommend regular exercise.
- Instruct the client to monitor weight.
- Teach the client about adverse effects (agitation, dizziness, sedation, sleep disruption) and instruct the client to notify his provider if they are present.

Ⓝ *NCLEX® Connection: Pharmacological and Parenteral Therapies, Adverse Effects/ Contraindications/Side Effects/Interactions*

UNIT 3   PSYCHOBIOLOGIC DISORDERS

CHAPTER 16 *Personality Disorders*

A client who has a personality disorder demonstrates pathological personality characteristics. A client who has a personality disorder exhibits impairments in self-identity or self-direction and interpersonal functioning.

The maladaptive behaviors of a personality disorder are not always perceived by the individual as dysfunctional, and some areas of personal functioning can be adequate.

Personality disorders often co-occur with other mental health diagnoses, such as depression, anxiety, and eating and substance use disorders.

DEFENSE MECHANISMS

Defense mechanisms used by clients who have personality disorders include repression, suppression, regression, undoing, and splitting.

- Of these, splitting, which is the inability to incorporate positive and negative aspects of oneself or others into a whole image, is frequently seen in the acute mental health setting. QEBP
- Splitting is commonly associated with borderline personality disorder.
- In splitting, the client tends to characterize people or things as all good or all bad at any particular moment. For example, the client might say, "You are the worst person in the world." Later that day, she might say, "You are the best, but the nurse from the last shift is absolutely terrible."

ASSESSMENT

RISK FACTORS

- Clients who have personality disorders often have comorbid substance use disorders, and can have a history of nonviolent and violent crimes, including sex offenses.
- Psychosocial influences, such as childhood abuse or trauma, and developmental factors with a direct link to parenting.
- Biological influences include genetic and biochemical factors.

EXPECTED FINDINGS

Clients who have a personality disorder exhibit one or more of the following common pathological personality characteristics.

- Inflexibility/maladaptive responses to stress
- Compulsiveness and lack of social restraint
- Inability to emotionally connect in social and professional relationships
- Tendency to provoke interpersonal conflict
- Ability to merge personal boundaries with others

THE 10 PERSONALITY DISORDERS

Cluster A (odd or eccentric traits)

- **Paranoid:** Characterized by distrust and suspiciousness toward others based on unfounded beliefs that others want to harm, exploit, or deceive the person
- **Schizoid:** Characterized by emotional detachment, disinterest in close relationships, and indifference to praise or criticism; often uncooperative
- **Schizotypal:** Characterized by odd beliefs leading to interpersonal difficulties, an eccentric appearance, and magical thinking or perceptual distortions that are not clear delusions or hallucinations

Cluster B (dramatic, emotional, or erratic traits)

- **Antisocial:** Characterized by disregard for others with exploitation, lack of empathy, repeated unlawful actions, deceit, and failure to accept personal responsibility; sense of entitlement, manipulative, impulsive, and seductive; nonadherence to traditional morals and values; verbally charming and engaging
- **Borderline:** Characterized by instability of affect, identity, and relationships, as well as splitting behaviors, manipulation, impulsiveness, and fear of abandonment; often self-injurious and potentially suicidal; ideas of reference are common; often accompanied by impulsivity
- **Histrionic:** Characterized by emotional attention-seeking behavior, in which the person needs to be the center of attention; often seductive and flirtatious
- **Narcissistic:** Characterized by arrogance, grandiose views of self-importance, the need for consistent admiration, and a lack of empathy for others that strains most relationships; often sensitive to criticism

Cluster C (anxious or fearful traits; insecurity and inadequacy)

- **Avoidant:** Characterized by social inhibition and avoidance of all situations that require interpersonal contact, despite wanting close relationships, due to extreme fear of rejection; often very anxious in social situations
- **Dependent:** Characterized by extreme dependency in a close relationship with an urgent search to find a replacement when one relationship ends
- **Obsessive-Compulsive:** Characterized by perfectionism with a focus on orderliness and control to the extent that the individual might not be able to accomplish a given task

PATIENT-CENTERED CARE

NURSING CARE

- Self-assessment is vital for nurses caring for clients who have personality disorders and should be performed prior to care.
  - Clients who have personality disorders can evoke intense emotions in the nurse.
  - Awareness of personal reactions to stress promotes effective nursing care.
  - Therapeutic communication and intervention are promoted when client behaviors are anticipated.
  - The nurse should repeat the self-assessment if experiencing a personal stress response to client behavior.
- Milieu management focuses on appropriate social interaction within a group context.
- Safety is always a priority concern because some clients who have a personality disorder are at risk for self-injury or violence. Qs

COMMUNICATION STRATEGIES

Developing a therapeutic relationship is often challenging due to the client's distrust or hostility toward others. Feelings of being threatened or having no control can cause a client to act out toward the nurse.

- A firm, yet supportive approach and consistent care will help build a therapeutic nurse-client relationship.
- Offer the client realistic choices to enhance the client's sense of control.
- Limit-setting and consistency are essential with clients who are manipulative, especially those who have borderline or antisocial personality disorders. QEBP
- Clients who have dependent and histrionic personality disorders often benefit from assertiveness training and modeling.
- Clients who have schizoid or schizotypal personality disorders tend to isolate themselves, and the nurse should respect this need.
- For clients who have histrionic personality disorder, who can be flirtatious, it is important for the nurse to maintain professional boundaries and communication at all times.
- When caring for clients who exhibit dependent behavior, self-assess frequently for countertransference reactions.

MEDICATIONS

Medications include the use of psychotropic agents to provide relief from manifestations. Antidepressant, anxiolytic, antipsychotic, or mood stabilizer medications may be prescribed.

INTERPROFESSIONAL CARE

PSYCHOBIOLOGICAL INTERVENTIONS

- Psychotherapy, group therapy, and cognitive and behavior therapy are effective treatment modalities for clients who have personality disorders.
- Dialectical behavior therapy is a cognitive-behavioral therapy used for clients who exhibit self-injurious behavior. It focuses on gradual behavior changes and provides acceptance and validation for these clients.
- Case management is beneficial for clients who have personality disorders and are persistently and severely impaired.
  - In acute care facilities, case management focuses on obtaining pertinent history from current or previous providers, supporting reintegration with the family, and ensuring appropriate referrals to outpatient care.
  - In long-term outpatient facilities, case management goals include reducing hospitalization by providing resources for crisis services and enhancing the social support system.

Application Exercises

1. A nurse manager is discussing the care of a client who has a personality disorder with a newly licensed nurse. Which of the following statements by the newly licensed nurse indicates an understanding of the teaching?

   A. "I can promote my client's sense of control by establishing a schedule."

   B. "I should encourage clients who have a schizoid personality disorder to increase socialization."

   C. "I should practice limit-setting to help prevent client manipulation."

   D. "I should implement assertiveness training with clients who have antisocial personality disorder."

2. A nurse is caring for a client who has avoidant personality disorder. Which of the following statements is expected from a client who has this type of personality disorder?

   A. "I'm scared that you're going to leave me."

   B. "I'll go to group therapy if you'll let me smoke."

   C. "I need to feel that everyone admires me."

   D. "I sometimes feel better if I cut myself."

3. A nurse is caring for a client who has borderline personality disorder. The client says, "The nurse on the evening shift is always nice! You are the meanest nurse ever!" The nurse should recognize the client's statement as an example of which of the following defense mechanisms?

   A. Regression

   B. Splitting

   C. Undoing

   D. Identification

4. A nurse is assisting with a court-ordered evaluation of a client who has antisocial personality disorder. Which of the following findings should the nurse expect? (Select all that apply.)

   A. Demonstrates extreme anxiety when placed in a social situation

   B. Has difficulty making even simple decisions

   C. Attempts to convince other clients to give him their belongings

   D. Becomes agitated if his personal area is not neat and orderly

   E. Blames others for his past and current problems

5. A charge nurse is preparing a staff education session on personality disorders. Which of the following personality characteristics associated with all of the personality disorders should the charge nurse include in the teaching? (Select all that apply.)

   A. Difficulty in getting along with other members of a group

   B. Belief in the ability to become invisible during times of stress

   C. Display of defense mechanisms when routines are changed

   D. Claiming to be more important than other persons

   E. Difficulty understanding why it is inappropriate to have a personal relationship with staff

---

PRACTICE Active Learning Scenario

A charge nurse is discussing self-assessment with a newly licensed nurse. Use the ATI Active Learning Template: Basic Concept to complete this item.

RELATED CONTENT: Identify how self-assessment relates to caring for a client who has a personality disorder.

UNDERLYING PRINCIPLES: Identify at least two concepts.

NURSING INTERVENTIONS: Identify who should perform self-assessment and when it is indicated.

Application Exercises Key

1. A. Rather than establishing a schedule, the nurse should ask for the client's input and offer realistic choices to promote the client's sense of control.

   B. The nurse should avoid trying to increase socialization for a client who has a schizoid personality disorder.

   C. **CORRECT:** When caring for a client who has a personality disorder, limit-setting is appropriate to help prevent client manipulation.

   D. The nurse should implement assertiveness training for clients who have dependent and histrionic personality disorders.

   Ⓝ *NCLEX® Connection: Psychosocial Integrity, Mental Health Concepts*

2. A. **CORRECT:** Clients who have avoidant personality disorder often have a fear of abandonment. This type of statement is expected.

   B. This statement indicates manipulation, which is expected from a client who has antisocial personality disorder.

   C. This statement indicates a need for admiration, which is expected from a client who has narcissistic personality disorder.

   D. This statement indicates a risk for self-injury, which is expected from a client who has borderline personality disorder.

   Ⓝ *NCLEX® Connection: Psychosocial Integrity, Mental Health Concepts*

3. A. Regression refers to resorting to an earlier way of functioning, such as having a temper tantrum.

   B. **CORRECT:** Splitting occurs when a person is unable to see both positive and negative qualities at the same time. The client who has borderline personality disorder tends to see a person as all bad one time and all good another time.

   C. Undoing is a behavior that is intended to undo or reverse unacceptable thoughts or acts, such as buying a gift for a spouse after having an extramarital affair.

   D. In identification, the person imitates the behavior of someone admired or feared.

   Ⓝ *NCLEX® Connection: Psychosocial Integrity, Mental Health Concepts*

4. A. Anxiety in social situations is an expected finding of clients who have avoidant personality disorder.

   B. Indecisiveness, due to a sensitivity to criticism, is an expected finding of clients who have narcissistic personality disorder.

   C. **CORRECT:** Exploitation and manipulation of others is an expected finding of antisocial personality disorder.

   D. Perfectionism with a focus on orderliness and control is an expected finding of clients who have obsessive-compulsive personality disorder.

   E. **CORRECT:** Failure to accept personal responsibility is an expected finding of clients who have antisocial personality disorder.

   Ⓝ *NCLEX® Connection: Psychosocial Integrity, Mental Health Concepts*

5. A. **CORRECT:** Difficulty with social and professional relationships is a personality characteristic that can be seen with all personality disorder types.

   B. Clients who have schizotypal personality disorder can display magical thinking or delusions. However, this is not associated with all personality disorder types.

   C. **CORRECT:** Maladaptive response to stress is a personality characteristic that can be seen with all personality disorder types.

   D. Clients who have narcissistic personality disorder can display grandiose thinking. However, this is not associated with all personality disorder types.

   E. **CORRECT:** Difficulty understanding personal boundaries is a personality characteristic that can be seen with all personality disorder types.

   Ⓝ *NCLEX® Connection: Psychosocial Integrity, Mental Health Concepts*

PRACTICE Answer

Using the ATI Active Learning Template: Basic Concept

RELATED CONTENT: Self-assessment is vital for nurses caring for clients who have personality disorders because of the intense emotions that can be elicited during client care.

UNDERLYING PRINCIPLES
- Self-assessment prepares the nurse for the personal emotions that can be experienced as a result of client care.
- The nurse can provide more effective nursing care when aware of personal reactions to stress.
- Therapeutic communication and intervention are promoted when client behaviors are anticipated.

NURSING INTERVENTIONS
- Who: Self-assessment should be performed by all nurses caring for a client who has a personality disorder.
- When: The nurse should perform a self-assessment prior to providing client care and whenever experiencing a personal stress response to client behavior.

Ⓝ *NCLEX® Connection: Psychosocial Integrity, Stress Management*

UNIT 3   PSYCHOBIOLOGIC DISORDERS

CHAPTER 17 *Neurocognitive Disorders*

Neurocognitive disorders are a group of conditions characterized by the disruption of thinking, memory, processing, and problem-solving. Treatment of clients who have neurocognitive disorders requires a compassionate understanding of both the client and family.

TYPES OF COGNITIVE DISORDERS

- Cognitive disorders recognized and defined by the DSM-5 include the following.
  - **Delirium**
  - **Mild neurocognitive disorder (NCD)**
  - **Major neurocognitive disorder** (commonly known as **dementia**)
- Major and mild NCD subtypes are further classified, such as NCD due to Alzheimer's disease, NCD due to Parkinson's disease, or NCD due to Huntington's disease.
- **Alzheimer's disease (AD)** is a subtype of NCD that is neurodegenerative, resulting in the gradual impairment of cognitive function. It is the most common type of major NCD.
- It is important to distinguish between a cognitive disorder and other mental health disorders that can have similar manifestations. Depression in the older adult can mimic the early stages of Alzheimer's disease. Ⓖ

ASSESSMENT

RISK FACTORS

- Risk factors for delirium include physiological changes, including neurological (Parkinson's disease, Huntington's disease); metabolic (hepatic or renal failure, fluid and electrolyte imbalances, nutritional deficiencies); and cardiovascular and respiratory diseases; infections (HIV/AIDS); surgery; and substance use or withdrawal.
- The best way to prevent and manage delirium is to minimize risk factors and promote early detection. Timely recognition is essential.
- Risk factors for neurocognitive disorder and AD include advanced age, prior head trauma, lifestyle factors, and a family history of AD. There is a strong genetic link in early-onset familial AD.

EXPECTED FINDINGS

- Delirium and neurocognitive disorder have some similarities and some important differences. **(17.1)**
- Clients who have NCD can also develop delirium.

STAGES OF ALZHEIMER'S DISEASE

Mild Alzheimer's (early stage)

- Memory lapses
- Losing or misplacing items
- Difficulty concentrating and organizing
- Unable to remember material just read
- Still able to perform ADLs
- Short-term memory loss noticeable to close relations

Moderate Alzheimer's (middle stage)

- Forgetting events of one's own history
- Difficulty performing tasks that require planning and organizing (paying bills, managing money)
- Difficulty with complex mental arithmetic
- Personality and behavioral changes: appearing withdrawn or subdued, especially in social or mentally challenging situations; compulsive; repetitive actions
- Changes in sleep patterns
- Can wander and get lost
- Can be incontinent
- Clinical findings that are noticeable to others

Severe Alzheimer's (late stage)

- Losing ability to converse with others
- Assistance required for ADLs
- Incontinence
- Losing awareness of one's environment
- Progressing difficulty with physical abilities (walking, sitting, and eventually swallowing)
- Eventually losses all ability to move; can develop stupor and coma
- Death frequently related to choking or infection

DEFENSE MECHANISMS

Assess for defense mechanisms used by the client to preserve self-esteem and to compensate when cognitive changes are progressive.

Denial: Both the client and family members can refuse to believe that changes, such as loss of memory, are taking place, even when those changes are obvious to others.

Confabulation: The client can make up stories when questioned about events or activities that she does not remember. This can seem like lying, but it is actually an unconscious attempt to save self-esteem and prevent admitting that she does not remember the occasion.

Perseveration: The client avoids answering questions by repeating phrases or behavior. This is another unconscious attempt to maintain self-esteem when memory has failed.

17.1 Delirium and neurocognitive disorder

Delirium	*Neurocognitive disorder*
ONSET	
Rapid over a short period of time (hours or days)	Gradual deterioration of function over months or years
MANIFESTATIONS	
Impairments in memory, judgment, ability to focus, and ability to calculate, which can fluctuate throughout the day. Disorientation and confusion often worse at night and early morning.	Impairments in memory, judgment, speech (aphasia), ability to recognize familiar objects (agnosia), executive functioning (managing daily tasks), and movement (apraxia); impairments do not change throughout the day.
Level of consciousness is usually altered and can rapidly fluctuate.	Level of consciousness is usually unchanged.
There are four types of delirium.	Restlessness and agitation are common; sundowning can occur.
• Hyperactive with agitation and restlessness	Personality change is gradual.
• Hypoactive with apathy and quietness	Vital signs are stable unless other illness is present.
• Mixed, having a combination of hyper and hypo manifestations	
• Unclassified for those whose manifestations do not classify into the other categories	
Restlessness, anxiety, motor agitation, and fluctuating moods are common. Personality change is rapid.	
Some perceptual disturbances can be present, such as hallucinations and illusions.	
Change in reality can cause fear, panic, and anger.	
Can cause vital signs to become unstable requiring intervention.	
Should be considered a medical emergency	
CAUSE	
Common problem associated with hospitalization of older adult clients.	Cognitive deficits are not related to another mental health disorder.
Caused secondary to another medical condition, such as infection, malnutrition, depression, electrolyte imbalance or substance use	Advanced age is the biggest risk factor. Other causes include genetics, sedentary lifestyle, metabolic syndrome, and diabetes.
Postoperative causes can include withdrawal from illegal substances or alcohol, or impaired respiratory function.	Subtypes of neurocognitive disorder can be related to:
Primary step to resolve is to determine the underlying cause.	• Alzheimer's disease
	• Traumatic brain injury
	• Parkinson's disease
	• Other disorders affecting the neurological system
OUTCOME	
Reversible if diagnosis and treatment are prompt	Irreversible and progressive

DIAGNOSTIC PROCEDURES Q$_{EBP}$

There is no specific laboratory or diagnostic testing to diagnose NCDs. Definitive diagnosis cannot be made until autopsy. Testing is done to rule out other pathologies that could be mistaken for NCDs.
- Chest and skull x-rays
- Electroencephalography (EEG)
- Electrocardiography (ECG)
- Liver function studies
- Thyroid function tests
- Neuroimaging (computer tomography and position emission tomography of the brain)
- Urinalysis
- Serum electrolytes
- Folate and vitamin B$_{12}$ levels
- Vision and hearing tests

SCREENING/ASSESSMENT TOOLS

Confusion Assessment Method (CAM): For delirium

Neelon/Champagne (NEECHAM) Confusion Scale: For delirium

Functional Dementia Scale: This tool will give the nurse information regarding the client's ability to perform self-care, extent of the client's memory loss, mood changes, and the degree of danger to self and/or others. Q$_{EBP}$

Brief Interview for Mental Status (BIMS): Used for clients in long-term care settings

Mini-mental status examination (MMSE)

Functional Assessment Screening Tool (FAST)

Global Deterioration Scale

Blessed Dementia Scale: This tool provides the nurse with client behavioral information based on an interview with a secondary source, such as a client's family member.

PATIENT-CENTERED CARE

NURSING CARE

- Perform self-assessment regarding possible feelings of frustration, anger, or fear when performing daily care for clients who have progressive cognitive decline.
- Nursing interventions are focused on protecting the client from injury, as well as promoting client dignity and quality of life.
- Provide for a safe and therapeutic environment. Qs
  - Assess for potential injury, such as falls or wandering.
  - Assign the client to a room close to the nurses' station for close observation.
  - Provide a room with a low level of visual and auditory stimuli.
  - Provide for a well-lit environment, minimizing contrasts and shadows.
  - Have the client sit in a room with windows to help with time orientation.
  - Have the client wear an identification bracelet. Use monitors and bed alarm devices as needed.
  - Use restraints only as an intervention of last resort.
  - Use caution when administering medications PRN for agitation or anxiety.
  - Assess the client's risk for injury and ensure safety in the physical environment, such as a lowered bed.

Cognitive support

- Provide compensatory memory aids, such as clocks, calendars, photographs, memorabilia, seasonal decorations, and familiar objects. Reorient as necessary.
- Keep a consistent daily routine.
- Maintain consistent caregivers.
- Cover or remove mirrors to decrease fear and agitation.

Physical needs

- Monitor neurological status.
- Identify disturbances in physiologic status which can contribute to the cause of delirium.
- Assess skin integrity which can be compromised due to poor nutrition, bed rest or incontinence.
- Monitor vital signs. Tachycardia, elevated blood pressure, sweating, dilated pupils can be associated with delirium.
- Implement measures to promote sleep.
- Monitor the client's level of comfort and assess for nonverbal indications of discomfort.
- Provide eyeglasses and assistive hearing devices as needed.
- Ensure adequate food and fluid intake. Underlying causes of delirium can result in electrolyte imbalance.

Communication

- Communicate in a calm, reassuring tone.
- Speak in positively worded phrases. Do not argue or question hallucinations or delusions.
- Reinforce reality.
- Reinforce orientation to time, place, and person.
- Introduce self to client with each new contact.
- Establish eye contact and use short, simple sentences when speaking to the client. Focus on one item of information at a time.
- Encourage reminiscence about happy times. Talk about familiar things.
- Break instructions and activities into short timeframes.
- Limit the number of choices when dressing or eating.
- Minimize the need for decision-making and abstract thinking to avoid frustration.
- Avoid confrontation.
- Approach slowly and from the front. Address the client by name.
- Encourage family visitation as appropriate.

MEDICATIONS

Use caution when administering medications PRN for agitation or anxiety. Qs

Delirium

Medications can be the underlying cause of delirium. Recognize medication reactions before delirium occurs.
- Pharmacological management focuses on the treatment of the underlying disorder.
- Antipsychotic or antianxiety medications may be prescribed.

Neurocognitive disorders

Cholinesterase inhibitor medications, such as donepezil, rivastigmine, and galantamine, increase acetylcholine at cholinergic synapses by inhibiting its breakdown by acetylcholinesterase, which increases the availability of acetylcholine at neurotransmitter receptor sites in the CNS.
- In some clients, these medications improve the ability to perform self-care and slow cognitive deterioration of Alzheimer's disease in the mild to moderate stages.
- ADVERSE EFFECTS
  - GI effects: Nausea, vomiting, and diarrhea
    - Monitor for gastrointestinal adverse effects and for fluid volume deficits.
    - Promote adequate fluid intake.
    - The provider may titrate the dosage to reduce gastrointestinal effects.
  - Bradycardia, syncope
    - Teach the family to monitor pulse rate for the client who lives at home.
    - The client should be screened for underlying heart disease.
- CONTRAINDICATIONS/PRECAUTIONS: Cholinesterase inhibitors should be used with caution in clients who have pre-existing asthma or other obstructive pulmonary disorders. Bronchoconstriction can be caused by an increase of acetylcholine.

- INTERACTIONS
  - **Concurrent use of NSAIDs, such as aspirin, can cause gastrointestinal bleeding.**
    - NURSING CONSIDERATIONS
      - Assess the use of over-the-counter NSAIDs.
      - Monitor for indications of gastrointestinal bleeding.
  - **Antihistamines, tricyclic antidepressants, and conventional antipsychotics (medications that block cholinergic receptors) can reduce the therapeutic effects of donepezil.**
    - NURSING CONSIDERATIONS: Use of cholinergic receptor blocking medications for clients taking any cholinesterase inhibitor is not recommended.
- NURSING ADMINISTRATION
  - Dosage should start low and gradually be increased until adverse effects are no longer tolerable or medication is no longer beneficial.
  - Monitor for adverse effects, and educate the client and family about these effects. Taper medication when discontinuing to prevent abrupt progression of clinical manifestations. QEBP
  - Monitor the client for the ability to swallow tablets. Most medications are available in tablets and oral solutions. Donepezil is available in an orally disintegrating tablet.
  - Administer with or without food.
  - Donepezil has a long half-life and is administered once daily at bedtime. The other cholinesterase inhibitors are usually administered twice daily.
  - Rivastigmine is available in oral form, and as a patch that is applied once daily.

Medications such as memantine block the entry of calcium into nerve cells, thus slowing down brain-cell death.
- Memantine is approved for moderate to severe stages of AD.
- NURSING CONSIDERATIONS
  - Memantine can be used concurrently with a cholinesterase inhibitor.
  - Administer the medication with or without food.
  - Monitor for common adverse effects, including dizziness, headache, confusion, and constipation.

Other medications that may be prescribed include selective serotonin reuptake inhibitors for depression and antianxiety agents as needed for agitation. Antipsychotics are reserved for clients who experience hallucinations or delusions, but are used as a last resort because these medications carry many side effects.

ALTERNATIVE/COMPLEMENTARY THERAPIES

Some vitamins and herbal products are currently under investigation for the treatment of neurocognitive disorders. There is currently no evidence that these products are effective.

CLIENT EDUCATION

CARE AFTER DISCHARGE
- Educate family/caregivers about the client's illness, methods of care, and adaptation of the home environment.
- Ensure a safe environment in the home.

QUESTIONS TO ASK Qs
- Will the client wander out into the street if doors are left unlocked?
- Is the client able to remember his address and his name?
- Does the client harm others when allowed to wander in a long-term care facility?

HOME SAFETY MEASURES Qs
- Remove scatter rugs.
- Install door locks that cannot be easily opened.
- Lock water heater thermostat and turn water temperature down to a safe level.
- Provide good lighting, especially on stairs.
- Install a handrail on stairs, and mark step edges with colored tape.
- Place mattresses on the floor.
- Remove clutter, keeping clear, wide pathways for walking through a room.
- Secure electrical cords to baseboards.
- Store cleaning supplies in locked cupboards.
- Install handrails in bathrooms.

SUPPORT FOR CAREGIVERS
- Encourage the client and family to seek legal counsel regarding advanced directives, guardianship, or durable power of attorney for health care.
- Determine teaching needs for the client and family members as the client's cognitive ability progressively declines.
- Review resources available to the family as the client's health declines. Include long-term care options. A variety of home care and community resources can be available in many areas of the country. These resources can allow the client to remain at home, rather than in a care facility. QTC
- Provide support for caregivers. Encourage caregivers to ask for help from friends and other family members for respite care, and to take advantage of local support groups.
- Encourage caregivers to take care of themselves and to take one day at a time.

Application Exercises

1. A nurse is caring for a client who has early stage Alzheimer's disease and a new prescription for donepezil. The nurse should include which of the following statements when teaching the client about the medication?

   A. "You should avoid taking over-the-counter acetaminophen while on donepezil."

   B. "You can expect the progression of cognitive decline to slow with donepezil."

   C. "You will be screened for underlying kidney disease prior to starting donepezil."

   D. "You should stop taking donepezil if you experience nausea or diarrhea."

2. A nurse in a long-term care facility is caring for a client who has major neurocognitive disorder and attempts to wander out of the building. The client states, "I have to get home." Which of the following statements should the nurse make?

   A. "You have forgotten that this is your home."

   B. "You cannot go outside without a staff member."

   C. "Why would you want to leave? Aren't you happy with your care?"

   D. "I am your nurse. Let's walk together to your room."

3. A home health nurse is making a visit to a client who has Alzheimer's disease to assess the home for safety. Which of the following suggestions should the nurse make to decrease the client's risk for injury?

   A. Install childproof door locks.

   B. Place rugs over electrical cords.

   C. Mark cleaning supplies with colored tape.

   D. Place the client's mattress on the floor.

   E. Install light fixtures above stairs.

4. A nurse is making a home visit to a client who is in the late stage of Alzheimer's disease. The client's partner, who is the primary caregiver, wishes to discuss concerns about the client's nutrition and the stress of providing care. Which of the following actions should the nurse take?

   A. Verify that a current power of attorney document is on file.

   B. Instruct the client's partner to offer finger foods to increase oral intake.

   C. Provide information on resources for respite care.

   D. Schedule the client for placement of an enteral feeding tube.

5. A nurse is performing an admission assessment for a client who has delirium related to an acute urinary tract infection. Which of the following findings should the nurse expect? (Select all that apply.)

   A. History of gradual memory loss

   B. Family report of personality changes

   C. Hallucinations

   D. Unaltered level of consciousness

   E. Restlessness

PRACTICE Active Learning Scenario

A nurse is planning care to promote a safe and therapeutic environment for a client who has severe cognitive decline due to Alzheimer's disease. Use the ATI Active Learning Template: System Disorder to complete this item.

ALTERATION IN HEALTH (DIAGNOSIS)

NURSING CARE: Identify five nursing actions.

Application Exercises Key

1. A. Clients taking donepezil should avoid NSAIDs, rather than acetaminophen, due to risk for gastrointestinal bleeding.

   B. **CORRECT:** Donepezil slows the cognitive deterioration of Alzheimer's disease.

   C. Clients should be screened for underlying heart and pulmonary disease, rather than kidney disease, prior to treatment.

   D. Gastrointestinal adverse effects are common with donepezil and can result in a dosage reduction. However, the client should not abruptly stop the medication without consulting a provider.

   Ⓝ *NCLEX® Connection: Pharmacological and Parenteral Therapies, Adverse Effects/Contraindications/Side Effects/Interactions*

2. A. The nurse should avoid statements that can be interpreted as argumentative or demeaning.

   B. The nurse should use positive, rather than negative, statements.

   C. Using a "why" question can promote a defensive reaction and does not reinforce reality.

   D. **CORRECT:** It is appropriate for the nurse to introduce herself with each new interaction and to promote reality in a calm, reassuring manner.

   Ⓝ *NCLEX® Connection: Psychosocial Integrity, Mental Health Concepts*

3. A. **CORRECT:** Door locks that are difficult to open are appropriate to reduce the risk of the client wandering outside without supervision.

   B. Rugs create a fall risk hazard and should be removed. Electrical cords should be secured to baseboards rather than covered.

   C. Cleaning supplies should be placed in locked cupboards. Marking the supplies with colored tape does not prevent the client's access to hazardous materials.

   D. **CORRECT:** Placing the client's mattress on the floor reduces the risk for falls out of bed.

   E. **CORRECT:** Stairs should have adequate lighting to reduce the risk for falls.

   Ⓝ *NCLEX® Connection: Safety and Infection Control, Accident/Error/Injury Prevention*

4. A. A power of attorney document does not address the client's care or the concerns of the caregiver.

   B. Clients in late-stage Alzheimer's disease are at risk for choking and are unable to eat without assistance. Offering finger foods is not an appropriate action.

   C. **CORRECT:** Providing information on resources for respite care is an appropriate action to provide the client's partner with a break from caregiving responsibilities.

   D. Placement of an enteral feeding tube is appropriate only with a prescription from the provider following a discussion that includes the provider, nurse, client's partner, and possibly social services and additional family members.

   Ⓝ *NCLEX® Connection: Management of Care, Referrals*

5. A. The client who has delirium can experience memory loss with sudden rather than gradual onset.

   B. **CORRECT:** The client who has delirium can experience rapid personality changes.

   C. **CORRECT:** The client who has delirium can have perceptual disturbances, such as hallucinations and illusions.

   D. The client who has delirium is expected to have an altered level of consciousness that can rapidly fluctuate.

   E. **CORRECT:** The client who has delirium commonly exhibits restlessness and agitation.

   Ⓝ *NCLEX® Connection: Psychosocial Integrity, Mental Health Concepts*

PRACTICE Answer

Using the ATI Active Learning Template: System Disorder

ALTERATION IN HEALTH (DIAGNOSIS):
Alzheimer's disease is a subtype of neurocognitive disorder that is neurodegenerative, resulting in the gradual impairment of cognitive function. A client who has severe cognitive decline has memory difficulties, loss of awareness to recent events and surroundings, inability to recall personal history, personality changes, wandering behavior, the need for assistance with ADLs, disruption of sleep/wake cycle, and violent tendencies.

NURSING CARE

- Assign a room close to the nurses' station
- Provide a room with a low level of visual and auditory stimuli.
- Provide for a well-lit environment, minimizing contrasts and shadows.
- Have the client sit in a room with windows to help with time orientation.
- Have the client wear an identification bracelet. Use monitors and bed alarm devices as needed.
- Monitor the client's level of comfort.

- Provide compensatory memory aids, such as clocks, calendars, photographs, memorabilia, seasonal decorations, and familiar objects. Reorient as necessary.
- Provide eyeglasses and assistive hearing devices as needed.
- Keep a consistent daily routine.
- Maintain consistent caregivers.
- Ensure adequate food and fluid intake.
- Allow for safe pacing and wandering.
- Cover or remove mirrors to decrease fear and agitation.

Ⓝ *NCLEX® Connection: Safety and Infection Control, Accident/Error/Injury Prevention*

UNIT 3 PSYCHOBIOLOGIC DISORDERS

CHAPTER 18 *Substance Use and Addictive Disorders*

Substance use disorders are related to alcohol, caffeine, cannabis, hallucinogens, inhalants, opioids, sedatives/hypnotics/anxiolytics, stimulants, tobacco, and other (or unknown) substances.

A substance use disorder involves repeated use of chemical substances, leading to clinically significant impairment during a 12-month period. Non-substance-related disorders (behavioral/process addictions) include gambling, sexual activity, shopping, social media, and Internet gaming.

Substance use and addictive disorders are characterized by loss of control due to the substance use or behavior, participation that continues despite continuing associated problems, and a tendency to relapse back into the substance use or behavior.

The defense mechanism of denial is commonly used by clients who have problems with a substance use or addictive disorder. For example, a person who has long-term tobacco use might say, "I can quit whenever I want to, but smoking really doesn't cause me any problems." Frequently, denial prevents a client from obtaining help with substance use or an addictive behavior.

ASSESSMENT

RISK FACTORS

- Genetics: predisposition to developing a substance use disorder due to family history
- Chronic stress: socioeconomic factors
- History of trauma: abuse, combat experience
- Lowered self-esteem
- Lowered tolerance for pain and frustration
- Few meaningful personal relationships
- Few life successes
- Risk-taking tendencies

SOCIOCULTURAL THEORIES

- Some cultures, such as Alaska natives and Native American groups, have a high percentage of members who have alcohol use disorder. Q EBP
  - Other cultures, such as Asian groups, have a low rate of alcohol use disorder.
  - Metabolism of alcohol and cultural views of alcohol use provide possible explanations for the incidence of alcohol use within a cultural group.
- Peer pressure and other sociological factors can increase the likelihood of substance use.
- Older adult clients can have a history of alcohol use or can develop a pattern of alcohol/substance use later in life due to life stressors, such as losing a partner or a friend, retirement, or social isolation. Ⓖ

EXPECTED FINDINGS

The nurse should use open-ended questions to obtain the following information for the nursing history. Q PCC
- Type of substance or addictive behavior
- Pattern and frequency of substance use
- Amount of substance used
- Age at onset of substance use
- Changes in occupational or school performance
- Changes in use patterns
- Periods of abstinence in history
- Previous withdrawal manifestations
- Date of last substance use or addictive behavior

REVIEW OF SYSTEMS
- Blackout or loss of consciousness
- Changes in bowel movements
- Weight loss or weight gain
- Experience of stressful situation
- Sleep problems
- Chronic pain
- Concern over substance use
- Cutting down on consumption or behavior

POPULATION-SPECIFIC CONSIDERATIONS

- The rate of substance use is highest in clients age 20 to 29.
- The younger the person is at the time of initial substance use, the higher the incidence of developing a substance use disorder.
- Cocaine use is decreased among adolescents. However, about half of adolescents report access to marijuana.
- According to 2013 data from the National Institute of Alcohol Abuse and Alcoholism, 86.8% of people over the age of 18 reported alcohol consumption at some point in their life with 56.4% reporting alcohol consumption in the past month.
- **OLDER ADULTS** who use substances are especially prone to falls and other injuries, memory loss, somatic reports (headaches), and changes in sleep patterns. ©
  - Indications of alcohol use in older adults can include a decrease in ability for self-care (functional status), urinary incontinence, and manifestations of dementia.
  - Older adults can show effects of alcohol use at lower doses than younger adults.
  - Polypharmacy (the use of multiple medications), the potential interaction between substances and medications, and age-related physiological changes raise the likelihood of adverse effects, such as confusion and falls in older adult clients. Q**QI**

STANDARDIZED SCREENING TOOLS

- Michigan Alcohol Screening Test (MAST) Q**EBP**
- Drug Abuse Screening Test (DAST) or DAST-A: Adolescent version
- CAGE Questionnaire: Asks questions of clients to determine how they perceive their current alcohol use
- Alcohol Use Disorders Identification Test (AUDIT)
- Clinical Institute Withdrawal Assessment of Alcohol Scale, Revised (CIWA-Ar)
- Clinical Opiate Withdrawal Scale

COMMONLY USED SUBSTANCES

- Designer or club drugs, such as ecstasy, can combine substances from different categories, producing varying effects of intoxication or withdrawal.
- Improper use of prescription medications, specifically opioids, CNS depressants, and CNS stimulants, can result in substance use disorder and drug-seeking behavior.

OPIOID AGONISTS

Opioid agonists attach to CNS receptors altering perception of and response to pain. This response can lead to generalized CNS depression. Prescribed opioid agonists are listed as Schedule II under the Controlled Substances Act.

Opioids

Heroin, morphine, and hydromorphone can be injected, smoked, and inhaled.

INTENDED EFFECTS: A rush of euphoria, relief from pain

EFFECTS OF INTOXICATION

- Slurred speech, impaired memory, pupillary changes.
- Decreased respirations and level of consciousness, which can cause death
- Maladaptive behavioral or psychological changes, including impaired judgment or social functioning
- An antidote, naloxone, available for IV use to relieve effects of overdose

WITHDRAWAL MANIFESTATIONS

- Abstinence syndrome begins with sweating and rhinorrhea progressing to piloerection (gooseflesh), tremors, and irritability followed by severe weakness, diarrhea, fever, insomnia, pupil dilation, nausea and vomiting, pain in the muscles and bones, and muscle spasms.

- Withdrawal is very unpleasant but not life-threatening.

CENTRAL NERVOUS SYSTEM DEPRESSANTS

CNS depressants can produce physiological and psychological dependence and can have cross-tolerance, cross-dependency, and an additive effect when take concurrently.

Alcohol (ethanol)

- A laboratory blood alcohol concentration (BAC) of 0.08% (80 g/dL) is considered legally intoxicated for adults operating automobiles in most U.S. states. Death could occur from acute toxicity in levels greater than about 0.4% (400 g/dL).
- BAC depends on many factors, including body weight, gender, concentration of alcohol in drinks, number of drinks, gastric absorption rate, and the individual's tolerance level.

INTENDED EFFECTS: Relaxation, decreased social anxiety, stress reduction

EFFECTS OF INTOXICATION

- **Effects of excess:** Slurred speech, nystagmus, memory impairment, altered judgment, decreased motor skills, decreased level of consciousness (which can include stupor or coma), respiratory arrest, peripheral collapse, and death (with large doses)
- **Chronic use:** Direct cardiovascular damage, liver damage (ranging from fatty liver to cirrhosis), erosive gastritis and gastrointestinal bleeding, acute pancreatitis, sexual dysfunction

WITHDRAWAL MANIFESTATIONS

- Manifestations include abdominal cramping; vomiting; tremors; restlessness and inability to sleep; increased heart rate; transient hallucinations or illusions; anxiety; increased blood pressure, respiratory rate, and temperature; and tonic-clonic seizures.
- Alcohol withdrawal delirium can occur 2 to 3 days after cessation of alcohol. This is considered a medical emergency. Manifestations include severe disorientation, psychotic manifestations (hallucinations), severe hypertension, cardiac dysrhythmias, and delirium. Alcohol withdrawal delirium can progress to death.

Sedatives/hypnotics/anxiolytics

Benzodiazepines like diazepam, **barbiturates** like pentobarbital, or **club drugs** like flunitrazepam ("date rape drug") can be taken orally or injected.

INTENDED EFFECTS: Decreased anxiety, sedation

EFFECTS OF INTOXICATION
- Increased drowsiness and sedation, agitation, slurred speech, uncoordinated motor activity, nystagmus, disorientation, nausea, vomiting
- Respiratory depression and decreased level of consciousness, which can be fatal
- An antidote, flumazenil, available for IV use for benzodiazepine toxicity
- No antidote to reverse barbiturate toxicity

WITHDRAWAL MANIFESTATIONS: Anxiety, insomnia, diaphoresis, hypertension, possible psychotic reactions, hand tremors, nausea, vomiting, hallucinations or illusions, psychomotor agitation, and possible seizure activity

Cannabis

Marijuana or hashish (which is more potent) can be smoked or orally ingested.

INTENDED EFFECTS: Euphoria, sedation, hallucinations, decrease of nausea and vomiting secondary to chemotherapy, management of chronic pain

EFFECTS OF INTOXICATION
- Chronic use: lung cancer, chronic bronchitis, and other respiratory effects
- In high doses: occurrence of paranoia, such as delusions and hallucinations
- Increased appetite, dry mouth, tachycardia

WITHDRAWAL MANIFESTATIONS: Irritability, aggression, anxiety, insomnia, lack of appetite, restlessness, depressed mood, abdominal pain, tremors, diaphoresis, fever, headache

CENTRAL NERVOUS SYSTEM STIMULANTS

The CNS stimulation seen in some CNS stimulants is dependent on the area of the brain and spinal cord affected.

Cocaine

Can be injected, smoked, or inhaled (snorted)

INTENDED EFFECTS: Rush of euphoria (extreme well-being) and pleasure, increased energy

EFFECTS OF INTOXICATION
- **Mild toxicity:** dizziness, irritability, tremor, blurred vision
- **Severe effects:** hallucinations, seizures, extreme fever, tachycardia, hypertension, chest pain, possible cardiovascular collapse and death

WITHDRAWAL MANIFESTATIONS
- Depression, fatigue, craving, excess sleeping or insomnia, dramatic unpleasant dreams, psychomotor retardation, agitation
- Not life-threatening, but possible occurrence of suicidal ideation

Amphetamines

Can be taken orally, injected intravenously, or smoked

INTENDED EFFECTS: Increased energy, euphoria similar to cocaine

EFFECTS OF INTOXICATION
- Impaired judgment, psychomotor agitation, hypervigilance, extreme irritability
- Acute cardiovascular effects (tachycardia, elevated blood pressure), which could cause death

WITHDRAWAL MANIFESTATIONS
- Craving, depression, fatigue, sleeping
- Not life-threatening

Inhalants

Amyl nitrate, nitrous oxide, and solvents are sniffed, huffed, or bagged, often by children or adolescents.

INTENDED EFFECTS: Euphoria

EFFECTS OF INTOXICATION: Depend on the substance, but generally can cause behavioral or psychological changes, dizziness, nystagmus, uncoordinated movements or gait, slurred speech, drowsiness, hyporeflexia, muscle weakness, diplopia, stupor or coma, respiratory depression, and possible death

WITHDRAWAL MANIFESTATIONS: None

Hallucinogens

Lysergic acid diethylamide (LSD), mescaline (peyote), and phencyclidine piperidine (PCP) are usually ingested orally, but can be injected or smoked.

INTENDED EFFECTS: Heightened sense of self and altered perceptions (colors being more vivid while under the influence)

EFFECTS OF INTOXICATION: Anxiety, depression, paranoia, impaired judgment, impaired social functioning, pupil dilation, tachycardia, diaphoresis, palpitations, blurred vision, tremors, incoordination, and panic attacks

WITHDRAWAL MANIFESTATIONS: **Hallucinogen persisting perception disorder:** Visual disturbances or flashback hallucinations can occur intermittently for years.

Caffeine

Includes cola drinks, coffee, tea, chocolate, energy drinks

INTENDED EFFECTS: Increased level of alertness and decreased fatigue

EFFECTS OF INTOXICATION: Intoxication commonly occurs with ingestion of greater than 250 mg. (One 2 oz high-energy drink can contain 215 to 240 mg caffeine.) Tachycardia and arrhythmias, flushed face, muscle twitching, restlessness, diuresis, GI disturbances, anxiety, insomnia.

WITHDRAWAL MANIFESTATIONS
- Can occur within 24 hr of last consumption
- Headache, nausea, vomiting, muscle pain, irritability, inability to focus, drowsiness

OTHER

icotine affects nicotinic receptors in the brain, the corotic body, aortic arch, and CNS. Activation of these receptors can simulate the action that occurs with cocaine and other addictive substances.

Tobacco (nicotine)

- Cigarettes and cigars are inhaled.
- Smokeless tobacco is snuffed or chewed.

INTENDED EFFECTS: Relaxation, decreased anxiety

EFFECTS OF INTOXICATION
- Highly toxic, but acute toxicity seen only in children or when exposure is to nicotine in pesticides
- Also contains other harmful chemicals that are highly toxic and have long-term effects
- **Long-term effects**
  - Cardiovascular disease (hypertension, stroke), respiratory disease (emphysema, lung cancer)
  - With smokeless tobacco (snuff or "chew"): irritation to oral mucous membranes and cancer

WITHDRAWAL MANIFESTATIONS: Abstinence syndrome evidenced by irritability, craving, nervousness, restlessness, anxiety, insomnia, increased appetite, difficulty concentrating, anger, and depressed mood

PATIENT-CENTERED CARE

NURSING CARE

- Personal views, culture, and history can affect the nurse's feelings regarding substance use and addictive disorders. Nurse must self-assess their own feelings because those feelings can be transferred to clients through body language and the terminology nurses can use in assessing clients. An objective, nonjudgmental nurse approach is imperative.
- Safety is the primary focus of nursing care during acute intoxication or withdrawal. Qs
  - Maintain a safe environment to prevent falls; implement seizure precautions as necessary.
  - Provide close observation for withdrawal manifestations, possibly one-on-one supervision. Physical restraint should be a last resort.
  - Orient the client to time, place, and person.
  - Maintain adequate nutrition and fluid balance.
  - Create a low-stimulation environment.
  - Administer medications as prescribed to treat the effects of intoxication or to prevent or manage withdrawal. This can include substitution therapy.
  - Monitor for covert substance use during the detoxification period.
- Provide emotional support and reassurance to the client and family. Educate the client and family about codependent behaviors.
- Begin to educate the client and family about addiction and the initial treatment goal of abstinence.
- Educate the client and family regarding removing any prescription medications in the home that are not being used. Encourage the client not to share medication with someone for whom that medication is not prescribed.

- Begin to develop motivation and commitment for abstinence and recovery (abstinence plus developing a program of personal growth and self-discovery).
- Encourage self-responsibility.
- Help the client develop an emergency plan: a list of things the client would need to do and people he would need to contact.
- Encourage attendance at self-help groups.

MEDICATIONS

Alcohol withdrawal: Diazepam, carbamazepine, clonidine, chlordiazepoxide, phenobarbital, naltrexone

Alcohol abstinence: Disulfiram, naltrexone, acamprosate

Opioid withdrawal: Methadone substitution, clonidine, buprenorphine, naltrexone, levo-alpha-acetylmethadol

Nicotine withdrawal from tobacco use: Bupropion, nicotine replacement therapy (nicotine gum and nicotine patch), varenicline, bupropion

Nicotine abstinence: Varenicline, rimonabant

NURSING CONSIDERATIONS
- Monitor vital signs and neurological status.
- Provide for client safety by implementing seizure precautions. Qs

CLIENT EDUCATION
- Encourage the client to adhere to the treatment plan.
- Advise clients taking disulfiram to avoid all alcohol.

INTERPROFESSIONAL CARE

Dual diagnosis, or comorbidity, means that an individual has both a mental health disorder, such as depression, and a substance use or addictive disorder. Both disorders need to be treated simultaneously and require a team approach.

INDIVIDUAL PSYCHOTHERAPIES
- Cognitive behavioral therapies, such as relaxation techniques or cognitive reframing, can be used to decrease anxiety and change behavior.
- Acceptance and commitment therapy (ACT) promotes acceptance of the client's experiences and promotes client commitment to positive behavior changes.
- Relapse prevention therapy assists clients in identifying the potential for relapse and promotes behavioral self-control.

GROUP THERAPY: Groups of clients who have similar diagnoses can meet in an outpatient setting or within mental health residential facilities.

FAMILY THERAPY

- This therapy identifies codependency, which is a common behavior demonstrated by the significant other/family/friends of an individual with substance or process dependency, and assists the family to change that behavior. The codependent person reacts in over-responsible ways that allow the dependent individual to continue the substance use or addiction disorder. For example, a partner can act as an enabler by calling the client's employer with an excuse of illness when the client is intoxicated.
- Families learn about use of specific substances.
- The client and family are educated regarding issues such as family coping, problem-solving, indications of relapse, and availability of support groups. Qpcc

CLIENT EDUCATION

- Teach the client to recognize indications of relapse and factors that contribute to relapse.
- Teach cognitive-behavioral techniques to help maintain sobriety and create feelings of pleasure from activities other than using substances or from process addictions.
- Assist the client to develop communication skills to communicate with coworkers and family members while sober.

- Encourage the client and family to attend a 12-step program, such as Alcoholics Anonymous (AA), Narcotics Anonymous, and Gambler's Anonymous, and family groups like Al-Anon or Ala-Teen. Qebp
  - These programs will teach clients the following.
    - Abstinence is necessary for recovery.
    - A higher power is needed to assist in recovery.
    - Clients are not responsible for their disease but are responsible for their recovery.
    - Other people cannot be blamed for the client's addictions, and they must acknowledge their feelings and problems.

PRACTICE Active Learning Scenario

A nurse is caring for a client who has cocaine use disorder and is experiencing severe effects of intoxication. Use the ATI Active Learning Template: System Disorder to complete this item.

ALTERATION IN HEALTH (DIAGNOSIS)

EXPECTED FINDINGS: Identify three expected findings.

NURSING CARE: Describe two nursing interventions.

INTERPROFESSIONAL CARE: Describe two forms of nonpharmacological therapy.

CLIENT EDUCATION: Identify two client outcomes.

Application Exercises

1. A nurse is planning a staff education program on substance use in older adults. Which of the following is appropriate for the nurse to include in the presentation?

    A. Older adults require higher doses of a substance to achieve a desired effect.

    B. Older adults commonly use rationalization to cope with a substance use disorder.

    C. Older adults are at an increased risk for substance use following retirement.

    D. Older adults develop substance use to mask manifestations of dementia.

2. A nurse is assessing a client who has alcohol use disorder and is experiencing withdrawal. Which of the following findings should the nurse expect? (Select all that apply.)

    A. Bradycardia

    B. Fine tremors of both hands

    C. Hypotension

    D. Vomiting

    E. Restlessness

3. A nurse is planning care for a client who is experiencing benzodiazepine withdrawal. Which of the following interventions should the nurse identify as the priority?

    A. Orient the client frequently to time, place, and person.

    B. Offer fluids and nourishing diet as tolerated.

    C. Implement seizure precautions.

    D. Encourage participation in group therapy sessions.

4. A nurse is caring for a client who has alcohol use disorder. The client is no longer experiencing withdrawal manifestations. Which of the following medications should the nurse anticipate administering to assist the client with maintaining abstinence from alcohol?

    A. Chlordiazepoxide

    B. Bupropion

    C. Disulfiram

    D. Carbamazepine

5. A nurse is providing teaching to the family of a client who has a substance use disorder. Which of the following statements by a family member indicate an understanding of the teaching? (Select all that apply.)

    A. "We need to understand that she is responsible for her disorder."

    B. "Eliminating any codependent behavior will promote her recovery."

    C. "She should participate in an Al-Anon group to help her recover."

    D. "The primary goal of her treatment is abstinence from substance use."

    E. "She needs to discuss her feelings about substance use to help her recover."

Application Exercises Key

1. A. Requiring higher doses of a substance to achieve a desired effect is a result of the length and severity of substance use rather than age.

   B. Denial, rather than rationalization, is a defense mechanism commonly used by substance users of all ages.

   C. **CORRECT:** Retirement and other life change stressors increase the risk for substance use in older adults, especially if there is a prior history of substance use.

   D. Substance use in the older adult can result in manifestations of dementia.

   Ⓝ *NCLEX® Connection: Psychosocial Integrity, Chemical and Other Dependencies/Substance Use Disorder*

2. A. An expected finding of alcohol withdrawal is tachycardia rather than bradycardia.

   B. **CORRECT:** Fine tremors of both hands is an expected finding of alcohol withdrawal.

   C. An expected finding of alcohol withdrawal is hypertension rather than hypotension.

   D. **CORRECT:** Vomiting is an expected finding of alcohol withdrawal.

   E. **CORRECT:** Restlessness is an expected finding of alcohol withdrawal.

   Ⓝ *NCLEX® Connection: Psychosocial Integrity, Chemical and Other Dependencies/Substance Use Disorder*

3. A. Reorienting the client is an appropriate intervention. However, it is not the priority.

   B. Providing hydration and nourishment is an appropriate intervention. However, it is not the priority.

   C. **CORRECT:** The greatest risk to the client is injury. Implementing seizure precautions is the priority intervention.

   D. Encouraging participation in therapy is an appropriate intervention. However, it is not the priority.

   Ⓝ *NCLEX® Connection: Safety and Infection Control, Accident/Error/Injury Prevention*

4. A. Chlordiazepoxide is indicated for acute alcohol withdrawal rather than to maintain abstinence from alcohol.

   B. Bupropion is indicated for nicotine withdrawal rather than to maintain abstinence from alcohol.

   C. **CORRECT:** The nurse should expect to administer disulfiram to help the client maintain abstinence from alcohol.

   D. Carbamazepine is indicated for acute alcohol withdrawal rather than to maintain abstinence from alcohol.

   Ⓝ *NCLEX® Connection: Pharmacological and Parenteral Therapies, Expected Actions/Outcomes*

5. A. Clients are not responsible for their disease but are responsible for their recovery.

   B. **CORRECT:** Families should be aware of codependent behavior, such as enabling, that can promote substance use rather than recovery.

   C. Al-Anon is a recovery group for the family of a client, rather than the client who has a substance use disorder.

   D. **CORRECT:** Abstinence is the primary treatment goal for a client who has a substance use disorder.

   E. **CORRECT:** Clients must acknowledge their feelings about substance use as part of a substance use recovery program.

   Ⓝ *NCLEX® Connection: Psychosocial Integrity, Chemical and Other Dependencies/Substance Use Disorder*

PRACTICE Answer

Using the ATI Active Learning Template: System Disorder

ALTERATION IN HEALTH (DIAGNOSIS):
Cocaine use disorder involves the repeated use of cocaine, leading to clinically significant impairment over a 12-month period.

EXPECTED FINDINGS
- Objective: Seizures, extreme fever, tachycardia, hypertension
- Subjective: Hallucinations, chest pain

NURSING CARE
- Perform a nursing self-assessment.
- Maintain a safe environment.
- Implement seizure precautions.
- Orient the client to time, place, and person.
- Create a low-stimulation environment.
- Monitor the client's vital signs and neurological status.

INTERPROFESSIONAL CARE
- Cognitive behavioral therapies decrease anxiety and promote a change in behavior.
- Acceptance and commitment therapy promotes acceptance of the client and promotes a commitment to change.
- Relapse prevention therapy assists clients in identifying relapse and promotes self-control.
- Group therapy allows clients who have similar diagnoses to work together toward recovery.
- Family therapy allows the client and family members to work together toward recovery.
- Narcotics Anonymous provides a 12-step program to promote recovery and abstinence from future substance use.

CLIENT EDUCATION: Client outcomes
- The client will verbalize coping strategies to use in times of stress.
- The client will remain substance-free.
- The client will remain free from injury.
- The client will attend a 12-step program regularly.

Ⓝ *NCLEX® Connection: Psychosocial Integrity, Chemical and Other Dependencies/Substance Use Disorder*

UNIT 3   PSYCHOBIOLOGIC DISORDERS

CHAPTER 19 *Eating Disorders*

The mortality rate for eating disorders is high, and suicide is also a risk. Treatment modalities focus on normalizing eating patterns and beginning to address the issues raised by the illness. Q̶EBP

Comorbidities include depression, personality disorders, substance use disorder, and anxiety. Various eating disorders are recognized and defined by the DSM-5.

Anorexia nervosa

- Persistent energy intake restriction leading to significantly low body weight in context of age, sex, developmental path, and physical health
- Fear of gaining weight or becoming fat
- Disturbance in self-perceived weight or shape

CHARACTERISTICS
- Clients are preoccupied with food and the rituals of eating, along with a voluntary refusal to eat.
- This condition occurs most often in female clients from adolescence to young adulthood.
- Onset can be associated with a stressful life event (e.g., college).
- Compared to clients who have restricting type, those who have binge-eating/purging type have higher rates of impulsivity and are more likely to abuse drugs and alcohol.

TYPES
- **Restricting type:** The individual drastically restricts food intake and does not binge or purge.
- **Binge-eating/purging type:** The individual engages in binge eating or purging behaviors.

Bulimia nervosa

- Clients recurrently eat large quantities of food over a short period of time (binge eating), which can be followed by inappropriate compensatory behaviors, such as self-induced vomiting (purging), to rid the body of the excess calories.
- Binge eating and inappropriate compensatory behavior both occur on average of once per week for 3 months.
- Binge eating is in a discrete period of time (usually less than 2 hours), and an amount of food definitely larger than what most individuals would eat in a similar period of time. Clients have a sense of lack of control over eating.

CHARACTERISTICS
- Most clients who have bulimia nervosa maintain a weight within a normal range or slightly higher. BMI is 18.5 to 30.
- The average age of onset in female clients is late adolescence or early adulthood.
- Bulimia nervosa occurs most commonly in female clients.
- Between binges, clients typically restrict caloric intake and select low-calorie "diet" foods.

TYPES
- **Purging type:** The client uses self-induced vomiting, laxatives, diuretics, and/or enemas to lose or maintain weight.
- **Nonpurging type:** The client can compensate for binge eating through other means, such as excessive exercise and the misuse of laxatives, diuretics, and/or enemas.

Binge eating disorder

- Clients recurrently eat large quantities of food over a short period of time without the use of compensatory behaviors associated with bulimia nervosa.
- An excessive food consumption must be accompanied by a sense of lack of control
- At least once per week for 3 months
- Binge eating disorder affects men and women of all ages, but is most common in adults age 46 to 55.
- The weight gain associated with binge eating disorder increases the client's risk for other disorders, including type 2 diabetes mellitus, hypertension, and cancer.

ASSESSMENT

RISK FACTORS

- Occupational choices that encourage thinness (fashion modeling)
- Individual history of being a "picky" eater in childhood
- Participation in athletics, especially at an elite level of competition or in a sport where lean body build is prized (bicycling) or where a specific weight is necessary (wrestling)
- A history of obesity

FAMILY GENETICS: more commonly seen in families who have a history of eating disorders

BIOLOGICAL: hypothalamic, neurotransmitter, hormonal, or biochemical imbalance, with disturbances of the serotonin neurotransmitter pathways seeming to be implicated

INTERPERSONAL RELATIONSHIPS: influenced by parental pressure and the need to succeed

PSYCHOLOGICAL INFLUENCES: rigidity, ritualism; separation and individuation conflicts; feelings of ineffectiveness, helplessness, and depression; distorted body image; internal or external locus of control or self-identity; and potential history of physical abuse

ENVIRONMENTAL FACTORS: media influence and pressure from society to have the "perfect body"

TEMPERAMENTAL: anxiety or obsessional traits in childhood

EXPECTED FINDINGS

Nursing history should include the following. Qpcc
- The client's perception of the issue
- Eating habits
- History of dieting
- Methods of weight control (restricting, purging, exercising)
- Value attached to a specific shape and weight
- Interpersonal and social functioning
- Difficulty with impulsivity, as well as compulsivity
- Family and interpersonal relationships (frequently troublesome and chaotic, reflecting a lack of nurturing)

MENTAL STATUS
- Cognitive distortions include the following.
  - **Overgeneralizations:** "Other girls don't like me because I'm fat."
  - **"All-or-nothing" thinking:** "If I eat any dessert, I'll gain 50 pounds."
  - **Catastrophizing:** "My life is over if I gain weight."
  - **Personalization:** "When I walk through the hospital hallway, I know everyone is looking at me."
  - **Emotional reasoning:** "I know I look bad because I feel bloated."
- Client demonstrates high interest in preparing food, but not eating.
- Client is terrified of gaining weight.
- Client perception is that she is severely overweight and sees this image reflected in the mirror.
- Client can exhibit low self-esteem, impulsivity, and difficulty with interpersonal relationships.
- Client can exhibit the need for an intense physical regimen.
- Client can experience guilt or shame due to binge eating behavior.
- Obsessive-compulsive features can be related and unrelated to food (collecting recipes, hoarding food, concerns about eating in public).

VITAL SIGNS
- Low blood pressure with possible orthostatic hypotension
- Decreased pulse and body temperature
- Hypertension can be present in clients who have binge eating disorder.

WEIGHT: Clients who have anorexia nervosa have a body weight that is less than 85% of expected normal weight.
- Most clients who have bulimia nervosa maintain a weight within the normal range or slightly higher.
- Clients who have binge eating disorder are typically overweight or obese.

INTEGUMENTARY: Skin, hair, and nails
- Clients who have anorexia nervosa can have fine, downy hair (lanugo) on the face and back; yellowed skin; mottled, cool extremities; and poor skin turgor.
- Clients who have bulimia can have calluses or scars on hand (Russell's sign).

HEAD, NECK, MOUTH, AND THROAT
- Clients who have bulimia can have enlargement of the parotid glands.
- Dental erosion and caries (if the client is purging)

CARDIOVASCULAR SYSTEM
- Irregular heart rate (dysrhythmias noted on cardiac monitor), heart failure, cardiomyopathy
- Peripheral edema
- Acrocyanosis

MUSCULOSKELETAL SYSTEM
- Muscle weakness
- Decreased energy
- Loss of bone density

GASTROINTESTINAL SYSTEM
- Constipation (dehydration)
- Diarrhea (laxative use)
- Abdominal pain
- Self-induced vomiting
- Excessive use of diuretics or laxatives
- Esophageal tears, gastric rupture (bulimia)

REPRODUCTIVE STATUS
- Amenorrhea can be seen in clients who have anorexia nervosa.
- Menstrual irregularities

PSYCHOSOCIAL
- Client can exhibit low self-esteem, impulsivity, and difficulty with interpersonal relationships
- Depressed mood
- Social withdrawal
- Irritability
- Insomnia

CRITERIA FOR ACUTE CARE TREATMENT

- Rapid weight loss or weight loss of greater than 30% of body weight over 6 months
- Unsuccessful weight gain in outpatient treatment, failure to adhere to treatment contract
- Vital signs demonstrating heart rate less than 40/min, systolic blood pressure less than 70 mm Hg, body temperature less than 36° C (96.8° F)
- ECG changes
- Electrolyte disturbances
- Psychiatric criteria: severe depression, suicidal behavior, family crisis, or psychosis

LABORATORY AND DIAGNOSTIC TESTS

COMMON LABORATORY ABNORMALITIES ASSOCIATED WITH ANOREXIA

- Hypokalemia, especially for those who have bulimia nervosa Qs
  - There is a direct loss of potassium due to purging (vomiting).
  - Dehydration stimulates increased aldosterone production, which leads to sodium and water retention and potassium excretion.
- Anemia and leukopenia with lymphocytosis; thrombocytopenia
- Possible impaired liver function, evidenced by increased enzyme levels
- Hypoalbuminemia
- Possible elevated cholesterol
- Elevated blood urea nitrogen (dehydration)
- Abnormal thyroid function tests
- Elevated carotene levels, which cause skin to appear yellow
- Decreased bone density (possible osteoporosis)
- Abnormal blood glucose level
- ECG changes (prolonged QT interval)
- Possible increase serum bicarbonate (metabolic alkalosis) related to self-induced vomiting
- Possible decrease serum bicarbonate (metabolic acidosis) related to laxative use

COMMON LABORATORY ABNORMALITIES ASSOCIATED WITH BULIMIA

Electrolyte imbalances can depend on the client's method of purging (laxatives, diuretics, vomiting).

- Hypokalemia
- Hyponatremia
- Hypochloremia
- Hypomagnesemia
- Hypophosphatemia
- Decreased estrogen (women)
- Decreased testosterone (men)

STANDARDIZED SCREENING TOOLS QEBP

- Eating Disorder Inventory
- Body Attitude Test
- Diagnostic Survey for Eating Disorders
- Eating Attitudes Test

PATIENT-CENTERED CARE

NURSING CARE

- Perform self-assessment regarding possible feelings of frustration regarding the client's eating behaviors, the belief that the disorder is self-imposed, or the need to nurture rather than care for the client.
- Provide a highly structured milieu in an acute care unit for the client requiring intensive therapy.
- Develop and maintain a trusting nurse/client relationship through consistency and therapeutic communication.
- Use a positive approach and support to promote client self-esteem and positive self-image.
- Encourage client decision making and participation in the plan of care to allow for a sense of control.
- Establish realistic goals for weight loss or gain.
- Promote cognitive-behavioral therapies. QEBP
  - Cognitive reframing
  - Relaxation techniques
  - Journal writing
  - Desensitization exercises
- Monitor the client's vital signs, intake and output, and weight (2 to 3 lb/week is medically acceptable).
- Use behavioral contracts to modify client behaviors.
- Reward the client for positive behaviors, such as completing meals or consuming a set number of calories.
- Closely monitor the client during and after meals to prevent purging, which can necessitate accompanying the client to the bathroom.
- Monitor the client for maintenance of appropriate exercise.
- Teach and encourage self-care activities.
- Incorporate the family when appropriate in client education and discharge planning.
- Work with a dietitian to provide nutrition education to include correcting misinformation regarding food, meal planning, and food selection. Qtc
  - Consider the client's preferences and ability to consume food when developing the initial eating plan.
  - A structured and inflexible eating schedule at the start of therapy, only permitting food during scheduled times, promotes new eating habits and discourages binge or binge-purge behavior.
  - Provide small, frequent meals, which are better tolerated and will help prevent the client from feeling overwhelmed.
  - Provide liquid supplement as prescribed.
  - Provide a diet high in fiber to prevent constipation.
  - Provide a diet low in sodium to prevent fluid retention.
  - Limit high-fat and gassy foods during the start of treatment.
  - Administer a multivitamin and mineral supplement.
  - Instruct the client to avoid caffeine to reduce the risk for increased energy, resulting in difficulty controlling eating disorder behaviors. Caffeine also can be used by clients as a substitute for healthy eating.
- Make arrangements for the client to attend individual, group, and family therapy to assist in resolving personal issues contributing to the eating disorder.

MEDICATIONS

Selective serotonin reuptake inhibitors

Such as fluoxetine

NURSING CONSIDERATIONS
- Instruct the client that medication can take 1 to 3 weeks for initial response, with up to 2 months for maximal response.
- Instruct the client to avoid hazardous activities (driving, operating heavy equipment/machinery) until individual side effects are known.
- Instruct the client to notify the provider if sexual dysfunction occurs and is intolerable.

INTERPROFESSIONAL CARE

- A registered dietitian should be involved to provide the client with nutritional and dietary guidance.
- Consistency of care among all staff is important.

CLIENT EDUCATION

CARE AFTER DISCHARGE
- Assist the client to develop and implement a maintenance plan related to weight management.
- Encourage follow-up treatment in an outpatient setting.
- Encourage client participation in a support group.
- Continue individual and family therapy as indicated.

COMPLICATIONS

Refeeding syndrome

Refeeding syndrome is the potentially fatal complication that can occur when fluids, electrolytes, and carbohydrates are introduced to a severely malnourished client.

NURSING ACTIONS
- Care for the client in a hospital setting.
- Consult with the provider and dietitian to develop a controlled rate of nutritional support during initial treatment. Qtc
- Monitor serum electrolytes, and administer fluid replacement as prescribed.

Cardiac dysrhythmias, severe bradycardia, and hypotension

NURSING ACTIONS
- Place the client on continuous cardiac monitoring.
- Monitor vital signs frequently.
- Report changes in the client's status to the provider.

Application Exercises

1. A nurse is preparing to obtain a nursing history from a client who has a new diagnosis of anorexia nervosa. Which of the following questions should the nurse to include in the assessment? (Select all that apply.)

   A. "What is your relationship like with your family?"

   B. "Why do you want to lose weight?"

   C. "Would you describe your current eating habits?"

   D. "At what weight do you believe you will look better?"

   E. "Can you discuss your feelings about your appearance?"

2. A nurse is caring for an adolescent client who has anorexia nervosa with recent rapid weight loss and a current weight of 90 lb. Which of the following statements indicates the client is experiencing the cognitive distortion of catastrophizing?

   A. "Life isn't worth living if I gain weight."

   B. "Don't pretend like you don't know how fat I am."

   C. "If I could be skinny, I know I'd be popular."

   D. "When I look in the mirror, I see myself as obese."

3. A nurse is performing an admission assessment of a client who has bulimia nervosa with purging behavior. Which of the following is an expected finding? (Select all that apply.)

   A. Amenorrhea

   B. Hypokalemia

   C. Mottling of the skin

   D. Slightly elevated body weight

   E. Presence of lanugo on the face

4. A nurse on an acute care unit is planning care for a client who has anorexia nervosa with binge-eating and purging behavior. Which of the following nursing actions should the nurse include in the client's plan of care?

   A. Allow the client to select preferred meal times.

   B. Establish consequences for purging behavior.

   C. Provide the client with a high-fat diet at the start of treatment.

   D. Implement one-to-one observation during meal times.

5. A nurse is caring for a client who has bulimia nervosa and has stopped purging behavior. The client tells the nurse that she is afraid she is going to gain weight. Which of the following response should the nurse make?

   A. "Many clients are concerned about their weight. However, the dietitian will ensure that you don't get too many calories in your diet."

   B. "Instead of worrying about your weight, try to focus on other problems at this time."

   C. "I understand you have concerns about your weight, but first, let's talk about your recent accomplishments."

   D. "You are not overweight, and the staff will ensure that you do not gain weight while you are in the hospital. We know that is important to you."

PRACTICE Active Learning Scenario

A nurse is caring for a client who has anorexia nervosa of the restricting type. The client refuses to eat and exhibits severe anxiety when food is offered. The nurse plans to use desensitization as a behavioral therapy. Use the ATI Active Learning Template: Therapeutic Procedure to complete this item.

DESCRIPTION OF PROCEDURE

INDICATIONS

OUTCOMES/EVALUATION

NURSING INTERVENTIONS: Identify at least two.

Application Exercises Key

1. A. **CORRECT:** A nursing history of a client who has anorexia nervosa should include an assessment of family and interpersonal relationships.

   B. Asking a "why" question promotes a defensive client response and is therefore nontherapeutic.

   C. **CORRECT:** A nursing history of a client who has anorexia nervosa should include an assessment of the client's current eating habits.

   D. This question promotes cognitive distortion, places the focus on weight, and implies that the client's current appearance is not acceptable.

   E. **CORRECT:** A nursing history of a client who has anorexia nervosa should include an assessment of the client's perception of the issue.

   Ⓝ *NCLEX® Connection: Psychosocial Integrity, Mental Health Concepts*

2. A. **CORRECT:** This statement reflects the cognitive distortion of catastrophizing because the client's perception of her appearance or situation is much worse than her current condition.

   B. This statement reflects the cognitive distortion of personalization rather than catastrophizing.

   C. This statement reflects the cognitive distortion of overgeneralization rather than catastrophizing.

   D. This statement reflects a perception of distorted body image commonly experienced by the client who has anorexia nervosa. However, it is not an example of catastrophizing.

   Ⓝ *NCLEX® Connection: Psychosocial Integrity, Sensory/Perceptual Alterations*

3. A. Amenorrhea is an expected finding of anorexia nervosa rather than bulimia nervosa.

   B. **CORRECT:** Hypokalemia is an expected finding of purging-type bulimia nervosa.

   C. Mottling of the skin is an expected finding of anorexia nervosa rather than bulimia nervosa.

   D. **CORRECT:** Most clients who have bulimia nervosa maintain a weight within a normal range or slightly higher.

   E. Lanugo is an expected finding of anorexia nervosa rather than bulimia nervosa.

   Ⓝ *NCLEX® Connection: Psychosocial Integrity, Mental Health Concepts*

4. A. The nurse should provide a highly structured milieu, including meal times, for the client requiring acute care for the treatment of anorexia nervosa.

   B. The nurse should use a positive approach to client care that includes rewards rather than consequences.

   C. The nurse should limit high-fat and gas-producing foods at the start of treatment.

   D. **CORRECT:** The nurse should closely monitor the client during and after meals to prevent purging.

   Ⓝ *NCLEX® Connection: Psychosocial Integrity, Behavioral Interventions*

5. A. This statement minimizes and generalizes the client's concern and is therefore a nontherapeutic response.

   B. This statement minimizes the client's concern and is therefore a nontherapeutic response.

   C. **CORRECT:** This statement acknowledges the client's concern and then focuses the conversation on the client's accomplishments, which can promote client self-esteem and self-image.

   D. This statement minimizes the client's concern and is therefore a nontherapeutic response.

   Ⓝ *NCLEX® Connection: Psychosocial Integrity, Mental Health Concepts*

PRACTICE Answer

Using the ATI Active Learning Template: Therapeutic Procedure

DESCRIPTION OF PROCEDURE:
Systematic desensitization is the planned, progressive, or graduated exposure to anxiety-provoking stimuli. During exposure, the anxiety response is suppressed through the use of relaxation techniques.

INDICATIONS: Systematic desensitization is appropriate for clients who have anorexia nervosa and anxiety related to food and eating.

OUTCOMES/EVALUATION: The client will effectively use relaxation techniques to suppress the anxiety response during meal times.

NURSING INTERVENTIONS
- Teach the client relaxation techniques.
- Gradually expose the client to food starting with small amounts of a food.
- Stay with the client during meals to assist with relaxation.
- Reward the client for food intake.
- Use a positive approach to communicate the procedure and expectations to the client.

Ⓝ *NCLEX® Connection: Psychosocial Integrity, Behavioral Interventions*

UNIT 3   PSYCHOBIOLOGIC DISORDERS

CHAPTER 20 *Somatic Symptom and Related Disorders*

Clients who have somatic symptom and related disorders are often encountered in primary care settings. It is important that nurses are familiar with these disorders, as well as their role when caring for these clients. Somatic symptom and related disorders include somatic symptom disorder, illness anxiety disorder, conversion disorder, psychological factors affecting other medical conditions, and factitious disorder.

Somatic symptom disorder

Somatization is the expression of psychological stress through physical manifestations. The physical manifestations of somatic symptom disorder cannot be explained by underlying pathology.

- Somatic symptoms cause distress for clients and often lead to long-term use of health care services. Manifestations can be vague or exaggerated. The course of the disease can be acute, but is often chronic, with periods of remission and exacerbation.
- Clients who have somatic symptom disorder spend a significant amount of time worrying about their physical manifestations to the point where it assumes a central role in the client's life and relationships. Clients often reject a psychological diagnosis as the cause for their physical manifestations. They seek care from several providers, increasing medical costs.
- Clients are usually seen initially in a primary or medical care setting rather than a mental health setting.

ASSESSMENT

RISK FACTORS

- First-degree relative who has somatic symptom disorder
- Decreased levels of neurotransmitters: serotonin and endorphins
- Depressive disorder, personality disorder, or anxiety disorder
- Childhood trauma, abuse, or neglect
- Learned helplessness
- Female gender (especially age 16 to 25)

EXPECTED FINDINGS

- Somatic symptoms that disrupt the client's daily life
- Excessive preoccupation with somatic symptoms
- Increased level of anxiety about somatic symptoms
- Somatic symptoms are usually present (though actual manifestations can vary) for longer than 6 months
- Remissions and exacerbations of somatic symptoms
- Probable alcohol or other substance use
- Client overmedication with analgesics and antianxiety medications

LABORATORY AND DIAGNOSTIC TESTS

Laboratory and diagnostic tests, such as CT scans and MRIs, can be performed to rule out underlying pathology.

ASSESSMENT TOOLS

Patient Health Questionnaire 15 (PHQ-15): Used to identify the presence of the 15 most commonly reported somatic symptoms: Q_{EBP}
- Abdominal pain
- Back pain
- Pain in the extremities/joints
- Menstrual problems or cramps
- Headaches
- Chest pain
- Dizziness
- Fainting
- Heart pounding or racing
- Dyspnea
- Problems or pain with sexual intercourse
- Problems with bowel elimination (constipation/diarrhea)
- Nausea, indigestion, or gas
- Lethargy
- Problems sleeping

PATIENT-CENTERED CARE

NURSING CARE

- Accept somatic symptoms as being real to the client.
- Assess for suicidal ideation and thoughts of self-harm.
- Identify the cultural impact on the client's view of health and illness.
- Identify secondary gains from somatic symptoms (attention, distraction from personal obligations or problems).
- Report new physical manifestations to the provider.
- Limit the amount of time allowed to discuss somatic symptoms.
- Encourage independence in self-care.
- Encourage verbalization of feelings.
- Educate the client on alternative coping mechanisms.
- Educate the client on assertiveness techniques.
- Encourage daily physical exercise.

Reattribution treatment

Work with the provider to provide reattribution treatment, which assists clients to identify the link between physical manifestations and psychological factors while promoting a sense of caring and understanding.

FOUR STAGES OF REATTRIBUTION TREATMENT ♡ᴛᴄ

- **Stage 1: Feeling understood:** Use therapeutic communication, active listening, and empathy to obtain a thorough history of manifestations while focusing on the client's perception of the manifestations and their cause. This stage also includes a brief physical assessment.
- **Stage 2: Broadening the agenda:** Provide acknowledgment of the client's concerns and provide feedback about assessment findings.
- **Stage 3: Making the link:** Use therapeutic communication to acknowledge the lack of a physical cause for the manifestations while allowing the client to maintain self-esteem.
- **Stage 4: Negotiating further treatment:** Work with the provider and client to develop a treatment plan that allows for regular follow-up visits.

MEDICATIONS

Administer medications as prescribed.
- Analgesics
- Antidepressants
- Anxiolytics

CLIENT EDUCATION

- Encourage client participation in individual and group therapy.
- Educate clients on prescribed medications.
- Assist a case manager to develop a follow-up appointment schedule with provider every 4 to 6 weeks. This strategy provides the client with set appointments and decreases the client's need for unscheduled health care, as well as medical costs associated with laboratory and diagnostic tests if the client seeks treatment from other providers. ♡ᴇʙᴘ

Illness anxiety disorder

Misinterprets physical manifestations as evidence of a serious disease process. Illness anxiety disorder, previously known as hypochondriasis, can lead to obsessive thoughts and fears about illness.

- Clients who have illness anxiety disorder are overly aware of bodily sensations and attribute them to a serious illness. Physical manifestations can be minimal or absent. However, clients still have a preoccupation about having an undiagnosed, serious illness.
- Clients research their suspected disease excessively and examine themselves repeatedly (e.g., examining throat in the mirror)
- Clients might either seek numerous medical opinions or avoid seeking health care so as not to increase their anxiety.
- Clients continue to have anxiety despite negative diagnostic tests and reassurance from the provider.

ASSESSMENT

RISK FACTORS

- First-degree relative who has illness anxiety disorder
- Previous losses or disappointments resulting in feelings of anger, guilt, or hostility
- Childhood trauma, abuse, or neglect
- Depressive disorder or anxiety disorder
- Major life stressor
- Low self-esteem

EXPECTED FINDINGS

- Excessive anxiety that a serious illness is present or will be acquired. This anxiety is present for more than 6 months though the actual illness the client fears can change.
- Preoccupation with performance of behaviors that are health-related, such as performing a daily breast self-exam due to fear of breast cancer
- Some clients have illness anxiety disorder that is the **health-seeking type** (frequently seeking medical care and diagnostic tests) while others exhibit the **care-avoidant type** (avoids all contact with providers due to the correlation with increased levels of anxiety).

LABORATORY AND DIAGNOSTIC TESTS

Laboratory and diagnostic tests, such as CT scans and MRIs, can be performed to rule out underlying pathology.

PATIENT-CENTERED CARE

NURSING CARE

- Build rapport and trust with client.
- Encourage independence in self-care.
- Encourage verbalization of feelings.
- Educate clients on alternative coping mechanisms.
- Educate clients on stress management techniques.

MEDICATIONS

Administer medications as prescribed.
- Antidepressants
- Anxiolytics

CLIENT EDUCATION

- Encourage client participation in individual and group therapy.
- Refer clients to community support groups.
- Educate clients on prescribed medications.
- Collaborate with the provider for the client to receive brief, frequent office visits.

Conversion disorder

Also known as functional neurological disorder, conversion disorder results when a client exhibits neurologic manifestations in the absence of a neurologic diagnosis. Clients who have conversion disorder transmit emotional or psychological stressors into physical manifestations.

- Neurologic manifestations can cause extreme anxiety and distress in some clients while others can exhibit a lack of emotional concern (la belle indifference).
- The neurologic manifestation causes a significant impairment in multiple aspects of the client's life.
- Clients who have conversion disorder have deficits in voluntary motor or sensory functions.

ASSESSMENT

RISK FACTORS

- First-degree relative who has conversion disorder
- Childhood physical or sexual abuse
- Comorbid psychiatric conditions
  - Depressive disorder
  - Anxiety disorder
  - Posttraumatic stress disorder
  - Personality disorder
  - Other somatic disorder
- Comorbid medical or neurological condition
- Recent acute stressful event
- Female gender
- Adolescent or young adult

EXPECTED FINDINGS

- Manifestations of an alteration in voluntary motor or sensory function
  - Motor: Paralysis, movement/gait disorders, seizure-like movements
  - Sensory: Blindness, inability to speak (aphonia), inability to smell (anosmia), numbness, deafness, tingling/burning sensations
- Clients who have an extreme desire to become pregnant can manifest a false pregnancy (pseudocyesis).

LABORATORY AND DIAGNOSTIC TESTS

Laboratory and diagnostic tests, such as CT scans and MRIs, can be performed to rule out underlying pathology.

PATIENT-CENTERED CARE

NURSING CARE

- Build rapport and trust with clients.
- Ensure safety of clients.
- Encourage verbalization of feelings. Assist the client to identify the psychological trigger of the manifestation. For example, a client's sudden blindness can be a conversion manifestation in response to seeing her partner being intimate with another woman.
- Educate client on alternative coping mechanisms.
- Educate client on stress management techniques.
- Understand the incidence of remissions and recurrence. Remission occurs without intervention in approximately 95% of clients, especially if the onset of manifestations is due to an acute stressful event.
  - Recurrence rate is approximately 25%, usually within 1 year of initial diagnosis.

MEDICATIONS

Administer medications as prescribed.
- Antidepressants
- Anxiolytics

CLIENT EDUCATION

- Encourage client participation in individual and group therapy.
- Refer clients to community support groups.
- Educate clients on prescribed medications.

Psychological factors affecting other medical conditions

Psychological and behavioral factors can play a role in any medical condition. The mind-body connection has been the subject of research, proving a link between a client's psychological state and their physical condition.

- The development of certain medical conditions, such as heart disease and cancer, has been linked to clients who have depressive and anxiety disorders.
- Psychological factors affecting other medical conditions indicate that the client has a medical diagnosis that is caused or perpetuated by a psychological or behavioral factor.

ASSESSMENT

RISK FACTORS

- Chronic stressors
- Depressive disorder or anxiety disorder
- Malfunction of neurotransmitters

EXPECTED FINDINGS

- A confirmed medical diagnosis
- A psychological or behavioral factor that is linked to the medical diagnosis in one of the following ways
  - Contributes to the development, exacerbation, or delayed recovery of the medical diagnosis
  - Interferes with the client's adherence to the treatment of the medical diagnosis
  - Places the client at increased risk for physical health problems
  - Causes or exacerbates physical manifestations or the client's need for medical treatment

PATIENT-CENTERED CARE

NURSING CARE

- Discuss the client's physical exam findings.
- Assess for suicidal ideation, thoughts of self-harm. Qs
- Explore the client's feelings and fears.
- Allow the client time to express feelings.
- Educate the client on alternative coping mechanisms.
- Educate the client on assertiveness techniques.
- Address both physical and psychological needs.
- Administer prescribed medications.

CLIENT EDUCATION

- Encourage client participation in treatment plan.
- Provide care that meets both the physical and psychological needs of the client.
- Educate the client on prescribed medications.

Factitious disorder

- Factitious disorder (previously known as Munchausen syndrome) is the conscious decision by the client to report physical or psychological manifestations. The falsification of manifestations is done in the absence of personal gain by the client other than possible fulfillment of an emotional need for attention. In some cases, clients inflict self-injury.
- **Factitious disorder imposed on another** (previously known as Munchausen syndrome by proxy) is present when the client deliberately causes injury or illness to a vulnerable person. The emotional need for attention or relief of responsibility remains a possible motivating factor.

- Clients often have an average or above-average IQ. The client is dramatic in the description of the illness, uses proper medical terminology, and is often hesitant for the provider to speak to family members or prior providers.
- The client often reports new manifestations following negative test results.
- Factitious disorder differs from **malingering**. Factitious disorder is a mental illness, while malingering is not. Malingering is consciously motivated and driven by personal gain (disability benefits, evading military service, etc.).

ASSESSMENT

RISK FACTORS

- History of emotional or physical distress, child abuse, or frequent/chronic childhood illnesses requiring hospitalizations
- Impaired neurological ability for information processing
- Dependent personality
- Borderline personality disorder

EXPECTED FINDINGS

- Report of false physical and psychological manifestations
- Possible evidence of self-injury (factitious disorder) or injury to others (factitious disorder imposed on another)

LABORATORY AND DIAGNOSTIC TESTS

Laboratory and diagnostic tests, such as CT scans and MRIs, can be performed to rule out underlying pathology.

PATIENT-CENTERED CARE

NURSING CARE

- Perform a self-assessment prior to care.
- Avoid confrontation.
- Build rapport and trust with client.
- Ensure safety of client and vulnerable persons affected by the client.
- Encourage verbalization of feelings.
- Educate client on alternative coping mechanisms.
- Educate client on stress management techniques.
- Communicate openly with the health care team any suspicions of factitious disorder or factitious disorder imposed on another. This action can help reduce medical costs and possible unnecessary treatments/surgical procedures. Qtc

CLIENT EDUCATION

- Encourage client participation in individual and group therapy.
- Refer client to community support groups.
- Educate client on prescribed medications.

Application Exercises

1. A nurse is discussing the risk factors for somatic symptom disorder with a newly licensed nurse. Which of the following risk factors should the nurse include? (Select all that apply.)

   A. Age older than 65 years

   B. Anxiety disorder

   C. Female gender

   D. Coronary artery disease

   E. Obesity

2. A nurse is reviewing the medical record of a client who has conversion disorder. Which of the following findings should the nurse identify as placing the client at risk for conversion disorder?

   A. Death of a child 2 months ago

   B. Recent weight loss of 30 lb

   C. Retirement 1 year ago

   D. History of migraine headaches

3. A nurse is assessing a client who has illness anxiety disorder. Which of the following findings should the nurse expect? (Select all that apply.)

   A. Obsessive thoughts about disease

   B. History of childhood abuse

   C. Avoidance of health care providers

   D. Depressive disorder

   E. Narcissistic personality

4. A nurse is developing a plan of care for a client who has conversion disorder. Which of the following actions should the nurse include?

   A. Encourage the client to spend time alone in his room.

   B. Monitor the client for self-harm once per day.

   C. Allow the client unlimited time to discuss physical manifestations.

   D. Discuss alternative coping strategies with the client.

5. A nurse is counseling a client who has factitious disorder imposed on another. Which of the following client statements should the nurse expect?

   A. "I had to pretend I was injured in order to get disability benefits."

   B. "I know that my abdominal pain is caused by a malignant tumor."

   C. "I needed to make my son sick so that someone else would take care of him for a while."

   D. "I became deaf when I heard that my husband was having an affair with my best friend."

PRACTICE Active Learning Scenario

A nurse is caring for a client who has psychological factors affecting other medical conditions. Use the ATI Active Learning Template: System Disorder to complete the following.

EXPECTED FINDINGS: Define psychological factors affecting other medical conditions.

RISK FACTORS: Identify the risk factors of psychological factors affecting other medical conditions.

NURSING CARE: Identify at least three nursing interventions for this client.

1. A. Age 16 to 25 years is a risk factor for somatic symptom disorder.

    B. **CORRECT:** Anxiety disorder is a risk factor for somatic symptom disorder.

    C. **CORRECT:** Female gender is a risk factor for somatic symptom disorder.

    D. Coronary artery disease is not a risk factor for somatic symptom disorder.

    E. Obesity is not a risk factor for somatic symptom disorder.

    Ⓝ *NCLEX® Connection: Health Promotion and Maintenance, Health Promotion/Disease Prevention*

2. A. **CORRECT:** The death of a child 2 months ago is an acute stressor that places the client at risk for conversion disorder.

    B. A recent weight loss of 30 lb does not place the client at risk for conversion disorder.

    C. Retiring 1 year ago does not place the client at risk for conversion disorder.

    D. A history of migraine headaches does not place the client at risk for conversion disorder.

    Ⓝ *NCLEX® Connection: Health Promotion and Maintenance, Health Promotion/Disease Prevention*

3. A. **CORRECT:** Obsessive thoughts about disease is an expected finding in a client who has illness anxiety disorder.

    B. **CORRECT:** A history of childhood abuse is an expected finding in a client who has illness anxiety disorder.

    C. **CORRECT:** Avoidance of health care providers is an expected finding in clients who have illness anxiety disorder of the care-avoidant type.

    D. **CORRECT:** A depressive disorder is an expected finding in a client who has illness anxiety disorder.

    E. Low self-esteem is an expected finding in a client who has illness anxiety disorder.

    Ⓝ *NCLEX® Connection: Psychosocial Integrity, Mental Health Concepts*

4. A. The nurse should encourage the client to communicate with others and participate in group therapy and support groups.

    B. The nurse should continuously monitor the client for risk of self-harm.

    C. The nurse should establish a time limit for discussion of physical manifestations.

    D. **CORRECT:** The nurse should discuss alternative coping strategies with the client.

    Ⓝ *NCLEX® Connection: Psychosocial Integrity, Mental Health Concepts*

5. A. INCORRECT: A client's falsification of an illness or injury for the purpose of personal gain is malingering, rather than factitious disorder.

    B. INCORRECT: Although clients who have factitious disorder often use proper medical terminology, a client's fear of a serious illness is expected with illness anxiety disorder rather than factitious disorder imposed on another.

    C. **CORRECT:** A client who has factitious disorder imposed on another often consciously injures another person or causes them to be sick due to a personal need for attention or relief of responsibility.

    D. Developing a sensory impairment due to an acute stressor is an expected finding of conversion disorder, rather than factitious disorder imposed on another.

    Ⓝ *NCLEX® Connection: Psychosocial Integrity, Mental Health Concepts*

PRACTICE Answer

Using the ATI Active Learning Template: System Disorder

EXPECTED FINDINGS

- Can play a role in any medical condition.
- Psychological factors affecting other medical conditions indicates that the client has a medical diagnosis that is caused or perpetuated by a psychological or behavioral factor.
- The mind-body connection has been the subject of research, proving a link between a client's psychological state and physical condition.
- The development of certain medical conditions, such as heart disease and cancer, has been linked to clients who have depressive disorders and anxiety disorders.
- Psychological stress can exacerbate manifestations of the physical illness, or make the illness more severe and difficult to treat. This, in turn, can increase psychological stress, leading to a cycle of illness.

Ⓝ *NCLEX® Connection: Psychosocial Integrity, Mental Health Concepts*

RISK FACTORS

- Include chronic stressors, depressive disorder or anxiety disorder, and imbalance of neurotransmitters.
- Clients experience both psychological and physical illness.

NURSING CARE

- Discuss physical exam findings with client.
- Assess for suicidal ideation and thoughts of self-harm.
- Explore the client's feelings and fears.
- Allow the client time to express feelings.
- Educate the client on alternative coping mechanisms.
- Educate the client on assertiveness techniques.
- Address both physical and psychological needs.
- Administer prescribed medications.

When reviewing the following chapters, keep in mind the relevant topics and tasks of the NCLEX outline, in particular:

Client Needs: Pharmacological and Parenteral Therapies

ADVERSE EFFECTS/CONTRAINDICATIONS/ SIDE EFFECTS/INTERACTIONS
Monitor for anticipated interactions among the client prescribed medications and fluids.

Provide information to the client on common side effects/ adverse effects/potential interactions of medications and inform the client when to notify the primary health care provider.

EXPECTED ACTIONS/OUTCOMES: Use clinical decision making/critical thinking when addressing expected effects/outcomes of medications.

MEDICATION ADMINISTRATION
Educate the client about medications.

Review pertinent data prior to medication administration.

Client Needs: Reduction of Risk Potential

CHANGES/ABNORMALITIES IN VITAL SIGNS: Assess and respond to changes in client vital signs.

LABORATORY VALUES
Monitor client laboratory values.

Notify primary health care provider about laboratory test results.

UNIT 4   PSYCHOPHARMACOLOGICAL THERAPIES

CHAPTER 21
Medications for Anxiety and Trauma- and Stressor-Related Disorders

MAJOR MEDICATIONS TO TREAT ANXIETY DISORDERS

BENZODIAZEPINE SEDATIVE HYPNOTIC ANXIOLYTICS:
Lorazepam, alprazolam, clonazepam, diazepam

ATYPICAL ANXIOLYTIC/NONBARBITURATE ANXIOLYTICS:
Buspirone

SELECTED ANTIDEPRESSANTS
- **Selective serotonin reuptake inhibitors (SSRIs):** Paroxetine, sertraline, fluoxetine, citalopram, escitalopram, fluvoxamine
- **Serotonin norepinephrine reuptake inhibitors (SNRIs):** Venlafaxine, duloxetine, desvenlafaxine

OTHER CLASSIFICATIONS THAT MAY BE USED
- **Other antidepressants**
  ○ Tricyclic antidepressants (TCAs): Amitriptyline, imipramine, clomipramine
  ○ Monoamine oxidase inhibitors (MAOIs): Phenelzine
  ○ Antihistamines: Hydroxyzine pamoate, hydroxyzine hydrochloride
  ○ Mirtazapine
  ○ Trazodone
- **Beta blockers:** Propranolol
- **Centrally acting alpha-blockers:** Prazosin
- **Anticonvulsants:** Gabapentin

MAJOR MEDICATIONS TO TREAT TRAUMA- AND STRESSOR-RELATED DISORDERS

ANTIDEPRESSANTS
- **Selective serotonin reuptake inhibitors:** Paroxetine, sertraline, fluoxetine
- **Serotonin norepinephrine reuptake inhibitor:** Venlafaxine
- **Tricyclic antidepressants:** Amitriptyline, imipramine
- **Monoamine oxidase inhibitor:** Phenelzine

BETA BLOCKERS: Propranolol

CENTRALLY ACTING ALPHA-BLOCKERS: Prazosin

Benzodiazepine sedative hypnotic anxiolytics

SELECT PROTOTYPE MEDICATION: **Alprazolam**

OTHER MEDICATIONS
- Diazepam
- Lorazepam
- Chlordiazepoxide
- Clorazepate
- Oxazepam
- Clonazepam

PURPOSE

EXPECTED PHARMACOLOGICAL ACTION

Benzodiazepines enhance the inhibitory effects of gamma-aminobutyric acid in the central nervous system. Relief from anxiety occurs rapidly following administration.

THERAPEUTIC USES

First-line treatment for generalized anxiety disorder and panic disorder

OTHER USES
- Seizure disorders
- Insomnia
- Muscle spasm
- Alcohol withdrawal (for prevention and treatment of acute manifestations)
- Induction of anesthesia
- Amnesic prior to surgery or procedures

COMPLICATIONS Qs

Central nervous system (CNS) depression

Such as sedation, lightheadedness, ataxia, and decreased cognitive function

CLIENT EDUCATION
- Advise the client to observe for manifestations. Instruct the client to notify the provider if effects occur.
- Advise the client to avoid hazardous activities (driving, operating heavy equipment/machinery).
- Advise clients to avoid concurrent use of alcohol and other CNS depressants.

Anterograde amnesia

Difficulty recalling events that occur after dosing

CLIENT EDUCATION: Advise the client to observe for manifestations. Instruct the client to notify the provider and withhold the medication if effects occur.

Acute toxicity

Oral toxicity: drowsiness, lethargy, confusion

IV toxicity: respiratory depression, severe hypotension, cardiac arrest
- Benzodiazepines for IV use include diazepam and lorazepam.

NURSING CONSIDERATIONS
- Advise the client and family to watch for manifestations of overdose. Notify the provider if these occur.
- For oral toxicity, gastric lavage is used, followed by the administration of activated charcoal or saline cathartics.
- Flumazenil is administered to counteract sedation and reverse the adverse effects.
- Monitor vital signs, maintain patent airway, and provide fluids to maintain blood pressure.
- Ensure availability of resuscitation equipment.

Paradoxical response

Insomnia, excitation, euphoria, anxiety, rage

CLIENT EDUCATION: Advise the client to observe for indications. Instruct the client to notify the provider if paradoxical response occurs.

Withdrawal effects

- Anxiety, insomnia, diaphoresis, tremors, and lightheadedness, delirium and seizures
- Occurs infrequently with short-term use

NURSING CONSIDERATIONS: After taking benzodiazepines regularly and in high doses, the client should taper the dose over several weeks using a prescribed tapered dosing schedule.

CONTRAINDICATIONS/PRECAUTIONS

- Benzodiazepines are Pregnancy Risk Category D medications and should be avoided in women who are pregnant or breastfeeding.
- Benzodiazepines are classified under Schedule IV of the Controlled Substances Act.
- Benzodiazepines are contraindicated in clients who have sleep apnea, respiratory depression, and/or glaucoma. Qs
- Use benzodiazepines cautiously in clients who have liver disease or a history of a substance use disorder.
- Benzodiazepines are generally used short-term due to the risk for dependence.

INTERACTIONS

CNS depressants, such as alcohol, barbiturates, and opioids can cause respiratory depression.
NURSING CONSIDERATIONS
- Advise the client to avoid alcohol and other substances that cause CNS depression.
- Advise the client to avoid hazardous activities (driving, operating heavy equipment/machinery).

NURSING ADMINISTRATION

- Advise the client to take the medication as prescribed, and to avoid abrupt discontinuation of treatment to prevent withdrawal manifestations. Do not change the dosage or frequency without approval of the prescriber.
- When discontinuing benzodiazepines that have been taken regularly for long periods and in higher doses, taper the dose over several weeks using a prescribed dosing schedule.
- Administer the medication with meals or snacks if GI upset occurs.
- Advise the client to swallow sustained-release tablets and to avoid chewing or crushing the tablets.
- Instruct the client about the potential for dependency during and after treatment and to notify the provider if indications of withdrawal occur. Qs
- Advise clients to keep benzodiazepines in a secure place due to abuse potential.

Atypical anxiolytic/ nonbarbiturate anxiolytics

SELECT PROTOTYPE MEDICATION: Buspirone

PURPOSE

EXPECTED PHARMACOLOGICAL ACTION

- The exact antianxiety mechanism is unknown. This medication binds to serotonin and dopamine receptors. There is less potential for dependency than with other anxiolytics. Use of buspirone does not result in sedation or potentiate the effects of other CNS depressants. It carries no risk of abuse.
- Antianxiety effects develop slowly. Initial responses take 1 week, and at least 2 to 6 weeks for it to reach its full effects. As a result of this pharmacological action, buspirone needs to be taken on a scheduled basis, and is not suitable for PRN usage.

THERAPEUTIC USES

- Panic disorder
- Obsessive-compulsive and related disorders
- Social anxiety disorder
- Generalized anxiety disorder

COMPLICATIONS

CNS effects

Dizziness, nausea, headache, lightheadedness, agitation

NURSING CONSIDERATIONS: This medication does not interfere with activities because it does not cause sedation.

CONTRAINDICATIONS/PRECAUTIONS

- Buspirone is a Pregnancy Risk Category B medication.
- Buspirone is not recommended for use by women who are breastfeeding. Qs
- Use buspirone cautiously in older adult clients, as well as clients who have liver or renal dysfunction.
- Buspirone is contraindicated for concurrent use with MAOI antidepressants, or for 14 days after MAOIs are discontinued. Hypertensive crisis can result.

INTERACTIONS

Erythromycin, ketoconazole, St. John's wort, and grapefruit juice can increase the effects of buspirone.
NURSING CONSIDERATIONS
- Advise the client to avoid the use of erythromycin and ketoconazole.
- Advise clients to avoid herbal preparations containing St. John's wort.
- Advise the client to avoid drinking grapefruit juice.

NURSING ADMINISTRATION

- Advise the client to take the medication with meals to prevent gastric irritation.
- Medication should be administered at the same time every day.
- Advise the client that effects do not occur immediately. It can take 1 week to notice first therapeutic effects, and 2 to 6 weeks to reach full therapeutic benefit. Medication should be taken on a regular basis, rather than an as-needed basis.
- Instruct clients that tolerance, dependence, or withdrawal manifestations are not an issue with this medication.

Selective serotonin reuptake inhibitors

SELECT PROTOTYPE MEDICATION: Paroxetine

OTHER MEDICATIONS
- Sertraline
- Citalopram
- Escitalopram
- Fluoxetine
- Fluvoxamine

PURPOSE

EXPECTED PHARMACOLOGICAL ACTION

- SSRIs selectively inhibit serotonin reuptake, allowing more serotonin to stay at the junction of the neurons.
- SSRIs do not block uptake of dopamine or norepinephrine.
- Paroxetine causes CNS stimulation, which can cause insomnia.
- As SSRIs have a long effective half-life, up to 4 weeks are necessary to produce therapeutic medication levels.

THERAPEUTIC USES QEBP

SSRI antidepressants are the first-line treatment for panic disorders and trauma- and stressor-related disorders.

Paroxetine
- Generalized anxiety disorder (GAD)
- Panic disorder: decreases both the frequency and intensity of panic attacks, and also prevents anticipatory anxiety about attacks
- Obsessive compulsive disorder (OCD): reduces manifestations by increasing serotonin
- Social anxiety disorder
- Trauma- and stressor-related disorders
- Depressive disorders
- Adjustment disorders
- Associated manifestations of dissociative disorders

Sertraline is indicated for panic disorder, OCD, social anxiety disorder, and PTSD.

Escitalopram is indicated for GAD and OCD.

Fluoxetine is used for panic disorder, OCD, and PTSD.

Fluvoxamine is used for OCD and social anxiety disorder.

COMPLICATIONS

Early adverse effects

First few days/weeks: nausea, diaphoresis, tremor, fatigue, drowsiness

CLIENT EDUCATION
- Instruct the client to report adverse effects to the provider.
- Instruct the client to take the medication as prescribed.
- Advise the client that these effects should soon subside
- Instruct client to avoid driving if these effects occur.

Later adverse effects

After 5 to 6 weeks of therapy: sexual dysfunction (e.g., impotence, delayed or absent orgasm, delayed or absent ejaculation, decreased sexual interest), weight gain, headache

CLIENT EDUCATION: Instruct the client to report problems with sexual function (managed with dose reduction, medication holiday, changing medications).

Weight changes

Occurrence of weight loss early in therapy that can be followed by weight gain with long-term treatment

NURSING CONSIDERATIONS
- Monitor the client's weight.
- Advise the client to follow a well-balanced diet and exercise regularly.

Gastrointestinal bleeding

NURSING CONSIDERATIONS
- Use cautiously in clients who have a history of gastrointestinal bleed, ulcers, and those taking other medications that affect blood coagulation.
- Advise clients to report indications of bleeding (dark stools, emesis that has the appearance of coffee grounds).

Hyponatremia

More likely in older adult clients taking diuretics

NURSING CONSIDERATIONS: Obtain baseline serum sodium, and monitor level periodically throughout treatment.

Serotonin syndrome

Can begin 2 to 72 hr after starting treatment and can be lethal.

MANIFESTATIONS
- Confusion, agitation, poor concentration, hostility
- Disorientation, hallucinations, delirium
- Seizures leading to status epilepticus
- Tachycardia leading to cardiovascular shock
- Labile blood pressure
- Diaphoresis
- Fever leading to hyperpyrexia
- Incoordination, hyperreflexia
- Nausea, vomiting, diarrhea, abdominal pain
- Coma leading to apnea (and death in severe cases)

CLIENT EDUCATION: Advise the client to observe for manifestations. If any occur, instruct the client to withhold the medication and notify the provider.

Bruxism

Grinding and clenching of teeth, usually during sleep

NURSING CONSIDERATIONS
Report bruxism to the provider, who may:
- Switch the client to another class of medication.
- Treat bruxism with low-dose buspirone.
- Advise the client to use a mouth guard during sleep.

Withdrawal syndrome

Nausea, sensory disturbances, anxiety, tremor, malaise, unease

CLIENT EDUCATION
- Advise the client that, after a long period of use, to taper the medication slowly according to a prescribed tapered dosing schedule to avoid withdrawal effects.
- Advise the client to avoid abrupt discontinuation of the medication.

CONTRAINDICATIONS/PRECAUTIONS Qs

- Paroxetine is a Pregnancy Risk Category D medication. Other SSRIs pose less risk during pregnancy.
- SSRIs are contraindicated in clients taking MAOIs or TCAs.
- Clients should avoid alcohol while taking SSRIs.
- Use cautiously in clients who have liver and renal dysfunction, seizure disorders, or a history of gastrointestinal bleeding.
- Use SSRIs cautiously in clients who have bipolar disorder, due to the risk for mania. Qs

INTERACTIONS

Concurrent use of MAOIs, TCAs, and St. John's wort can cause serotonin syndrome.
NURSING CONSIDERATIONS
- Discontinue MAOIs 14 days prior to starting an SSRI. Fluoxetine should be discontinued 5 weeks before starting an MAOI.
- Advise the client against concurrent use of TCAs and St. John's wort with SSRIs.

Concurrent use with warfarin can displace warfarin from bound protein and result in increased warfarin levels.
NURSING CONSIDERATIONS
- Monitor prothrombin time (PT)) and INR levels.
- Assess for indications of bleeding and the need for dosage adjustment.

Concurrent use with TCAs and lithium can result in increased levels of these medications.
NURSING CONSIDERATIONS: Advise the client to avoid concurrent use.

Concurrent use with NSAIDs and anticoagulants can further suppress platelet aggregation, thereby increasing the risk of bleeding.
NURSING CONSIDERATIONS: Advise the client to monitor for indications of bleeding (bruising, hematuria) and to notify the provider if they occur.

NURSING ADMINISTRATION

- Advise the client that SSRIs may be taken with food. Sleep disturbances are minimized by taking the medication in the morning. Q EBP
- Instruct the client to take the medication on a daily basis to establish therapeutic plasma levels.
- Assist the client with medication regimen adherence by informing the client that it can take up to 4 weeks to achieve therapeutic effects.

Serotonin norepinephrine reuptake inhibitors

SELECT PROTOTYPE MEDICATION: Venlafaxine

OTHER MEDICATIONS
- Duloxetine
- Desvenlafaxine

PURPOSE

EXPECTED PHARMACOLOGICAL ACTION: Inhibit the uptake of serotonin and norepinephrine; minimal inhibition of dopamine

THERAPEUTIC USES: Used for major depression, panic disorders, and generalized anxiety disorder

COMPLICATIONS

Headache, nausea, agitation, anxiety, dry mouth, and sleep disturbances

NURSING CONSIDERATIONS: Instruct the client to report adverse effects to the provider.

Hyponatremia, especially in older adult clients taking diuretics

NURSING CONSIDERATIONS: Obtain baseline serum sodium, and monitor level periodically throughout treatment

Anorexia resulting in weight loss

NURSING CONSIDERATIONS
- Monitor the client's weight.
- Advise the client to follow a well-balanced diet and exercise regularly.

Hypertension

NURSING CONSIDERATIONS: Monitor for increases in blood pressure.

Sexual dysfunction

NURSING CONSIDERATIONS: Instruct the client to report problems with sexual function (managed with dose reduction, medication holiday, changing medications).

CONTRAINDICATIONS/PRECAUTIONS

- SNRIs are Pregnancy Risk Category C.
- SNRIs are contraindicated in clients taking MAOIs.
- Advise the client to avoid abrupt cessation of the medication.
- Clients should avoid alcohol while taking SNRIs.
- Duloxetine should not be used in clients who have hepatic disease or in those who consume large amounts of alcohol.

INTERACTIONS

Concurrent use of MAOIs and St. John's wort can cause serotonin syndrome.
NURSING CONSIDERATIONS
- Discontinue MAOIs 14 days prior to starting an SNRI.
- Advise the client against concurrent use of St. John's wort along with SNRIs.

CNS depression with alcohol, opioids, antihistamines, sedative/hypnotics
NURSING CONSIDERATIONS: Avoid concurrent use.

Concurrent use with NSAIDs and anticoagulants can further suppress platelet aggregation, thereby increasing the risk of bleeding.
NURSING CONSIDERATIONS: Advise the client to monitor for indications of bleeding (bruising, hematuria) and to notify the provider if they occur.

NURSING ADMINISTRATION

- Advise the client to avoid abrupt cessation of the medication. Q EBP
- Duloxetine should not be used in clients who have hepatic disease or in those who consume large amounts of alcohol.
- Advise the client that SNRIs may be taken with food.
- Instruct the client to take the medication on a daily basis to establish therapeutic plasma levels.
- Assist the client with medication regimen adherence by informing the client that it can take up to 4 weeks to achieve therapeutic effects.

For all medication classifications in this chapter

NURSING EVALUATION OF MEDICATION EFFECTIVENESS

Depending on therapeutic intent, effectiveness is evidenced by the following.
- Verbalized feeling of less anxiety
- Description of improved mood
- Improved memory retrieval
- Maintenance of a normal sleep pattern
- Greater ability to participate in social and occupational interactions
- Improved ability to cope with manifestations and identified stressors
- Ability to perform activities of daily living
- Report of increased well-being

Application Exercises

1. A nurse working in a mental health clinic is providing teaching to a client who has a new prescription for diazepam for generalized anxiety disorder. Which of the following information should the nurse provide?

   A. Three to six weeks of treatment is required to achieve therapeutic benefit.

   B. Combining alcohol with diazepam will produce a paradoxical response.

   C. Diazepam has a lower risk for dependence than other antianxiety medications.

   D. Report confusion as a potential indication of toxicity.

2. A nurse working in an emergency department is caring for a client who has benzodiazepine toxicity due to an overdose. Which of the following actions is the nurse's priority?

   A. Administer flumazenil.

   B. Identify the client's level of orientation.

   C. Infuse IV fluids.

   D. Prepare the client for gastric lavage.

3. A nurse is caring for a client who is to begin taking fluoxetine for treatment of generalized anxiety disorder. Which of the following statements indicates the client understands the use of this medication?

   A. "I will take the medication at bedtime."

   B. "I will follow a low-sodium diet while taking this medication."

   C. "I will need to discontinue this medication slowly."

   D. "I will be at risk for weight loss with long-term use of this medication."

4. A nurse is assessing a client 4 hr after receiving an initial dose of fluoxetine Which of the following findings should the nurse report to the provider as indications of serotonin syndrome? (Select all that apply.)

   A. Hypothermia

   B. Hallucinations

   C. Muscular flaccidity

   D. Diaphoresis

   E. Agitation

5. A nurse is caring for a client who takes paroxetine to treat posttraumatic stress disorder. The client states that he grinds his teeth during the night, which causes pain in his mouth. The nurse should identify which of the following interventions as possible measures to manage the client's bruxism? (Select all that apply.)

   A. Concurrent administration of buspirone

   B. Administration of a different SSRI

   C. Use of a mouth guard

   D. Changing to a different class of antianxiety medication

   E. Increasing the dose of paroxetine

PRACTICE Active Learning Scenario

A nurse is providing teaching for a client who has a new prescription for buspirone. Use the ATI Active Learning Template: Medication to complete this item.

THERAPEUTIC USES: Identify at least three therapeutic uses for this medication.

COMPLICATIONS: List at least three adverse effects of this medication.

INTERACTIONS: Identify two medication interactions and one food interaction.

CLIENT EDUCATION: Describe two things to teach the client to reduce the risk of medication/food interactions.

Application Exercises Key

1. A. Buspirone, rather than diazepam, requires 3 to 6 weeks to achieve therapeutic benefit.

   B. Combining alcohol with diazepam can produce CNS and respiratory depression rather than a paradoxical response.

   C. Diazepam is preferably used for short-term treatment because of the increased risk of dependence.

   D. **CORRECT:** Confusion is a potential indication of diazepam toxicity that the client should report to the provider.

   Ⓝ *NCLEX® Connection: Pharmacological and Parenteral Therapies, Medication Administration*

2. A. Administering flumazenil is an appropriate action. However it is not the priority when taking the nursing process approach to client care.

   B. **CORRECT:** When taking the nursing process approach to client care, the initial step is assessment. Identifying the client's level of orientation is the priority action.

   C. Infusing IV fluids is an appropriate action. However, it is not the priority when taking the nursing process approach to client care.

   D. Gastric lavage is an appropriate action. However, it is not the priority when taking the nursing process approach to client care.

   Ⓝ *NCLEX® Connection: Pharmacological and Parenteral Therapies, Dosage Calculation*

3. A. The client should take fluoxetine in the morning to minimize sleep disturbances.

   B. The client is at risk for hyponatremia while taking fluoxetine.

   C. **CORRECT:** When discontinuing fluoxetine, the client should taper the medication slowly according to a prescribed tapered dosing schedule to reduce the risk of withdrawal syndrome.

   D. The client is at risk for weight gain, rather than loss, with long-term use of fluoxetine.

   Ⓝ *NCLEX® Connection: Pharmacological and Parenteral Therapies, Expected Actions/Outcomes*

4. A. Fever, rather than hypothermia, is an indication of serotonin syndrome.

   B. **CORRECT:** Hallucinations are an indication of serotonin syndrome.

   C. Muscle tremors, rather than flaccidity, are an indication of serotonin syndrome.

   D. **CORRECT:** Diaphoresis is an indication of serotonin syndrome.

   E. **CORRECT:** Agitation is an indication of serotonin syndrome.

   Ⓝ *NCLEX® Connection: Pharmacological and Parenteral Therapies, Adverse Effects/Contraindications/Side Effects/Interactions*

5. A. **CORRECT:** Concurrent administration of a low-dose of buspirone is an effective measure to manage the adverse effect of paroxetine.

   B. Other SSRIs will also have bruxism as an adverse effect therefore this is not an effective measure.

   C. **CORRECT:** Using a mouth guard during sleep can decrease the risk for oral damage resulting from bruxism.

   D. **CORRECT:** Changing to a different class of antianxiety medication that does not have the adverse effect of bruxism is an effective measure.

   E. Increasing the dose of paroxetine can cause the adverse effect of bruxism to worsen therefore this is not an effective measure.

   Ⓝ *NCLEX® Connection: Pharmacological and Parenteral Therapies, Expected Actions/Outcomes*

PRACTICE Answer

Using the ATI Active Learning Template: Medication

THERAPEUTIC USES	COMPLICATIONS	INTERACTIONS	CLIENT EDUCATION
• Panic disorder	• Dizziness	Medication Interactions	• Buspirone is contraindicated for concurrent use with MAOI antidepressants, or for 14 days after MAOIs are discontinued due to the risk for hypertensive crisis.
• Obsessive-compulsive and related disorders	• Nausea	• MAOI antidepressants	
• Social anxiety disorder	• Headache	• Erythromycin	• Avoid the use of erythromycin or ketoconazole, which can increase the effects of buspirone.
• Trauma- and stressor-related disorders	• Lightheadedness	• Ketoconazole	
	• Agitation	Food Interaction: Grapefruit juice	• Avoid drinking grapefruit juice, which can increase the effects of buspirone.

Ⓝ *NCLEX® Connection: Pharmacological and Parenteral Therapies, Medication Administration*

CHAPTER 22 # Medications for Depressive Disorders

Depressive disorders affect many clients and are a leading cause of disability. Advise clients starting antidepressant medication therapy for a depressive disorder that relief is not immediate, and it can take several weeks or longer to reach full therapeutic benefits. Encourage continued compliance. Clients who have major depression can require hospitalization with the implementation of close observation and suicide precautions until antidepressant medications reach their peak effect.

Antidepressant medications are classified into four main groups: tricyclic antidepressants (TCAs), selective serotonin reuptake inhibitors (SSRIs), monoamine oxidase inhibitors (MAOIs), atypical antidepressants. A combination of antidepressant medications can be required to alleviate all symptoms. QEBP

Tricyclic antidepressants

SELECT PROTOTYPE MEDICATION: Amitriptyline

OTHER MEDICATIONS
- Imipramine
- Doxepin
- Nortriptyline
- Amoxapine
- Trimipramine

PURPOSE

EXPECTED PHARMACOLOGICAL ACTION

These medications block reuptake of norepinephrine and serotonin in the synaptic space, thereby intensifying the effects of these neurotransmitters.

THERAPEUTIC USES

Depressive disorders

OTHER USES
- Neuropathic pain
- Fibromyalgia
- Anxiety disorders
- Insomnia
- Bipolar disorder

COMPLICATIONS

Orthostatic hypotension

NURSING CONSIDERATIONS: Monitor blood pressure and heart rate for orthostatic changes. If a significant decrease in blood pressure or increase in heart rate is noted, do not administer the medication. Notify the provider. Qs

CLIENT EDUCATION
- Instruct the client about the indications of postural hypotension (lightheadedness, dizziness). If these occur, advise the client to sit or lie down. Orthostatic hypotension is minimized by getting up or changing positions slowly.
- Advise the client to avoid dehydration, which increases the risk for hypotension.

Anticholinergic effects

- Dry mouth
- Blurred vision
- Photophobia
- Urinary hesitancy or retention
- Constipation
- Tachycardia

CLIENT EDUCATION
- Instruct the client on ways to minimize anticholinergic effects.
  - Chewing sugarless gum
  - Sipping on water
  - Wearing sunglasses when outdoors
  - Eating foods high in fiber
  - Exercising regularly to promote peristalsis
  - Increasing fluid intake to at least 2 L/day from beverage and food sources
  - Voiding just before taking the medication
- Advise the client to notify the provider if adverse effects persist.

Sedation

NURSING CONSIDERATIONS: This adverse effect usually diminishes over time.

CLIENT EDUCATION
- Advise the client to avoid hazardous activities, such as driving, if sedation is excessive.
- Advise the client to take medication at bedtime to minimize daytime sleepiness and to promote sleep. Taking the medication at bedtime minimizes experiencing side effects during the day.

Toxicity

Results in cholinergic blockade and cardiac toxicity evidenced by dysrhythmias, mental confusion, and agitation, which are followed by seizures, coma, and possible death

NURSING CONSIDERATIONS
- Give no more than a 1-week supply of medication to clients who are acutely ill due to the high risk of lethality with overdose.
- Obtain baseline ECG.
- Monitor vital signs frequently.
- Monitor for signs of toxicity.
- Notify the provider if signs of toxicity occur.

Decreased seizure threshold

NURSING CONSIDERATIONS: Monitor clients who have seizure disorders.

Excessive sweating

NURSING CONSIDERATIONS: Inform clients of this adverse effect. Assist clients with frequent linen changes.

Increased appetite

CLIENT EDUCATION
- Instruct client to weigh weekly.
- Encourage good nutrition and exercise to decrease risk of weight gain.

CONTRAINDICATIONS/PRECAUTIONS

- Amitriptyline is a Pregnancy Risk Category C medication.
- This medication is contraindicated for clients who have seizure disorders.
- Use this medication cautiously in clients who have coronary artery disease; diabetes; liver, kidney, and respiratory disorders; urinary retention and obstruction; angle closure glaucoma; benign prostatic hypertrophy; and hyperthyroidism.
- TCAs can increase suicide risk. Qs

INTERACTIONS

Concurrent use with MAOIs can cause severe hypertension.
NURSING CONSIDERATIONS: Avoid concurrent use of TCAs and MAOIs.

Concurrent use with antihistamines and other anticholinergic agents can result in additive anticholinergic effects.
NURSING CONSIDERATIONS: Avoid concurrent use of TCAs and antihistamines.

Concurrent use with direct-acting sympathomimetics can result in increased effects of these medications, because uptake is blocked by TCAs.
NURSING CONSIDERATIONS: Avoid concurrent use of TCAs with these medications.

Concurrent use with indirect-acting sympathomimetics can result in decreased effect of these medications, due to the inhibition of their uptake and inability to get to the site of action in the nerve terminal.
NURSING CONSIDERATIONS: Avoid concurrent use of TCAs with these medications.

Concurrent use with alcohol, benzodiazepines, opioids, and antihistamines can result in additive CNS depression.
NURSING CONSIDERATIONS: Advise the client to avoid other CNS depressants.

Selective serotonin reuptake inhibitors

SELECT PROTOTYPE MEDICATION: Fluoxetine

OTHER MEDICATIONS
- Citalopram
- Escitalopram
- Paroxetine
- Sertraline
- Vilazodone

PURPOSE

EXPECTED PHARMACOLOGICAL ACTION

- SSRIs selectively block reuptake of the monoamine neurotransmitter serotonin in the synaptic space, thereby intensifying the effects of serotonin. Qebp
- First line treatment for depression.

THERAPEUTIC USES

- Major depression
- Obsessive compulsive disorder
- Bulimia nervosa
- Premenstrual dysphoric disorders
- Panic disorders
- Posttraumatic stress disorder (PTSD)
- Bipolar disorder

COMPLICATIONS

Sexual dysfunction

Anorgasmia, impotence, decreased libido

CLIENT EDUCATION
- Warn the client of possible adverse effects, and to notify the provider if they become intolerable. Qs
- Instruct the client on ways to manage sexual dysfunction, which can include lowering the dosage, discontinuing the medication temporarily (medication holiday), and using adjunct medications to improve sexual function.
- Inform the client that the provider can prescribe an atypical antidepressant with fewer sexual dysfunction adverse effects, such as bupropion.

CNS stimulation: insomnia, agitation, anxiety

CLIENT EDUCATION
- Advise the client to notify the provider for a possible dosage reduction.
- Advise the client to take this medication in the morning.
- Advise the client to avoid caffeinated beverages.
- Teach the client relaxation techniques to promote sleep.

Weight changes

Occurrence of weight loss early in therapy that can be followed by weight gain with long-term treatment

NURSING CONSIDERATIONS: Monitor the client's weight.

CLIENT EDUCATION: Encourage the client to participate in regular exercise and to follow a healthy, well-balanced diet.

Serotonin syndrome

Can begin 2 to 72 hr after the start of treatment, and it can be lethal.

MANIFESTATIONS
- Mental confusion, difficulty concentrating
- Abdominal pain
- Diarrhea
- Agitation
- Fever
- Anxiety
- Hallucinations
- Hyperreflexia, incoordination
- Diaphoresis
- Tremors

CLIENT EDUCATION: Advise the client to observe for manifestations. If any occur, instruct the client to withhold the medication and notify the provider. Qs

Withdrawal syndrome

Headache, nausea, visual disturbances, anxiety, dizziness, and tremors

CLIENT EDUCATION: Instruct the client to taper the dose gradually when discontinuing the medication using a prescribed tapered dosing schedule.

Hyponatremia

More likely to occur in older adult clients taking diuretics

NURSING CONSIDERATIONS: Obtain baseline serum sodium, and monitor the level periodically throughout treatment.

Rash

CLIENT EDUCATION: Advise the client that a rash is treatable with an antihistamine or discontinuation of the medication.

Sleepiness, faintness, lightheadedness

CLIENT EDUCATION
- Advise the client that these adverse effects are not common, but can occur.
- The client should avoid driving if these effects occur.

Gastrointestinal bleeding

NURSING CONSIDERATIONS: Use cautiously in clients who have a history of gastrointestinal bleeding and ulcers, and in those taking other medications that affect blood coagulation.

Bruxism

CLIENT EDUCATION
- Advise the client to report this to the provider.
- Advise the client to use a mouth guard, and that changing to a different classification of antidepressants, or adding a low dose of buspirone, can decrease this adverse effect.

CONTRAINDICATIONS/PRECAUTIONS

- Fluoxetine is a Pregnancy Risk Category C medication.
- Fluoxetine and paroxetine can increase the risk of birth defects. Other SSRIs are recommended. Late in pregnancy, use of SSRIs can increase the risk of withdrawal effects or pulmonary hypertension in the newborn. Qs
- These medications are contraindicated in clients taking MAOIs or TCAs.
- Use cautiously in clients who have liver and/or renal dysfunction, cardiac disease, seizure disorders, diabetes, ulcers, and a history of gastrointestinal bleeding. Qs

INTERACTIONS

Concurrent use with MAOIs, TCAs, or St. John's wort increases the risk of serotonin syndrome.
NURSING CONSIDERATIONS
- Discontinue MAOIs 14 days prior to starting an SSRI. Fluoxetine should be discontinued 5 weeks before starting an MAOI.
- Advise the client against concurrent use of TCAs and St. John's wort along with SSRIs.

Concurrent use with warfarin can displace warfarin from bound protein and result in increased warfarin levels.
NURSING CONSIDERATIONS
- Monitor prothrombin time (PT) and INR levels.
- Assess for indications of bleeding and the need for dosage adjustment.

Concurrent use with tricyclic antidepressants and lithium can result in increased levels of these medications.
NURSING CONSIDERATIONS: Advise the client to avoid concurrent use.

Concurrent use with NSAIDs and anticoagulants can further suppress platelet aggregation, thereby increasing the risk of bleeding.
NURSING CONSIDERATIONS: Advise the client to monitor for indications of bleeding (bruising, hematuria) and to notify the provider if they occur.

Monoamine oxidase inhibitors

SELECT PROTOTYPE MEDICATION: Phenelzine

OTHER MEDICATIONS
- Isocarboxazid
- Tranylcypromine
- Selegiline: transdermal patch

PURPOSE

EXPECTED PHARMACOLOGICAL ACTION

These medications block MAO in the brain, thereby increasing the amount of norepinephrine, dopamine, and serotonin available for transmission of impulses. An increased amount of those neurotransmitters at nerve endings intensifies responses and relieves depression. Q EBP

THERAPEUTIC USES

- Depression
- Bulimia nervosa
- First-line treatment for atypical depression.

COMPLICATIONS

CNS stimulation

Anxiety, agitation, hypomania, mania

CLIENT EDUCATION: Advise the client to observe for effects and to notify the provider if they occur.

Orthostatic hypotension

NURSING CONSIDERATIONS
- Monitor blood pressure and heart rate for orthostatic changes.
- Hold the medication, and notify the provider regarding significant changes.

CLIENT EDUCATION: Advise the client to change positions slowly. Qs

Hypertensive crisis

Resulting from intake of dietary tyramine: severe hypertension as a result of intensive vasoconstriction and stimulation of the heart.

MANIFESTATIONS
- Headache
- Nausea and vomiting
- Increased heart rate
- Increased blood pressure
- Diaphoresis
- Change in level of consciousness

NURSING CONSIDERATIONS
- Administer phentolamine IV, a rapid-acting alpha-adrenergic blocker, or nifedipine.
- Provide continuous cardiac monitoring and respiratory support as indicated.

CLIENT EDUCATION: Educate client on foods to avoid.

Local rash associated with transdermal preparation

NURSING CONSIDERATIONS
- Choose a clean, dry area for each application.
- Apply a topical glucocorticoid on the affected areas if rash occurs.

CONTRAINDICATIONS/PRECAUTIONS

- Phenelzine is a Pregnancy Risk Category C medication.
- MAOIs are contraindicated in clients taking SSRIs.
- MAOIs are contraindicated in clients who have pheochromocytoma, heart failure, cardiovascular and cerebral vascular disease, or severe renal insufficiency. Qs
- Use cautiously in clients who have diabetes or seizure disorders, or those taking TCAs.
- Transdermal selegiline is contraindicated for clients taking carbamazepine or oxcarbazepine. Concurrent use of these medications can increase blood levels of the MAOI.

INTERACTIONS

Concurrent use with indirect-acting sympathomimetic medications (ephedrine, amphetamine) can promote the release of norepinephrine and lead to hypertensive crisis.
CLIENT EDUCATION: Instruct the client that over-the-counter (OTC) decongestants and cold remedies frequently contain medications with sympathomimetic action and therefore should be avoided.

Concurrent use with TCAs can lead to hypertensive crisis.
NURSING CONSIDERATIONS: Avoid concurrent use of MAOIs and TCAs.

Concurrent use with SSRIs can lead to serotonin syndrome.
NURSING CONSIDERATIONS: Avoid concurrent use.

Concurrent use with antihypertensives can cause additive hypotensive effects.
NURSING CONSIDERATIONS
- Monitor blood pressure.
- Notify the provider if there is a significant drop in the client's blood pressure, as the dosage of antihypertensive can need to be reduced.

Concurrent use with meperidine can lead to hyperpyrexia.
NURSING CONSIDERATIONS: Alternative analgesic should be used.

Hypertensive crisis (severe hypertension as a result of intensive vasoconstriction and stimulation of the heart) can result from intake of dietary tyramine.

- MANIFESTATIONS
  - Headache
  - Nausea
  - Increase heart rate
  - Increased blood pressure
- NURSING CONSIDERATIONS: Assess the client for ability to follow strict adherence to dietary restrictions.
- CLIENT EDUCATION
  - Inform the client of indications and to notify the provider if they occur.
  - Provide the client with written instructions regarding foods and beverages to avoid. Tyramine-rich foods include aged cheese, pepperoni, salami, avocados, figs, bananas, smoked fish, protein, some dietary supplements, some beers, and red wine.
  - Advise the client to avoid taking any medications (prescription or OTC) without approval from the provider.

Concurrent use with vasopressors (caffeine, phenylethylamine) can result in hypertension.
CLIENT EDUCATION: Advise the client to avoid foods that contain these agents (caffeinated beverages, chocolate, fava beans, ginseng).

Atypical antidepressants

SELECT PROTOTYPE MEDICATION: Bupropion

PURPOSE

EXPECTED PHARMACOLOGICAL ACTION

This medication acts by inhibiting dopamine uptake. Q**EBP**

THERAPEUTIC USES

- Treatment of depression
- Alternative to SSRIs for clients unable to tolerate the sexual dysfunction side effects
- Aid to quit smoking
- Prevention of seasonal pattern depression

COMPLICATIONS

Headache, dry mouth, GI distress, constipation, increased heart rate, nausea, restlessness, insomnia

NURSING CONSIDERATIONS: Treat headaches with a mild analgesic.

CLIENT EDUCATION
- Advise the client to observe for effects and to notify the provider if they become intolerable.
- Advise the client to sip water to treat dry mouth, and to increase dietary fiber to prevent constipation.

Suppression of appetite resulting in weight loss

NURSING CONSIDERATIONS: Monitor the client's food intake and weight.

Seizures, especially at higher dose ranges

NURSING CONSIDERATIONS
- Avoid administering to clients at risk for seizures, such as a client who has a head injury. Q**s**
- Monitor for seizures, and treat accordingly.

CONTRAINDICATIONS/PRECAUTIONS

- Bupropion is a Pregnancy Risk Category B medication.
- This medication is contraindicated in clients who have a seizure disorder. Q**s**
- This medication is contraindicated in clients taking MAOIs.
- Bupropion is contraindicated in clients who have anorexia nervosa or bulimia nervosa.

INTERACTIONS

Concurrent use with MAOIs, such as phenelzine, can increase the risk for toxicity.
NURSING CONSIDERATIONS: MAOIs should be discontinued 2 weeks prior to beginning treatment with bupropion.

There is an increased risk of seizures with concurrent use of SSRIs.
NURSING CONSIDERATIONS: Do not use medications together.

Other atypical antidepressants

Venlafaxine, duloxetine, desvenlafaxine, levomilnacipran

PHARMACOLOGICAL ACTION: These agents, known as serotonin norepinephrine reuptake inhibitors (SNRIs), increase the amount of these neurotransmitters available in the brain for impulse transmission. SNRIs have little effect on other neurotransmitters and receptors.

NURSING CONSIDERATIONS
- Adverse effects include headache, nausea, agitation, anxiety, dry mouth, and sleep disturbances.
- Monitor for hyponatremia, especially in older adult clients.
- Monitor for weight loss.
- Monitor for increases in blood pressure.
- Discuss ways to manage interference with sexual functioning.
- Advise the client to avoid abrupt cessation of the medication.
- Duloxetine should not be used in clients who have hepatic disease or who consume large amounts of alcohol.

Mirtazapine

PHARMACOLOGICAL ACTION: This agent increases the release of serotonin and norepinephrine, thereby increasing the amount of these neurotransmitters available for impulse transmission.

NURSING CONSIDERATIONS

- Therapeutic effects can occur sooner, and with less sexual dysfunction, than with SSRIs.
- This medication is generally well tolerated. Adverse effects include sleepiness that can be exacerbated by other CNS depressants, increased appetite and weight gain, and elevated cholesterol.

Trazodone

PHARMACOLOGICAL ACTION: This agent has moderate selective blockade of serotonin receptors, thereby increasing the amount of that neurotransmitter available for impulse transmission.

NURSING CONSIDERATIONS

- This agent is usually used with another antidepressant agent. Sedation can be an issue, so it can be indicated for a client who has insomnia caused by an SSRI. Advise the client to take at bedtime.
- Priapism can be a serious adverse effect. Instruct to seek medical attention immediately if this occurs.
- This medication should be used with caution in clients who have cardiac disease.

NURSING ADMINISTRATION

- Instruct the client to take antidepressant medication as prescribed on a daily basis to establish therapeutic plasma levels. Qᴘᴄᴄ
- Assist with medication regimen compliance by informing the client that therapeutic effects might not be experienced for 1 to 3 weeks. Full therapeutic effects can take 2 to 3 months.
- Instruct the client to continue therapy after improvement in manifestations. Sudden discontinuation of the medication can result in relapse or major withdrawal effects.
- Advise the client that therapy usually continues for 6 months after resolution of manifestations, and it can continue for 1 year or longer.

> **!** Suicide prevention is facilitated by prescribing only 1 week of medication for an acutely ill client, and following that, only prescribing 1 month of medication at a time, especially with TCAs, which have a high risk for lethality with overdose. Assess clients for suicide risk. Antidepressant medications can increase the client's risk for suicide particularly during initial treatment. Antidepressant-induced suicide is mainly associated with clients under the age of 25. Qs

FOR TCAS

- Monitor for cardiac dysrhythmias, which are an indication of toxicity.
- Administer at bedtime due to sedation and risk for orthostatic hypotension.

FOR SSRIS

- Advise clients to take these medications in the morning to minimize sleep disturbances.
- Advise clients to take these medications with food to minimize gastrointestinal disturbances.
- Obtain baseline sodium levels for older adult clients taking diuretics. Monitor these clients periodically. ⓒ

FOR MAOIS

- Provide clients with a list of foods containing tyramine to reduce the risk of hypertensive crisis.
- Instruct the client to avoid taking any other prescription or nonprescription medications unless approved by the provider.

FOR ATYPICAL ANTIDEPRESSANTS

- Advise clients who have seasonal pattern depression to begin taking bupropion in autumn each year and gradually taper dose and discontinue by spring.
- Avoid concurrent use with MAOIs.

NURSING EVALUATION OF MEDICATION EFFECTIVENESS

Effectiveness of antidepressant medication can be evidenced by the following.

- Verbalizing improvement in mood
- Ability to perform ADLs
- Improved sleeping and eating habits
- Increased interaction with peers

Application Exercises

1. A nurse is providing teaching to a client who has a new prescription for amitriptyline. Which of the following statements by the client indicates an understanding of the teaching?

    A. "While taking this medication, I'll need to stay out of the sun to avoid a skin rash."

    B. "I may feel drowsy for a few weeks after starting this medication."

    C. "I cannot eat my favorite pizza with pepperoni while taking this medication."

    D. "This medication will help me lose the weight that I have gained over the last year."

2. A nurse is caring for a client who is taking phenelzine For which of the following adverse effects should the nurse monitor? (Select all that apply.)

    A. Elevated blood glucose level

    B. Orthostatic hypotension

    C. Priapism

    D. Headache

    E. Bruxism

3. A nurse is reviewing the medical record of a client who has a new prescription for bupropion for depression. Which of the following findings is the priority for the nurse to report to the provider?

    A. The client has a family history of seasonal pattern depression.

    B. The client currently smokes 1.5 packs of cigarettes per day.

    C. The client had a motor vehicle crash last year and sustained a head injury.

    D. The client has a BMI of 25 and has gained 10 lb over the last year.

4. A nurse is teaching a client who has a new prescription for imipramine how to minimize anticholinergic effects. Which of the following instructions should the nurse include in the teaching? (Select all that apply.)

    A. Void just before taking the medication.

    B. Increase the dietary intake of potassium.

    C. Wear sunglasses when outside.

    D. Change positions slowly when getting up.

    E. Chew sugarless gum.

5. A charge nurse is discussing mirtazapine with a newly licensed nurse. Which of the following statements by the newly licensed nurse indicates understanding?

    A. "This medication increases the release of serotonin and norepinephrine."

    B. "I will need to monitor the client for hyponatremia while taking this medication."

    C. "This medication is contraindicated for clients who have an eating disorder."

    D. "Sexual dysfunction is a common adverse effect of this medication."

PRACTICE Active Learning Scenario

A nurse is providing teaching for a client who has a new prescription for sertraline for the treatment of depression. Use the ATI Active Learning Template: Medication to complete this item.

COMPLICATIONS: Identify at least four adverse effects of sertraline.

INTERACTIONS: Identify at least two interactions.

NURSING INTERVENTIONS: Identify two nursing administration interventions.

Application Exercises Key

1. A. Skin rash is associated with SSRIs rather than TCAs like amitriptyline.

   B. **CORRECT:** Sedation is an adverse effect of amitriptyline during the first few weeks of therapy.

   C. Foods such as pepperoni should be avoided if the client is prescribed an MAOI rather than a TCA like amitriptyline.

   D. Weight gain, rather than weight loss, is expected with TCAs.

   Ⓝ *NCLEX® Connection: Pharmacological and Parenteral Therapies, Medication Administration*

2. A. An elevated blood glucose level is not an adverse effect of phenelzine.

   B. **CORRECT:** The nurse should observe for orthostatic hypotension, which is an adverse effect of phenelzine.

   C. Priapism is an adverse effect of trazodone rather than phenelzine.

   D. **CORRECT:** The nurse should observe for a headache which is an adverse effect of phenelzine.

   E. Bruxism is an adverse effect of SSRIs rather than phenelzine.

   Ⓝ *NCLEX® Connection: Pharmacological and Parenteral Therapies, Adverse Effects/Contraindications/Side Effects/Interactions*

3. A. The nurse should report family history information. However, this does not address the greatest risk to the client and is not the priority.

   B. The nurse should report the client's current smoking status. However, this does not address the greatest risk to the client and is not the priority.

   C. **CORRECT:** The greatest risk to the client is development of seizures. Bupropion can lower the seizure threshold and should be avoided by clients who have a history of a head injury. This information is the highest priority to report to the provider.

   D. The nurse should report the client's BMI and change in weight. However, this does not address the greatest risk to the client and is not the priority.

   Ⓝ *NCLEX® Connection: Pharmacological and Parenteral Therapies, Adverse Effects/Contraindications/Side Effects/Interactions*

4. A. **CORRECT:** Voiding just before taking the medication will help minimize the anticholinergic effects of urinary hesitancy or retention.

   B. The anticholinergic effects of imipramine do not affect the client's potassium level.

   C. **CORRECT:** Wearing sunglasses when outside will help minimize the anticholinergic effect of photophobia.

   D. The client should change positions slowly to avoid orthostatic hypotension. However, this is not an anticholinergic effect.

   E. **CORRECT:** Chewing sugarless gum will help minimize the anticholinergic effect of dry mouth.

   Ⓝ *NCLEX® Connection: Pharmacological and Parenteral Therapies, Adverse Effects/Contraindications/Side Effects/Interactions*

5. A. **CORRECT:** Mirtazapine provides relief from depression by increasing the release of serotonin and norepinephrine.

   B. Hyponatremia is an adverse effect of venlafaxine, rather than mirtazapine.

   C. Bupropion, rather than mirtazapine, is contraindicated in clients who have an eating disorder.

   D. Sexual dysfunction is an adverse effect of SSRIs rather than mirtazapine.

   Ⓝ *NCLEX® Connection: Pharmacological and Parenteral Therapies, Adverse Effects/Contraindications/Side Effects/Interactions*

PRACTICE Answer

Using the ATI Active Learning Template: Medication

COMPLICATIONS

- Sexual dysfunction
- CNS stimulation
- Weight changes
- Serotonin syndrome
- Hyponatremia
- Rash
- Gastrointestinal bleeding
- Bruxism

INTERACTIONS

- MAOIs
- TCAs
- St. John's wort
- Warfarin
- NSAIDs

NURSING INTERVENTIONS

- Administer SSRIs in the morning to minimize sleep disturbances.
- Administer SSRIs with food to minimize gastrointestinal disturbances.
- Instruct the client to take this medication on a daily basis.
- Inform the client that therapeutic effects can take several weeks.

Ⓝ *NCLEX® Connection: Pharmacological and Parenteral Therapies, Medication Administration*

CHAPTER 23 *Medications for Bipolar Disorders*

Bipolar disorder is primarily managed with mood-stabilizing medications, such as lithium carbonate. Bipolar disorder also can be treated with certain antiepileptic medications.

ANTIEPILEPTIC MEDICATIONS FOR BIPOLAR DISORDER Q̣EBP

- Valproic acid
- Carbamazepine
- Lamotrigine
- Oxcarbazepine
- Topiramate

OTHER MEDICATIONS USED FOR BIPOLAR DISORDER

Antipsychotics: These can be useful in early treatment to promote sleep and to decrease anxiety and agitation. These medications also demonstrate mood-stabilizing properties.

Anxiolytics: Clonazepam and lorazepam can be useful in treating acute mania and managing the psychomotor agitation often seen in mania.

Antidepressants: Medications such as bupropion, venlafaxine, and selective serotonin reuptake inhibitors (SSRIs) are useful during the depressive phase. These are typically prescribed in combination with a mood stabilizer to prevent rebound mania.

Mood stabilizer

SELECT PROTOTYPE MEDICATION: Lithium carbonate

PURPOSE

EXPECTED PHARMACOLOGICAL ACTION

- Lithium produces neurochemical changes in the brain, including serotonin receptor blockade.
- There is evidence that lithium decreases neuronal atrophy and/or increases neuronal growth.

THERAPEUTIC USES

Lithium is used in the treatment of bipolar disorders. Lithium controls episodes of acute mania, helps to prevent the return of mania or depression, and decreases the incidence of suicide.

COMPLICATIONS

Advise the client that some adverse effects resolve within a few weeks of starting the medication. Q̣s

Gastrointestinal distress

Nausea, diarrhea, abdominal pain

NURSING CONSIDERATIONS
- Advise the client that GI distress is usually transient.
- Administer medication with meals or milk.

Fine hand tremors

Can interfere with purposeful motor skills and can be exacerbated by factors such as stress and caffeine

NURSING CONSIDERATIONS
- Administer beta-adrenergic blocking agents, such as propranolol.
- Adjust dosage to be as low as possible; give in divided doses; or use long-acting formulations.
- Advise the client to report an increase in tremors, which could be a manifestation of lithium toxicity.

Polyuria, mild thirst

NURSING CONSIDERATIONS
- Use a potassium-sparing diuretic, such as spironolactone.
- Instruct the client to maintain adequate fluid intake by consuming at least 1.5 to 3 L/day fluid from beverages and food sources.

Weight gain

NURSING CONSIDERATIONS: Assist the client to follow a healthy diet and regular exercise regimen.

Renal toxicity

NURSING CONSIDERATIONS
- Monitor I&O.
- Adjust dosage, and keep dose at the lowest level necessary.
- Assess baseline BUN and creatinine, and monitor kidney function periodically.

Goiter and hypothyroidism

With long-term treatment

NURSING CONSIDERATIONS
- Obtain baseline T_3, T_4, and TSH levels prior to starting treatment, and then annually.
- Advise the client to monitor for indications of hypothyroidism (cold, dry skin; decreased heart rate; weight gain).
- Administer levothyroxine.

Bradydysrhythmias, hypotension, and electrolyte imbalances

NURSING CONSIDERATIONS: Encourage the client to maintain adequate fluid and sodium intake.

Lithium toxicity

Early indications
- LITHIUM LEVEL: Less than 1.5 mEq/L
- MANIFESTATIONS: Diarrhea, nausea, vomiting, thirst, polyuria, muscle weakness, fine hand tremors, slurred speech, lethargy
- NURSING CONSIDERATIONS
  - Instruct the client to withhold the medication, and notify the provider.
  - Administer new dosage based on serum lithium and sodium levels. Qᴇʙᴘ

Advanced indications
- LITHIUM LEVEL: 1.5 to 2.0 mEq/L
- MANIFESTATIONS: Mental confusion, sedation, poor coordination, coarse tremors, and ongoing GI distress, including nausea, vomiting, and diarrhea
- NURSING CONSIDERATIONS
  - Instruct the client to withhold the medication, and notify the provider.
  - Administer new dosage based on serum lithium and sodium levels.
  - Excretion can need to be promoted.

Severe toxicity
- LITHIUM LEVEL: 2.0 to 2.5 mEq/L
- MANIFESTATIONS: Extreme polyuria of dilute urine, tinnitus, giddiness, jerking movements, blurred vision, ataxia, seizures, severe hypotension and stupor leading to coma, and possible death from respiratory complications
- NURSING CONSIDERATIONS
  - Administer an emetic to alert clients, or administer gastric lavage.
  - Urea, mannitol, or aminophylline may be prescribed to increase the rate of excretion.

Greater than 2.5 mEq/L
- MANIFESTATIONS: Rapid progression of manifestations leading to coma and death
- NURSING CONSIDERATIONS: Hemodialysis can be warranted.

CONTRAINDICATIONS/PRECAUTIONS

- Lithium is a Pregnancy Risk Category D medication. It is considered teratogenic, especially during the first trimester of pregnancy.
- Discourage clients from breastfeeding if lithium therapy is necessary.
- Lithium is contraindicated in clients who have hepatic disease, severe renal or cardiac disease, hypovolemia, and schizophrenia.
- Use cautiously in older adult clients and clients who have thyroid disease, seizure disorder, or diabetes. Qꜱ

INTERACTIONS

Diuretics

Sodium is excreted with the use of diuretics. With decreased serum sodium, lithium excretion is decreased, which can lead to toxicity.

NURSING CONSIDERATIONS
- Monitor for indications of toxicity.
- Advise the client to observe for indications of toxicity and to notify the provider.
- Encourage the client to maintain a diet adequate in sodium, and to drink 1.5 to 3 L/day of water.

NSAIDs

Concurrent use increases renal reabsorption of lithium, leading to toxicity.

NURSING CONSIDERATIONS
- Avoid use of NSAIDs to prevent toxic accumulation of lithium.
- Use aspirin as a mild analgesic, as it does not lead to toxicity.

Anticholinergics (antihistamines, tricyclic antidepressants)

Abdominal discomfort can result from anticholinergic-induced urinary retention and polyuria.

NURSING CONSIDERATIONS: Advise the client to avoid medications that have anticholinergic effects.

NURSING ADMINISTRATION

- Monitor plasma lithium levels while undergoing treatment. At initiation of treatment, monitor levels every 2 to 3 days until stable and then every 1 to 3 months. Closely monitor levels after any dosage change. Lithium blood levels should be obtained in the morning, 8 to 12 hr after last dose.
  - During initial treatment of a manic episode, levels should be 0.8 to 1.4 mEq/L.
  - Maintenance level range is 0.4 to 1.0 mEq/L.
  - Plasma levels greater than 1.5 mEq/L can result in toxicity.
- Older adult clients are at an increased risk for toxicity and require more frequent monitoring of serum lithium levels. Ⓖ
- Care for a client who has a toxic plasma lithium level should take place in an acute care setting with supportive measures provided. Hemodialysis can be indicated.
- Advise the client that effects begin within 5 to 7 days. Maximum benefits might not be seen for 2 to 3 weeks.
- Advise the client to take lithium as prescribed. This medication must be administered in 2 to 3 doses daily due to a short half-life. Taking lithium with food will help decrease GI distress.
- Encourage the client to adhere to laboratory appointments needed to monitor lithium effectiveness and adverse effects. Emphasize the high risk of toxicity due to the narrow therapeutic range. Qꜱ

- Provide nutritional counseling. Stress the importance of adequate fluid and sodium intake.
- Instruct the client to monitor for indications of toxicity and when to contact the provider. The client should withhold the medication and seek medical attention if she is experiencing diarrhea, vomiting, or excessive sweating.

Mood-stabilizing antiepileptic drugs

SELECT PROTOTYPE MEDICATIONS
- Carbamazepine
- Valproate
- Lamotrigine

PURPOSE

EXPECTED PHARMACOLOGICAL ACTION

Antiepileptic drugs help treat and manage bipolar disorder through various mechanisms.
- Slowing the entrance of sodium and calcium back into the neuron, thus extending the time it takes for the nerve to return to its active state
- Potentiating the inhibitory effects of gamma butyric acid (GABA)
- Inhibiting glutamic acid (glutamate), which in turn suppresses central nervous system (CNS) excitation Q**EBP**

THERAPEUTIC USES

These medications are used to treat and prevent relapse of manic and depressive episodes. They are particularly useful for clients who have mixed mania and rapid-cycling bipolar disorders.

COMPLICATIONS

CARBAMAZEPINE

Minimal effect on cognitive function

CNS effects

- Nystagmus
- Double vision
- Vertigo
- Staggering gait
- Headache

NURSING CONSIDERATIONS
- Administer in low doses initially, and then gradually increase dosage.
- Advise the client that effects should subside within a few weeks.
- Administer dose at bedtime.

Blood dyscrasias

Leukopenia, anemia, thrombocytopenia

NURSING CONSIDERATIONS
- Obtain baseline CBC and platelets. Perform ongoing monitoring of these.
- Observe for indications of thrombocytopenia, including bruising and bleeding of gums.
- Monitor for indications of infection, such as fever or lethargy.
- Advise the client to notify the provider if indications of blood dyscrasias are present.

Teratogenesis

NURSING CONSIDERATIONS: Advise the client to avoid use in pregnancy.

Hypoosmolarity

Promotes secretion of antidiuretic hormone, which inhibits water excretion by the kidneys, and places the client who has heart failure at risk for fluid overload

NURSING CONSIDERATIONS
- Monitor serum sodium.
- Monitor for edema, decrease in urine output, and hypertension.

Skin disorders

Includes dermatitis, rash (Stevens–Johnson syndrome)

NURSING CONSIDERATIONS
- Treat mild reactions with anti-inflammatory or antihistamine medications.
- Advise the client to wear sunscreen.
- Instruct the client to withhold the medication and notify the provider if Stevens–Johnson syndrome occurs.

LAMOTRIGINE

Double or blurred vision, dizziness, headache, nausea, vomiting

NURSING CONSIDERATIONS: Caution the client about performing activities that require concentration or visual acuity. Q**s**

Serious skin rashes

Includes Stevens–Johnson syndrome

NURSING CONSIDERATIONS: Instruct the client to withhold the medication, and notify the provider if a rash occurs.

VALPROATE

GI effects (nausea, vomiting, indigestion)

NURSING CONSIDERATIONS
- Advise the client that these effects are generally self-limiting.
- Advise the client to take medication with food, or switch to enteric-coated formulations.

Hepatotoxicity

Evidenced by anorexia, nausea, vomiting, fatigue, abdominal pain, jaundice

NURSING CONSIDERATIONS
- Assess baseline liver function, and monitor liver function regularly (minimum of every 2 months during the first 6 months of treatment).
- Advise the client to observe for indications of hepatotoxicity and to notify the provider immediately if they occur.
- Avoid using in children younger than 2 years old.
- Administer the lowest effective dose.

Pancreatitis

Evidenced by nausea, vomiting, abdominal pain

NURSING CONSIDERATIONS
- Advise the client to observe for manifestations of pancreatitis and to notify the provider immediately if they occur.
- Monitor amylase levels.
- Discontinue the medication if pancreatitis develops.

Thrombocytopenia

NURSING CONSIDERATIONS
- Advise the client to observe for indications, such as bruising, and to notify the provider if these occur.
- Monitor platelet counts.

Teratogenesis

NURSING CONSIDERATIONS
- Advise the client to avoid use during pregnancy.
- Advise the client to talk to the provider if she is considering pregnancy to discuss other treatment options.

Weight gain

NURSING CONSIDERATIONS: Assist the client to follow a healthy diet and regular exercise regimen

CONTRAINDICATIONS/PRECAUTIONS

- These medications are Pregnancy Risk Category D medications. They can result in birth defects.
- Carbamazepine is contraindicated in clients who have bone marrow suppression or bleeding disorders.
- Monitor plasma levels of valproate and carbamazepine while undergoing treatment.
- Lamotrigine needs to be slowly titrated to prevent adverse effects.

INTERACTIONS

Carbamazepine

Oral contraceptives, warfarin
- Concurrent use of carbamazepine causes a decrease in the effects of these medications due to stimulation of hepatic and drug-metabolizing enzymes.
- NURSING CONSIDERATIONS
  - Advise the client to use an alternate form of birth control.
  - Monitor for therapeutic effects of warfarin. Dosage can need to be adjusted.

Grapefruit juice inhibits metabolism of carbamazepine, thereby increasing blood levels of the medication.
NURSING CONSIDERATIONS: Advise the client to avoid intake of grapefruit juice.

Concurrent use of other anticonvulsants decreases the effects of carbamazepine by stimulating metabolism.
NURSING CONSIDERATIONS: Monitor carbamazepine levels, and adjust dosages as prescribed.

Lamotrigine

Carbamazepine, phenytoin, phenobarbital: Concurrent use decreases the effect of lamotrigine.
NURSING CONSIDERATIONS: Monitor for therapeutic effects, and adjust dosages as prescribed.

Concurrent use of valproate inhibits drug-metabolizing enzymes, thereby increasing the half-life of lamotrigine.
NURSING CONSIDERATIONS: Monitor for adverse effects, and adjust dosages as prescribed.

Concurrent use of oral contraceptives decreases the effectiveness of both medications.
NURSING CONSIDERATIONS: Advise the client to use an alternate form of birth control.

Valproate

Concurrent use of other anticonvulsants affects serum levels of valproate.
NURSING CONSIDERATIONS: Monitor valproate levels, and adjust dosages as prescribed.

NURSING EVALUATION OF MEDICATION EFFECTIVENESS

Depending on therapeutic intent, effectiveness can be evidenced by the following.
- Relief of acute manic manifestations (flight of ideas, excessive talking, agitation) or depressive manifestations (fatigue, poor appetite, psychomotor retardation)
- Verbalization of improvement in mood
- Ability to perform ADLs
- Improved sleeping and eating habits
- Appropriate interaction with peers

Application Exercises

1. A nurse is caring for a client who is prescribed lithium therapy. The client states that he wants to take ibuprofen for osteoarthritis pain relief. Which of the following statements should the nurse make?

   A. "That is a good choice. Ibuprofen does not interact with lithium."

   B. "Regular aspirin would be a better choice than ibuprofen."

   C. "Lithium decreases the effectiveness of ibuprofen."

   D. "The ibuprofen will make your lithium level fall too low."

2. A nurse is discussing early indications of toxicity with a client who has a new prescription for lithium carbonate for bipolar disorder. The nurse should include which of the following manifestations in the teaching? (Select all that apply.)

   A. Constipation

   B. Polyuria

   C. Rash

   D. Muscle weakness

   E. Tinnitus

3. A nurse is discussing routine follow-up needs with a client who has a new prescription for valproate. The nurse should inform the client of the need for routine monitoring of which of the following?

   A. AST/ALT and LDH

   B. Creatinine and BUN

   C. WBC and granulocyte counts

   D. Serum sodium and potassium

4. A nurse is caring for a client who is experiencing extreme mania due to bipolar disorder. Prior to administration of lithium carbonate, the client's lithium blood level is 1.2 mEq/L. Which of the following actions should the nurse take?

   A. Administer the next dose of lithium carbonate as scheduled.

   B. Prepare for administration of aminophylline.

   C. Notify the provider for a possible increase in the dosage of lithium carbonate.

   D. Request a stat repeat of the client's lithium blood level.

5. A nurse is admitting a client who has a new diagnosis of bipolar disorder and is scheduled to begin lithium therapy. When collecting a medical history from the client's adult daughter, which of the following statements is the priority to report to the provider?

   A. "My mother has diabetes that is controlled by her diet."

   B. "My mother recently completed a course of prednisone for acute bronchitis."

   C. "My mother received her flu vaccine last month."

   D. "My mother is currently on furosemide for her congestive heart failure."

PRACTICE Active Learning Scenario

A nurse is providing teaching to a client who has rapid cycling bipolar disorder and a new prescription for carbamazepine. Use the ATI Active Learning Template: Medication to complete this item.

THERAPEUTIC USES: Discuss the use of carbamazepine as it relates to bipolar disorder.

COMPLICATIONS: Identify at least four adverse effects.

NURSING INTERVENTIONS: Describe at least four nursing interventions or client education points.

Application Exercises Key

1. A. Ibuprofen is not recommended for clients taking lithium.

   B. **CORRECT:** Aspirin is recommended as a mild analgesic rather than ibuprofen due to the risk for lithium toxicity.

   C. Lithium does not decrease the effectiveness of ibuprofen. However, concurrent use is not recommended due to the risk of toxicity.

   D. Ibuprofen increases the risk for a toxic, rather than low, lithium level.

   Ⓝ *NCLEX® Connection: Pharmacological and Parenteral Therapies, Adverse Effects/Contraindications/Side Effects/Interactions*

2. A. Diarrhea, rather than constipation, is an early indication of lithium toxicity.

   B. **CORRECT:** Polyuria is an early indication of lithium toxicity.

   C. A rash is not indication of lithium toxicity.

   D. **CORRECT:** Muscle weakness is an early indication of lithium toxicity.

   E. Tinnitus is an indication of severe, rather than early, toxicity.

   Ⓝ *NCLEX® Connection: Pharmacological and Parenteral Therapies, Adverse Effects/Contraindications/Side Effects/Interactions*

3. A. **CORRECT:** Routine monitoring of liver function tests is necessary due to the risk for hepatotoxicity.

   B. Baseline levels can be drawn. However, routine monitoring of creatinine and BUN is not necessary.

   C. Baseline levels can be drawn. However, routine monitoring of WBC and granulocyte counts is not necessary.

   D. Baseline levels can be drawn. However, routine monitoring of serum sodium and potassium is not necessary.

   Ⓝ *NCLEX® Connection: Reduction of Risk Potential, Medication Administration*

4. A. **CORRECT:** During a manic episode, the lithium blood level should be 0.8 to 1.4 mEq/L. It is appropriate to administer the next dose as scheduled.

   B. Aminophylline can be prescribed for treatment of severe toxicity for levels greater than 1.5 mEq/L.

   C. A dosage increase would place the client at risk for toxicity and is therefore not an appropriate action.

   D. A lithium level of 1.2 mEq/L is an expected finding for a client who is experiencing a manic episode. It is not necessary to request a stat repeat of the laboratory test.

   Ⓝ *NCLEX® Connection: Reduction of Risk Potential, Expected Actions/Outcomes*

5. A. It is important to notify the provider of the client's medical history. However, this information does not pose the greatest risk to the client and is therefore not the priority.

   B. It is important to notify the provider of the client's medical history. However, this information does not pose the greatest risk to the client and is therefore not the priority.

   C. It is important to notify the provider of the client's medical history. However, this information does not pose the greatest risk to the client and is therefore not the priority.

   D. **CORRECT:** Diuretics, such as furosemide, are contraindicated for use with lithium due to the risk for toxicity. This is the greatest risk for the client and is therefore the highest priority to report to the provider.

   Ⓝ *NCLEX® Connection: Pharmacological and Parenteral Therapies, Adverse Effects/Contraindications/Side Effects/Interactions*

PRACTICE Answer

Using ATI Active Learning Template: Medication

THERAPEUTIC USES:
Carbamazepine is used to treat manic and depressive episodes, as well as to prevent relapse of mania and depressive episodes of bipolar disorder. This type of medication is particularly useful for clients who have mixed mania and rapid cycling bipolar disorders.

COMPLICATIONS
- CNS effects
- Nystagmus
- Diplopia
- Vertigo
- Staggering gait
- Headache
- Blood dyscrasias
- Teratogenesis
- Hypoosmolarity
- Dermatitis
- Rash

NURSING INTERVENTIONS
- Advise the client that CNS effects should subside within a few weeks.
- Administer carbamazepine at bedtime to minimize CNS effects.
- Advise the client of the need for routine monitoring of CBC, platelets, and serum sodium levels.
- Monitor for indications of bleeding.
- Advise the client to avoid use in pregnancy.
- Monitor the client for indications of fluid retention.
- Advise the client to wear sunscreen.
- Instruct the client to notify the provider if a rash occurs.

Ⓝ *NCLEX® Connection: Pharmacological and Parenteral Therapies, Medication Administration*

CHAPTER 24

Medications for Psychotic Disorders

Schizophrenia spectrum disorders are the primary reason for the administration of antipsychotic medications. The clinical course of schizophrenia usually involves acute exacerbations with intervals of semiremission in which manifestations remain present but are less severe.

MANIFESTATIONS

Medications are used to treat the following.

POSITIVE SYMPTOMS related to behavior, thought, perception, and speech: Agitation, bizarre behavior, delusions, hallucinations, flight of ideas, loose associations

NEGATIVE SYMPTOMS: Social withdrawal, lack of emotion, lack of energy, flattened affect, decreased motivation, decreased pleasure in activities

GOALS OF TREATMENT

The goals of psychopharmacological treatment for schizophrenia and other psychotic disorders include the following.
- Suppression of acute episodes
- Prevention of acute recurrence
- Maintenance of the highest possible level of functioning

FIRST-GENERATION ANTIPSYCHOTICS

- First-generation (conventional) antipsychotic medications are used mainly to control positive symptoms of psychotic disorders.
- Due to adverse effects, first-generation antipsychotic medications are reserved for clients who are
  - Using them successfully and can tolerate the adverse effects.
  - Concerned about the cost associated with second-generation antipsychotic medications.
- First-generation agents are classified as either low-, medium-, or high-potency depending on their association with extrapyramidal symptoms (EPSs), level of sedation, and anticholinergic adverse effects.
  - Low potency: low EPSs, high sedation, and high anticholinergic adverse effects
  - Medium potency: moderate EPSs, moderate sedation, and low anticholinergic adverse effects
  - High potency: high EPSs, low sedation, and low anticholinergic adverse effects

SECOND-GENERATION ANTIPSYCHOTICS

Second-generation (atypical) antipsychotic agents are often chosen as first-line treatment for schizophrenia. They are the current medications of choice for clients receiving initial treatment, and for treating breakthrough episodes in clients on conventional medication therapy, because they are more effective with fewer adverse effects.

ADVANTAGES
- Relief of both positive and negative symptoms
- Decrease in affective findings (depression, anxiety) and suicidal behaviors
- Improvement of neurocognitive defects, such as poor memory
- Fewer or no EPSs, including tardive dyskinesia, due to less dopamine blockade
- Fewer anticholinergic effects, with the exception of clozapine, which has a high incidence of anticholinergic effects. This is because most of the atypical antipsychotics cause little or no blockade of cholinergic receptors.
- Less relapse

THIRD-GENERATION ANTIPSYCHOTICS

Third-generation antipsychotic agents are used to treat both positive and negative symptoms while improving cognitive function.

ADVANTAGES
- Decreased risk of EPSs or tardive dyskinesia
- Lower risk for weight gain and anticholinergic effects

Antipsychotics: First-generation (conventional)

SELECT PROTOTYPE MEDICATION: Chlorpromazine, low potency

OTHER MEDICATIONS
- Haloperidol, high potency
- Fluphenazine, high potency
- Loxapine, medium potency
- Thioridazine, low potency
- Thiothixene, high potency
- Perphenazine, medium potency
- Trifluoperazine, high potency

PURPOSE

EXPECTED PHARMACOLOGICAL ACTION

- First-generation antipsychotic medications block dopamine (D_2), acetylcholine, histamine, and norepinephrine receptors in the brain and periphery.
- Inhibition of psychotic symptoms is believed to be a result of D_2 blockade in the brain.

THERAPEUTIC USES

- Treatment of acute and chronic psychotic disorders
- Schizophrenia spectrum disorders
- Bipolar disorder: primarily the manic phase
- Tourette disorder
- Agitation
- Prevention of nausea/vomiting through blocking of dopamine in the chemoreceptor trigger zone of the medulla

COMPLICATIONS

Agranulocytosis

NURSING CONSIDERATIONS
- Advise clients to observe for indications of infection (fever, sore throat), and to notify the provider if these occur.
- If indications of infection appear, obtain a CBC. Medication should be discontinued if WBC count is less than 3,000 mm³.

Anticholinergic effects

MANIFESTATIONS
- Dry mouth
- Blurred vision
- Photophobia
- Urinary hesitancy or retention
- Constipation
- Tachycardia

NURSING CONSIDERATIONS: Suggest the following strategies to decrease anticholinergic effects.
- Chewing sugarless gum
- Sipping on water
- Avoiding hazardous activities
- Wearing sunglasses when outdoors
- Eating foods high in fiber
- Participating in regular exercise
- Maintaining fluid intake of 2 to 3 L/day from beverages and food sources
- Voiding just before taking medication

EXTRAPYRAMIDAL SIDE EFFECTS

Acute dystonia

MANIFESTATIONS
- Severe spasm of the tongue, neck, face, and back
- Crisis situation that requires rapid treatment

NURSING CONSIDERATIONS
- Begin to monitor for acute dystonia anywhere between 1 to 5 days after administration of first dose.
- Treat with an antiparkinsonian agents such as benztropine.
- IM or IV administration diphenhydramine can also be beneficial.
- Stay with the client and monitor the airway until spasms subside (usually 5 to 15 min).

Pseudoparkinsonism

MANIFESTATIONS
- Bradykinesia
- Rigidity
- Shuffling gait
- Drooling
- Tremors

NURSING CONSIDERATIONS
- Observe for pseudoparkinsonism for the first month after the initiation of therapy. Can occur in as little as 5 hr following the first dose.
- Treat with an antiparkinsonian agent, such as benztropine or trihexyphenidyl.
- Implement interventions to reduce the risk for falling.

Akathisia

MANIFESTATIONS
- Inability to sit or stand still
- Continual pacing and agitation

NURSING CONSIDERATIONS
- Observe for akathisia for the first 2 months after the initiation of treatment. Can occur in as little as 2 hr following the first dose.
- Manage with antiparkinsonian agents, beta blockers, or lorazepam/diazepam.
- Monitor for increased risk for suicide in clients who have severe akathisia.

Tardive dyskinesia (TD)

MANIFESTATIONS
- Late EPSs, which can require months to years of medication therapy for TD to develop
- Involuntary movements of the tongue and face, such as lip smacking and tongue fasciculations
- Involuntary movements of the arms, legs, and trunk

NURSING CONSIDERATIONS
- Evaluate the client every 3 months. If TD appears, dosage should be lowered, or the client should be switched to another type of antipsychotic agent.
- Once TD develops, it usually does not decrease, even with discontinuation of the medication.
- There is not a treatment for TD.
- Teach client that purposeful muscle movement helps to control the involuntary TD.

Neuroendocrine effects

MANIFESTATIONS
- Gynecomastia
- Weight gain
- Menstrual irregularities

NURSING CONSIDERATIONS
- Monitor weight. Some clients gain 100 lb or more.
- Advise the client to observe for these manifestations and to notify the provider if they occur.

Neuroleptic malignant syndrome

MANIFESTATIONS
- Sudden high fever
- Blood pressure fluctuations
- Diaphoresis
- Tachycardia
- Muscle rigidity
- Drooling
- Decreased level of consciousness
- Coma
- Tachypnea

NURSING CONSIDERATIONS
- This life-threatening medical emergency can occur within the first week of treatment or any time thereafter.
- Stop antipsychotic medication.
- Monitor vital signs.
- Apply cooling blankets.
- Administer antipyretics
- Increase the client's fluid intake.
- Administer dantrolene or bromocriptine to induce muscle relaxation.
- Administer medication as prescribed to treat arrhythmias.
- Assist with immediate transfer to an ICU.

Orthostatic hypotension

NURSING CONSIDERATIONS
- The client should develop tolerance in 1 to 2 weeks.
- Monitor blood pressure and heart rate for orthostatic changes. Hold medication until the provider is notified if systolic blood pressure is less than 80 mm Hg.
- Instruct clients about the indications of orthostatic hypotension (lightheadedness, dizziness). If these occur, advise the client to sit or lie down. Orthostatic hypotension can be minimized by getting up or changing positions slowly.
- Encourage the client to increase fluid intake to maintain hydration.

Sedation

NURSING CONSIDERATIONS
- Inform the client that effects should diminish after about 1 week.
- Instruct the client to take the medication at bedtime to avoid daytime sleepiness.
- Advise the client not to drive until sedation has subsided.

Seizures

INDICATIONS: Greatest risk in clients who have an existing seizure disorder

NURSING CONSIDERATIONS
- Advise the client to report seizure activity to the provider.
- An increase in antiseizure medication can be necessary.

Severe dysrhythmias

NURSING CONSIDERATIONS
- Obtain baseline ECG and potassium level prior to treatment, and periodically throughout the treatment period.
- Avoid concurrent use with other medications that prolong QT interval.

Sexual dysfunction

Note: Common in both males and females

NURSING CONSIDERATIONS
- Advise the client of possible adverse effects.
- Encourage that the client report effects to the provider.
- The client can need dosage lowered or be switched to a high-potency agent.

Skin effects

MANIFESTATIONS
- Photosensitivity that can result in severe sunburn
- Contact dermatitis from handling medications

NURSING CONSIDERATIONS
- Advise clients to avoid excessive exposure to sunlight, to use sunscreen, and to wear protective clothing.
- Advise clients to avoid direct contact with the medication.

Liver impairment

NURSING CONSIDERATIONS
- Assess baseline liver function, and monitor periodically.
- Educate clients to observe for indications (anorexia, nausea, vomiting, fatigue, abdominal pain, jaundice) and to notify the provider.

CONTRAINDICATIONS/PRECAUTIONS

- These medications are contraindicated in clients who are in a coma or have Parkinson's disease, liver damage, or severe hypotension.
- Use of conventional antipsychotic medications is contraindicated in older adult clients who have dementia. Ⓖ
- Use cautiously in clients who have prostate enlargement, heart disorders, kidney disease, or seizure disorders.

INTERACTIONS

Concurrent use with other anticholinergic medications increases effects.
NURSING CONSIDERATIONS: Advise the client to avoid over-the-counter medications that contain anticholinergic agents, such as sleep aids and antihistamines.

Additive CNS depressant effects with concurrent use of alcohol, opioids, and antihistamines.
NURSING CONSIDERATIONS
- Advise the client to avoid alcohol and other medications that cause CNS depression.
- Advise the client to avoid hazardous activities, such as driving.

By activating dopamine receptors, levodopa counteracts effects of antipsychotic agents.
NURSING CONSIDERATIONS: Advise the client to avoid concurrent use of levodopa and other direct dopamine receptor agonists.

NURSING ADMINISTRATION

- Use the Abnormal Involuntary Movement Scale (AIMS) to screen for the presence of EPSs.
- Assess the client to differentiate between EPSs and worsening of a psychotic disorder.
- Administer anticholinergics, beta-blockers, and benzodiazepines to control early EPS. If adverse effects are intolerable, a client can be switched to a low-potency or atypical antipsychotic agent.
- Advise clients that antipsychotic medications rarely cause physical or psychological dependence.
- Advise clients to take medication as prescribed and on a regular schedule.
- Advise clients that some therapeutic effects can be noticeable within a few days, but significant improvement can take 2 to 4 weeks, and possibly several months for full effects.
- Consider depot preparations (haloperidol decanoate, fluphenazine decanoate), administered IM once every 3 to 4 weeks, for clients who have difficulty maintaining a medication regimen. Inform the client that lower doses can be used with depot preparations, which will decrease the risk of adverse effects and the development of tardive dyskinesia. Qpcc
- Begin administration with twice-daily dosing, but switch to daily dosing at bedtime to decrease daytime drowsiness and promote sleep.

Antipsychotics: Second- and third-generation (atypical)

SELECT PROTOTYPE MEDICATION: Risperidone

OTHER MEDICATIONS
- Asenapine
- Clozapine
- Iloperidone
- Lurasidone
- Olanzapine
- Paliperidone
- Quetiapine
- Ziprasidone
- Aripiprazole (third generation)

PURPOSE

EXPECTED PHARMACOLOGICAL ACTION

These antipsychotic agents work mainly by blocking serotonin, and to a lesser degree, dopamine receptors. These medications also block receptors for norepinephrine, histamine, and acetylcholine.

THERAPEUTIC USES

- Negative and positive symptoms of schizophrenia spectrum disorders
- Psychosis induced by levodopa therapy
- Relief of psychotic manifestations in other disorders, such as bipolar disorder
- Impulse control disorders

COMPLICATIONS

Metabolic syndrome

- New onset of diabetes mellitus or loss of glucose control in clients who have diabetes
- Dyslipidemia with increased risk for hypertension and other cardiovascular disease
- Weight gain

NURSING CONSIDERATIONS
- Obtain baseline fasting blood glucose, and monitor the value periodically throughout treatment.
- Instruct the client to report indications, such as increased thirst, urination, and appetite, to the provider.
- Advise the client to follow a healthy, low-calorie diet, engage in regular exercise, and monitor weight gain.
- Monitor cholesterol, triglycerides, and blood glucose if weight gain is greater than 14 kg (31 lb).

Orthostatic hypotension

NURSING CONSIDERATIONS
- Monitor blood pressure and heart rate for orthostatic changes.
- Hold medication while notifying the provider of significant changes.

Anticholinergic effects

Such as urinary hesitancy or retention, dry mouth

NURSING CONSIDERATIONS
- Monitor for these adverse effects, and report their occurrence to the provider.
- Encourage the client to use measures to relieve dry mouth, such as sipping water throughout the day.

Agitation, dizziness, sedation, sleep disruption

NURSING CONSIDERATIONS
- Monitor for these adverse effects, and report their occurrence to the provider.
- Administer an alternative medication if prescribed.

Mild EPS, such as tremor

NURSING CONSIDERATIONS
- Monitor for and teach clients to recognize EPS.
- Use AIMS test to screen for EPS.

Elevated prolactin levels

NURSING CONSIDERATIONS
- Advise clients to observe for galactorrhea, gynecomastia, and amenorrhea, and to notify the provider if these occur.
- Obtain prolactin level if indicated.

Sexual dysfunction

Anorgasmia, impotence, low libido

NURSING CONSIDERATIONS
- Advise clients to observe for possible sexual side effects.
- Encourage clients to notify provider if intolerable.
- Instruct client on ways to manage sexual dysfunction, which can include using adjunct medications to improve sexual function (e.g., sildenafil).

CONTRAINDICATIONS/PRECAUTIONS

Risperidone

- Risperidone is a Pregnancy Risk Category C medication.
- These medications should not be used for clients who have dementia. Use of these medications can cause death related to cerebrovascular accident or infection. Qs
- Clients should avoid the concurrent use of alcohol.
- Use cautiously in clients who have cardiovascular or cerebrovascular disease, seizures, or diabetes mellitus. Clients who have diabetes mellitus should have a baseline fasting blood sugar, and blood glucose should be monitored carefully.

OTHER ATYPICAL ANTIPSYCHOTIC AGENTS

Aripiprazole (third-generation antipsychotic)

- Tablets
- Orally disintegrating tablets
- Oral solution
- Short-acting injectable
- Long-acting injectable

NURSING CONSIDERATIONS
- Low or no risk of EPS
- Low or no risk of diabetes, weight gain, dyslipidemia, orthostatic hypotension, and anticholinergic effects

ADVERSE EFFECTS
- Sedation
- Headache
- Anxiety
- Insomnia
- Gastrointestinal upset

Asenapine

Sublingual tablets

NURSING CONSIDERATIONS: Low risk of diabetes, weight gain, dyslipidemia, and anticholinergic effects

OTHER ADVERSE EFFECTS
- Drowsiness
- Prolonged QT interval
- EPS (higher doses)
- Causes temporary numbing of the mouth

Clozapine

The first atypical antipsychotic developed, it is no longer considered a first-line medication for schizophrenia spectrum disorders due to its adverse effects.
- Tablets
- Orally disintegrating tablets

NURSING CONSIDERATIONS
- Low risk of EPS
- High risk of weight gain, diabetes, and dyslipidemia
- Risk for fatal agranulocytosis
- Baseline and regular monitoring of WBC per protocol (weekly, bi-weekly, then monthly) required
- Notification of the provider of indications of infection (fever, sore throat, mouth lesions) is necessary

OTHER ADVERSE EFFECTS
- Sedation
- Orthostatic hypotension
- Hypersalivation
- Anticholinergic effects

Iloperidone

Tablets

NURSING CONSIDERATIONS
- Significant risk for weight gain, prolonged QT interval, and orthostatic hypotension
- Advise clients to follow titration schedule during initial therapy to minimize hypotension.
- Low risk for diabetes, dyslipidemia, and EPS

COMMON ADVERSE EFFECTS
- Dry mouth
- Sedation
- Fatigue
- Nasal congestion

Lurasidone

Tablets

NURSING CONSIDERATIONS
- Low risk for diabetes, weight gain, and dyslipidemia.
- Does not cause anticholinergic effects

COMMON ADVERSE EFFECTS
- Sedation
- Akathisia
- Parkinsonism
- Agitation and anxiety
- Nausea

Olanzapine

- Tablets
- Short-acting injectable
- Extended-release injection

NURSING CONSIDERATIONS
- Low risk of EPS
- High risk of diabetes, weight gain, and dyslipidemia

OTHER ADVERSE EFFECTS
- Sedation
- Orthostatic hypotension
- Anticholinergic effects

! Following administration of extended-release injection, the client requires observation for at least 3 hr to monitor for adverse effects.

Paliperidone

- Extended-release tablets
- Extended-release injections

NURSING CONSIDERATIONS: Significant risk for diabetes, weight gain, and dyslipidemia

OTHER ADVERSE EFFECTS
- Sedation
- Prolonged QT interval
- Orthostatic hypotension
- Anticholinergic effects
- Mild EPS

Quetiapine

- Tablets
- Extended-release tablets

NURSING CONSIDERATIONS
- Low risk of EPS
- Moderate risk of diabetes, weight gain, and dyslipidemia

OTHER ADVERSE EFFECTS
- Cataracts
- Sedation
- Orthostatic hypotension
- Anticholinergic effects

Ziprasidone

This medication affects both dopamine and serotonin, so it can be used for clients who have concurrent depression.
- Capsules
- Short-acting injectable

NURSING CONSIDERATIONS
- Low risk of EPS
- Low risk of diabetes, weight gain, and dyslipidemia

OTHER ADVERSE EFFECTS
- Sedation
- Orthostatic hypotension
- Anticholinergic effects
- ECG changes and QT prolongation that can lead to *torsades de pointes*

INTERACTIONS

Immunosuppressive medications, such as anticancer medications, can further suppress immune function.
NURSING CONSIDERATIONS: Avoid use in clients who are taking clozapine.

Additive CNS depressant effects can occur with concurrent use of alcohol, opioids, antihistamines, and other CNS depressants.
NURSING CONSIDERATIONS
- Advise clients to avoid alcohol and other medications that cause CNS depression.
- Advise clients to avoid hazardous activities, such as driving.

By activating dopamine receptors, levodopa counteracts the effects of antipsychotic agents.
NURSING CONSIDERATIONS: Avoid concurrent use of levodopa and other direct dopamine receptor agonists.

Tricyclic antidepressants, amiodarone, and clarithromycin prolong QT intervals, thereby increasing the risk of cardiac dysrhythmias.
NURSING CONSIDERATIONS: Atypical antipsychotics that prolong the QT interval should not be used concurrently with other medications that have the same effect.

Barbiturates and phenytoin stimulate hepatic medication-metabolizing enzymes, thereby decreasing medication levels of aripiprazole, quetiapine, and ziprasidone.
NURSING CONSIDERATIONS: Monitor medication effectiveness.

Fluconazole inhibits hepatic medication-metabolizing enzymes, thereby increasing medication levels of aripiprazole, quetiapine, and ziprasidone.
NURSING CONSIDERATIONS: Monitor medication effectiveness.

NURSING ADMINISTRATION

Risperidone also is available as a depot injection administered IM once every 2 weeks, and the extended-release injection of paliperidone is administered every 28 days. Aripiprazole also has a long-acting injectable which is administered on a monthly basis. This method of administration is a good option for clients who have difficulty adhering to a medication schedule. Therapeutic effect occurs 2 to 6 weeks after first depot injection.
- Advise clients that low doses of medication are given initially, and dosages are then gradually increased. ("Start low and go slow.")
- Use oral disintegrating tablets for clients who can attempt to "cheek" or "pocket" tablets, or for those who have difficulty swallowing them.
- Advise clients taking asenapine to avoid eating or drinking for 10 min after each dose.
- Administer lurasidone and ziprasidone with food to increase absorption.
- The cost of antipsychotic medications can be a factor for some clients. Assess the need for case management intervention. Qᴛᴄ

NURSING EVALUATION OF MEDICATION EFFECTIVENESS

Depending on therapeutic intent, effectiveness can be evidenced by the following.
- Improvement and/or prevention of acute psychotic manifestations, absence of hallucinations, delusions, anxiety, hostility
- Improvement in ability to perform ADLs
- Improvement in ability to interact socially with peers
- Improvement of sleeping and eating habits

Application Exercises

1. A nurse is caring for a client who has schizophrenia and exhibits a lack of grooming and a flat affect. The nurse should anticipate a prescription of which of the following medications?

   A. Chlorpromazine

   B. Thiothixene

   C. Risperidone

   D. Haloperidol

2. A nurse is caring for a client who takes ziprasidone. The client reports difficulty swallowing the oral medication and becomes extremely agitated with injectable administration. The nurse should contact the provider to discuss a change to which of the following medications? (Select all that apply.)

   A. Olanzapine

   B. Quetiapine

   C. Aripiprazole

   D. Clozapine

   E. Asenapine

3. A charge nurse is discussing manifestations of schizophrenia with a newly licensed nurse. Which of the following manifestations should the charge nurse identify as being effectively treated by first-generation antipsychotics? (Select all that apply.)

   A. Auditory hallucinations

   B. Withdrawal from social situations

   C. Delusions of grandeur

   D. Severe agitation

   E. Anhedonia

4. A nurse is assessing a client who is currently taking perphenazine. Which of the following findings should the nurse identify as an extrapyramidal symptom (EPS)? (Select all that apply.)

   A. Decreased level of consciousness

   B. Drooling

   C. Involuntary arm movements

   D. Urinary retention

   E. Continual pacing

5. A nurse is providing discharge teaching for a client who has schizophrenia and a new prescription for iloperidone. Which of the following client statements indicates understanding of the teaching?

   A. "I will be able to stop taking this medication as soon as I feel better."

   B. "If I feel drowsy during the day, I will stop taking this medication and call my provider."

   C. "I will be careful not to gain too much weight while taking this medication."

   D. "This medication is highly addictive and must be withdrawn slowly."

PRACTICE Active Learning Scenario

A nurse is providing teaching to a client who has a new prescription for clozapine. Use the ATI Active Learning Template: Medication to complete this item.

THERAPEUTIC USES: Identify two.

COMPLICATIONS: Identify at least four adverse effects.

EVALUATION OF MEDICATION EFFECTIVENESS: Identify at least two outcomes.

Application Exercises Key

1. A. First-generation antipsychotics, such as chlorpromazine, are used mainly to control positive, rather than negative, symptoms of schizophrenia.

   B. First-generation antipsychotics, such as thiothixene, are used mainly to control positive symptoms of schizophrenia.

   C. **CORRECT:** Second-generation antipsychotics, such as risperidone, are effective in treating negative symptoms of schizophrenia, such as lack of grooming and flat affect.

   D. First-generation antipsychotics, such as haloperidol, are used mainly to control positive symptoms of schizophrenia.

   Ⓝ *NCLEX® Connection: Pharmacological and Parenteral Therapies, Expected Actions/Outcomes*

2. A. Olanzapine is available only in tablet or injectable form and will therefore not address the current concerns with medication administration.

   B. Quetiapine is available only in tablets or extended-release tablets and will therefore not address the current concerns with medication administration.

   C. **CORRECT:** Aripiprazole is available in an orally disintegrating tablet, which is appropriate for clients who have difficulty swallowing oral tablets. This route also decreases the risk for agitation associated with an injection.

   D. **CORRECT:** Clozapine is available in an orally disintegrating tablet, which is appropriate for clients who have difficulty swallowing oral tablets. This route also decreases the risk for agitation associated with an injection.

   E. **CORRECT:** Asenapine is available in a sublingual tablet, which is appropriate for clients who have difficulty swallowing oral tablets. This route also decreases the risk for agitation associated with an injection.

   Ⓝ *NCLEX® Connection: Pharmacological and Parenteral Therapies, Expected Actions/Outcomes*

3. A. **CORRECT:** Positive symptoms of schizophrenia, such as auditory hallucinations, are effectively treated with first-generation antipsychotics.

   B. First-generation antipsychotics have minimal effectiveness with negative symptoms of schizophrenia, such as social withdrawal.

   C. **CORRECT:** Positive symptoms of schizophrenia, such as delusions of grandeur, are effectively treated with first-generation antipsychotics.

   D. **CORRECT:** Positive symptoms of schizophrenia, such as severe agitation, are effectively treated with first-generation antipsychotics.

   E. First-generation antipsychotics have minimal effectiveness with negative symptoms of schizophrenia, such as anhedonia.

   Ⓝ *NCLEX® Connection: Pharmacological and Parenteral Therapies, Expected Actions/Outcomes*

4. A. Decreased level of consciousness is an indication of neuroleptic malignant syndrome rather than an EPS.

   B. **CORRECT:** Drooling is an indication of pseudoparkinsonism, which is an EPS.

   C. **CORRECT:** Involuntary arm movements are an indication of tardive dyskinesia, which is an EPS.

   D. Urinary retention is an anticholinergic effect rather than an EPS.

   E. **CORRECT:** Continual pacing is an indication of akathisia, which is an EPS.

   Ⓝ *NCLEX® Connection: Pharmacological and Parenteral Therapies, Adverse Effects/Contraindications/Side Effects/Interactions*

5. A. Antipsychotic medications are considered a long-term treatment for schizophrenia. Discontinuing the medication can result in an exacerbation of manifestations.

   B. Drowsiness is a common adverse effect of antipsychotic medications. However, it is not appropriate to discontinue the medication.

   C. **CORRECT:** Antipsychotic medications, such as iloperidone, have a high risk for significant weight gain.

   D. Antipsychotic medications are not considered addictive, and it is not necessary to titrate iloperidone when discontinuing treatment.

   Ⓝ *NCLEX® Connection: Pharmacological and Parenteral Therapies, Medication Administration*

PRACTICE Answer

Using the ATI Active Learning Template: Medication

THERAPEUTIC USES
- Treatment of negative and positive symptoms of schizophrenia spectrum disorders
- Psychosis induced by levodopa therapy
- Relief of psychotic manifestations in nonpsychotic disorders, such as bipolar disorder

COMPLICATIONS
- Weight gain
- Diabetes mellitus
- Dyslipidemia
- Agranulocytosis
- Sedation
- Orthostatic hypotension
- Anticholinergic effects

EVALUATION OF MEDICATION EFFECTIVENESS
- Improvement of positive and negative symptoms
- Improvement in ability to perform ADLs
- Improvement in ability to interact socially with peers
- Improvement in sleeping and eating habits

Ⓝ *NCLEX® Connection: Pharmacological and Parenteral Therapies, Medication Administration*

CHAPTER 25 *Medications for Children and Adolescents Who Have Mental Health Issues*

Various medications are used to manage behavioral disorders in children and adolescents. Parents should understand that pharmacological management is most effective when accompanied by techniques to modify behavior.

Medications include central nervous system (CNS) stimulants, selective reuptake inhibitors (SNRIs), tricyclic antidepressants (TCAs), alpha$_2$-adrenergic agonists, atypical antipsychotics, and selective serotonin reuptake inhibitors (SSRIs).

Other medications used to treat the manifestations of intermittent explosive disorder include lithium, mood-stabilizing antiepileptics, and beta-adrenergic blockers.

CNS stimulants

SELECT PROTOTYPE MEDICATION: Methylphenidate

OTHER MEDICATIONS
- Amphetamine mixture
- Dextroamphetamine

PURPOSE QEBP

EXPECTED PHARMACOLOGICAL ACTION: These medications raise the levels of norepinephrine, serotonin, and dopamine into the central nervous system.

THERAPEUTIC USES
- ADHD in children and adults

COMPLICATIONS

CNS stimulation (insomnia, restlessness)

NURSING CONSIDERATIONS
- Advise the client to observe for effects, and if they occur, instruct the client to notify the provider.
- Decrease dosage as prescribed.
- Administer the last dose of the day before 4 p.m.
- Advise client to decrease use of items that contain caffeine (coffee, tea, cola, chocolate)

Weight loss related to reduced appetite; growth suppression

NURSING CONSIDERATIONS
- Monitor the client's height and weight and compare to baseline height and weight.
- Administer medication right before or after meals.
- Encourage children to eat at regular meal times and to avoid unhealthy food choices.

Cardiovascular effects

- Dysrhythmias, chest pain, high blood pressure
- Can increase the risk of sudden death in clients who have heart abnormalities

NURSING CONSIDERATIONS
- Monitor vital signs and ECG.
- Advise clients to observe for effects and to notify the provider if they occur.

Development of psychotic manifestations, such as hallucinations and paranoia

NURSING CONSIDERATIONS: Instruct the client to report manifestations immediately and discontinue the medication.

Withdrawal reaction

NURSING CONSIDERATIONS: Advise the client to avoid abrupt cessation of the medication, as it could lead to depression and severe fatigue.

Hypersensitivity skin reaction to transdermal methylphenidate: hives, papules

NURSING CONSIDERATIONS: Advise the client to remove the patch and notify the provider.

CONTRAINDICATIONS/PRECAUTIONS

- Contraindicated in clients who have a history of substance use disorder, cardiovascular disorders, severe anxiety, and psychosis.
- CNS stimulants are Pregnancy Risk Category C.

INTERACTIONS

MAOIs

Concurrent use can cause hypertensive crisis.

NURSING CONSIDERATIONS: Avoid concurrent use.

Caffeine

Concurrent use can cause an increase in CNS stimulant effects.

NURSING CONSIDERATIONS: Instruct the client to avoid foods and beverages that contain caffeine.

Phenytoin warfarin and phenobarbital

Methylphenidate inhibits metabolism of these medications, leading to increased serum levels.

NURSING CONSIDERATIONS
- Monitor for adverse effects (CNS depression, signs of bleeding).
- Caution with concurrent use of these medications.

OTC cold and decongestant medications

Concurrent use can lead to increased CNS stimulation.

NURSING CONSIDERATIONS: Instruct the client to avoid the use of these OTC medications.

NURSING ADMINISTRATION Qpcc

- Advise clients to swallow sustained-release tablets whole and to not chew or crush them.
- Teach the client the importance of administering the medication on a regular schedule. Medications are available in regular or extended-release formulas.
- Oral medication should be given 30 to 45 min before meals, with the last dose of the day given by 4 p.m.
- Teach clients who use transdermal medication to place the patch on one hip daily in the morning, and leave it in place no longer than 9 hr. Alternate hips daily. Flush the patch down the toilet after removal.
- Advise parents that full response to medications can take up to 6 weeks.
- Teach client to avoid use of all OTC medications unless approved by the provider.
- Advise client to avoid alcohol use while taking this medication.
- Instruct parents and clients that ADHD is not cured by the medication. Management in conjunction with an overall treatment plan that includes family and cognitive therapy will improve outcomes. Qebp
- Instruct parents that these medications have special handling procedures controlled by federal law. Handwritten prescriptions are required for medication refills.
- Instruct parents regarding safety and storage of medications.
- Advise parents that use of these medications causes a high potential for development of a substance use disorder, especially in adolescents.

NURSING EVALUATION OF MEDICATION EFFECTIVENESS

Depending on therapeutic intent, effectiveness can be evidenced by improvement of manifestations of ADHD, such as an increased ability to focus and complete tasks, interact with peers, and manage impulsivity.

Selective norepinephrine reuptake inhibitor

SELECT PROTOTYPE MEDICATION: Atomoxetine

PURPOSE Qebp

EXPECTED PHARMACOLOGICAL ACTION: Block reuptake of norepinephrine at synapses in the CNS. Atomoxetine is not a stimulant medication.

THERAPEUTIC USES: ADHD in children and adults

COMPLICATIONS Qs

Usually tolerated well with minimal side effects

Appetite/growth suppression, weight loss

NURSING CONSIDERATIONS
- Monitor height and weight and compare to baseline.
- Administer medication right before meals.
- Encourage children to eat at regular meal times and avoid unhealthy food choices.

GI effects (nausea, vomiting, upper abdominal pain)

CLIENT EDUCATION: Advise the client to take the medication with food if GI effects occur.

Suicidal ideation (in children and adolescents)

NURSING CONSIDERATIONS
- Monitor the client for indications of depression.
- Advise the client to report changes in mood, excessive sleeping, agitation, and irritability.

Hepatotoxicity

CLIENT EDUCATION: Advise the client to report indications of liver damage, such as flu-like manifestations, yellowing skin, abdominal pain.

CNS effects (headache, insomnia, irritability)

NURSING CONSIDERATIONS
- Advise the client to observe for effects, instruct the client to notify the provider if they occur.
- Decrease dosage as prescribed.
- Administer the last dose of the day before 4 p.m.
- Advise client to decrease use of items that contain caffeine (coffee, tea, cola, chocolate).

CONTRAINDICATIONS/PRECAUTIONS

- Use cautiously in clients who have cardiovascular disorders. Qs
- Contraindicated in clients who have suicidal ideation.

INTERACTIONS

MAOIs

Concurrent use can cause hypertensive crisis.

NURSING CONSIDERATIONS
- Advise the client to avoid concurrent use.

Paroxetine, fluoxetine, or quinidine gluconate

These medications inhibit metabolizing enzymes, thereby increasing levels of atomoxetine.

NURSING CONSIDERATIONS
- Instruct the client to watch for and report increased adverse effects of atomoxetine.
- Concurrent use can require a reduction in the dosage of atomoxetine.

NURSING ADMINISTRATION

- Note any changes in the client related to dosing and timing of medications.
- Administer the medication in one daily dose in the morning or in two divided doses, morning and afternoon, with or without food.
- Instruct the client that therapeutic effect can take 1 to 3 weeks to fully develop.
- Advise client to avoid alcohol use while taking this medication.
- Teach client to avoid use of all OTC medications unless approved by provider.

NURSING EVALUATION OF MEDICATION EFFECTIVENESS

Depending on therapeutic intent, effectiveness can be evidenced by improvement of the manifestations of ADHD, such as increase in ability to focus and complete tasks, interact with peers, and manage impulsivity.

Tricyclic antidepressants

SELECT PROTOTYPE MEDICATION: Desipramine

OTHER MEDICATIONS
- Imipramine
- Clomipramine

PURPOSE

EXPECTED PHARMACOLOGICAL ACTION: These medications block reuptake of norepinephrine and serotonin in the synaptic space, thereby intensifying the effects of these neurotransmitters.

THERAPEUTIC USES IN CHILDREN
- Depression
- Autism spectrum disorder
- ADHD
- Panic disorder, separation anxiety disorder
- Social phobia, school phobia
- OCD

COMPLICATIONS Qs

Orthostatic hypotension

NURSING CONSIDERATIONS
- Monitor blood pressure with first dose.
- If orthostatic hypotension occurs, instruct the client to change positions slowly.

Anticholinergic effects

- Dry mouth
- Blurred vision
- Photophobia
- Urinary hesitancy or retention
- Constipation
- Tachycardia

CLIENT EDUCATION
- Instruct the client regarding ways to minimize anticholinergic effects.
  - Chewing sugarless gum
  - Sipping water
  - Avoiding hazardous activities
  - Wearing sunglasses when outdoors
  - Eating foods high in fiber
  - Participating in regular exercise
  - Increasing fluid intake to at least 2 to 3 L/day from beverages and other food sources
  - Voiding just before taking the medication
- Advise the client to notify the provider if effects become intolerable.

Weight gain related to increased appetite

CLIENT EDUCATION: Instruct the client to weigh weekly. Encourage the client to participate in regular exercise and to follow a healthy, low-calorie diet.

Sedation

CLIENT EDUCATION

- Advise the client that sedative effects should diminish over time.
- Advise the client to avoid hazardous activities, such as driving if sedation is excessive.
- Advise the client to take the medication at bedtime to minimize daytime sleepiness and to promote sleep. Taking the medication at bedtime minimizes side effects during the day.

Toxicity

Resulting in cholinergic blockade and cardiac toxicity evidenced by dysrhythmias, mental confusion, and agitation followed by seizures, coma, and possible death

NURSING CONSIDERATIONS

- Give a client who is acutely ill a 1-week supply of medication.
- Obtain baseline ECG.
- Monitor vital signs frequently.
- Monitor for toxicity.
- Notify the provider if indications of toxicity occur.

Decreased seizure threshold

NURSING CONSIDERATIONS: Monitor clients who have seizure disorders.

Excessive sweating

CLIENT EDUCATION: Inform the client of this adverse effect, and assist with frequent linen changes.

CONTRAINDICATIONS/PRECAUTIONS

- Desipramine and clomipramine are Pregnancy Risk Category C medications. Imipramine is a Pregnancy Risk Category D medication. Qs
- This medication is contraindicated for clients who have seizure disorders.
- Use this medication cautiously in clients who have coronary artery disease; diabetes; liver, kidney, and respiratory disorders; urinary retention and obstruction; angle closure glaucoma; benign prostatic hypertrophy; and hyperthyroidism.
- TCAs can increase suicide risk.

INTERACTIONS

MAOIs

Concurrent use can cause severe hypertension.

NURSING CONSIDERATIONS: Do not administer concurrently with MAOIs.

Antihistamines and other anticholinergic agents

Concurrent use can cause additive anticholinergic effects.

NURSING CONSIDERATIONS: Do not administer concurrently with antihistamines.

Epinephrine and dopamine (direct-acting sympathomimetics)

Concurrent use can cause hypertensive effect.

NURSING CONSIDERATIONS: Do not administer these medications concurrently with TCAs.

Alcohol, benzodiazepines, opioids, and antihistamines

Concurrent use can cause additive CNS depression.

NURSING CONSIDERATIONS: Advise the client to avoid other CNS depressants while taking a TCA.

NURSING ADMINISTRATION Qpcc

- Instruct the client's parents to administer this medication as prescribed on a daily basis to establish therapeutic plasma levels.
- Assist with medication regimen adherence by informing the client and parents that it can take 1 to 3 weeks to experience therapeutic effects. Full therapeutic effects can take 2 to 3 months.
- Instruct the client and parents on the importance of continuing therapy after improvement in manifestations. Sudden discontinuation of the medication can result in relapse.
- Due to high suicide potential, give only a 1-week supply of medication for a client who is acutely ill, and then only give a 1-month supply of medication at a time. Qs

NURSING EVALUATION OF MEDICATION EFFECTIVENESS

Depending on therapeutic intent, effectiveness can be evidenced by the following.

FOR CLIENTS WHO HAVE DEPRESSION

- Verbalization of improvement in mood.
- Improved sleeping and eating habits
- Increased interaction with peers

FOR CLIENTS WHO HAVE AUTISM SPECTRUM DISORDER

- Decreased anger
- Decreased compulsive behavior

FOR CLIENTS WHO HAVE ADHD

- Decreased hyperactivity
- Greater ability to pay attention

FOR CLIENTS WHO HAVE OCD, PANIC, AND ANXIETY DISORDERS

- Reduced levels of anxiety
- Increased ability to recognize symptoms and triggers of disorder
- Ability to manage episodes of disorder
- Ability to perform self-care
- Increased interaction with peers
- Ability to assume usual role

Alpha₂-adrenergic agonists

SELECT PROTOTYPE MEDICATION: **Guanfacine**

OTHER MEDICATION: Clonidine

PURPOSE Q EBP

EXPECTED PHARMACOLOGICAL ACTION: The action of alpha₂-adrenergic agonists is not completely understood, however they are known to activate presynaptic alpha₂-adrenergic receptors within the brain.

THERAPEUTIC USES: ADHD

COMPLICATIONS

CNS effects (sedation, drowsiness, fatigue)

NURSING CONSIDERATIONS
- Monitor for these adverse effects and report their occurrence to the provider.
- Advise clients to avoid hazardous activities

Cardiovascular effects (hypotension, bradycardia)

NURSING CONSIDERATIONS
- Monitor blood pressure and pulse, especially during initial treatment.
- Advise clients not to abruptly discontinue medication, which can cause rebound hypertension.

Weight gain

NURSING CONSIDERATIONS
- Monitor clients' weight.
- Encourage clients to participate in regular exercise and to follow a healthy, well-balanced diet.

GI effects

Nausea, vomiting, constipation, dry mouth

NURSING CONSIDERATIONS
- Monitor for these adverse effects and report their occurrence to the provider.
- Suggest that the client use the following strategies to prevent or minimize GI effects.
  - Chewing sugarless gum
  - Sipping water
  - Eating foods high in fiber
  - Participating in regular exercise
  - Increasing fluid intake to at least 2 to 3 L/day from beverages and other food sources

CONTRAINDICATIONS/PRECAUTIONS

- Extended-release clonidine is contraindicated for children younger than 6 years old.
- Use cautiously in clients who have cardiac disease. Q S

INTERACTIONS

CNS depressants, including alcohol, can increase CNS effects.
NURSING CONSIDERATIONS: Avoid concurrent use.

Antihypertensives can worsen hypotension.
NURSING CONSIDERATIONS: Avoid concurrent use.

Foods with high-fat content increase guanfacine absorption.
NURSING CONSIDERATIONS: Advise clients to avoid taking medication with a high-fat meal.

NURSING ADMINISTRATION

- Assess use of alcohol and CNS depressants, especially with adolescent clients. Q PCC
- Instruct clients to not chew, crush, or split extended-release preparations.
- Monitor blood pressure and pulse at baseline, with initial treatment, and with each dosage change.
- Advise clients to avoid abrupt discontinuation of medication, which can result in rebound hypertension. Medication should be tapered according to a prescribed dosage schedule when discontinuing treatment.

NURSING EVALUATION OF MEDICATION EFFECTIVENESS

Depending on therapeutic intent, effectiveness can be evidenced by improvement of manifestations of ADHD such as increase in ability to focus and complete tasks, interact with peers, and manage impulsivity.

Atypical antipsychotics

SELECT PROTOTYPE MEDICATION: Risperidone

OTHER MEDICATION: Olanzapine

PURPOSE Q EBP

EXPECTED PHARMACOLOGICAL ACTION

These antipsychotic agents work mainly by blocking serotonin, and to a lesser degree, dopamine receptors. These medications also block receptors for norepinephrine, histamine, and acetylcholine.

THERAPEUTIC USES

- Pervasive development disorders (PDD), including autism spectrum disorder
- Conduct disorder
- OCD
- Relief of psychotic manifestations

COMPLICATIONS

Diabetes mellitus

New onset of diabetes or loss of glucose control in clients who have diabetes

NURSING CONSIDERATIONS
- Obtain baseline fasting blood glucose, and monitor periodically throughout treatment.
- Instruct the client to report indications such as increased thirst, urination, and appetite.

Weight gain

CLIENT EDUCATION: Advise the client to follow a healthy, low-calorie diet; engage in regular exercise; and monitor weight gain.

Hypercholesterolemia

With increased risk for hypertension and other cardiovascular disease

NURSING CONSIDERATIONS: Monitor cholesterol, triglycerides, and blood glucose if weight gain is more than 14 kg (30 lb).

Orthostatic hypotension

NURSING CONSIDERATIONS: Monitor blood pressure with first dose, and instruct the client to change positions slowly if orthostatic hypotension occurs.

Anticholinergic effects

Urinary retention or hesitancy, dry mouth

NURSING CONSIDERATIONS
- Monitor for these adverse effects, and report their occurrence to the provider.
- Encourage clients to use measures to relieve dry mouth, such as sipping fluids throughout the day.

Agitation, dizziness, sedation, and sleep disruption

NURSING CONSIDERATIONS
- Monitor for these adverse effects and report their occurrence to the provider.
- Administer an alternative medication if prescribed.

Mild extrapyramidal side effects, such as tremor

NURSING CONSIDERATIONS: Monitor for and teach clients to recognize EPS. These effects are usually dose related.

CONTRAINDICATIONS/PRECAUTIONS

- Be aware of possible alcohol use in the adolescent client. Instruct clients to avoid the use of alcohol. Qs
- Use cautiously in clients who have cardiovascular disease, seizures, or diabetes. Clients who have diabetes should have a baseline fasting blood sugar, and blood glucose should be monitored carefully.

INTERACTIONS

CNS depressants
- Additive CNS depression occurs with concurrent use of alcohol, opioids, antihistamines.
- NURSING CONSIDERATIONS
  - Advise the client to avoid alcohol and other medications that cause CNS depression.
  - Advise the client to avoid hazardous activities, such as driving.

Levodopa
- By activating dopamine receptors, levodopa counteracts the effects of antipsychotic agents.
- NURSING CONSIDERATIONS: Avoid concurrent use of levodopa and other direct dopamine receptor agonists.

TCAs, amiodarone, and clarithromycin prolong QT interval, thereby increasing the risk of cardiac dysrhythmias.
NURSING CONSIDERATIONS: Avoid concurrent use of these medications.

Barbiturates and phenytoin promote hepatic drug-metabolizing enzymes, thereby decreasing drug levels of quetiapine.
NURSING CONSIDERATIONS: Monitor medication for effectiveness.

Fluconazole inhibits hepatic drug-metabolizing enzymes, thereby increasing drug levels of aripiprazole, quetiapine, and ziprasidone.
NURSING CONSIDERATIONS: Monitor for adverse medication effects.

NURSING ADMINISTRATION Qpcc

- Administer by oral or IM route.
  - Risperidone is available in an oral solution and quick-dissolving tablets for ease in administration.
  - Olanzapine is available in an orally disintegrating tablet for ease in administration.
- Advise clients that low doses of medication are given initially and are then gradually increased.
- Medications may be taken without regard to food.

NURSING EVALUATION OF MEDICATION EFFECTIVENESS

Depending on therapeutic intent, effectiveness can be evidenced by the following.

FOR CLIENTS WHO HAVE PPD
- Reduction of hyperactivity
- Improvement in mood

FOR CLIENTS WHO HAVE CONDUCT DISORDER: Decreased aggressiveness

FOR CLIENTS WHO HAVE OCD
- Reduced levels of anxiety
- Ability to manage compulsive actions
- Ability to perform self-care
- Increased interaction with peers
- Ability to assume usual role

Selective serotonin reuptake inhibitors

SELECT PROTOTYPE MEDICATION: Fluoxetine

PURPOSE Q_{EBP}

EXPECTED PHARMACOLOGICAL ACTION: SSRIs work by blocking the synaptic reuptake of serotonin, allowing more serotonin to stay at the junction of the neurons.

THERAPEUTIC USE: Intermittent explosive disorder

COMPLICATIONS

Agitation, anxiety, sleep disturbance, tremors, and tension headache

NURSING CONSIDERATIONS: Monitor for these adverse effects and report their occurrence to the provider.

Weight loss

NURSING CONSIDERATIONS
- Instruct the client to weigh weekly and report any significant weight loss to the provider.
- Encourage the client to follow a healthy diet.

GI effects

Nausea, constipation or diarrhea, dry mouth

NURSING CONSIDERATIONS
- Monitor for these adverse effects and report their occurrence to the provider.
- Encourage client to use measures to relieve dry mouth, such as sipping fluids throughout the day, chewing sugarless gum.

CONTRAINDICATIONS/PRECAUTIONS

- Paroxetine can increase suicidal ideation in children and adolescents. Q_s
- Abrupt withdrawal of medication can lead to discontinuation syndrome (dizziness, insomnia, nervousness, irritability, agitation). Dose should be tapered.

INTERACTIONS

Concurrent use of MAOIs or St. John's wort can cause serotonin syndrome.
NURSING CONSIDERATIONS
- Advise the client to avoid concurrent use
- Advise client to allow 2 weeks between fluoxetine and MAOI use.

NURSING ADMINISTRATION

- Advise the client that SSRIs may be taken with food. Sleep disturbances are minimized by taking the medication in the morning. Q_{EBP}
- Instruct the client to take the medication on a daily basis to establish therapeutic plasma levels.
- Assist the client with medication regimen adherence by informing the client that it can take up to 4 weeks to achieve therapeutic effects.
- Sustained-release tablets should be taken whole and not chewed or crushed.

NURSING EVALUATION OF MEDICATION EFFECTIVENESS

Depending on therapeutic intent, effectiveness can be evidenced by the following.

FOR CLIENTS WHO HAVE INTERMITTENT EXPLOSIVE DISORDER
- Reduction of hyperactivity
- Improvement in mood

FOR CLIENTS WHO HAVE CONDUCT DISORDER:
Decreased aggressiveness

Application Exercises

1. A nurse is teaching the parents of a child who has autism spectrum disorder and a new prescription for imipramine about indications of toxicity. Which of the following should the nurse include in the teaching? (Select all that apply.)

   A. Seizures

   B. Agitation

   C. Photophobia

   D. Dry mouth

   E. Irregular pulse

2. A nurse is providing teaching to an adolescent client who has a new prescription for clomipramine for OCD. Which of the following information should the nurse provide?

   A. Eat a diet high in fiber.

   B. Check temperature daily.

   C. Take medication first thing in the morning before eating.

   D. Add extra calories to the diet as between-meal snacks.

3. A nurse is providing teaching to an adolescent client who is to begin taking atomoxetine for ADHD. The nurse should instruct the client to monitor for which of the following adverse effects? (Select all that apply.)

   A. Somnolence

   B. Yellowing skin

   C. Increased appetite

   D. Fever

   E. Malaise

4. A nurse is caring for a school age child who has conduct disorder and a new prescription for methylphenidate transdermal patches. Which of the following information should the nurse provide about the medication?

   A. Apply the patch once daily at bedtime.

   B. Place the patch carefully in a trash can after removal.

   C. Apply the transdermal patch to the anterior waist area.

   D. Remove the patch each day after 9 hr.

5. A nurse is teaching a client who has intermittent explosive disorder about a new prescription for fluoxetine. Which of the following information should the nurse provide? (Select all that apply.)

   A. An adverse effect of this medication is CNS depression.

   B. Administer the medication in the morning.

   C. Monitor for weight loss while taking this medication.

   D. Therapeutic effects of this medication will take 1 to 3 weeks to fully develop.

   E. This medication blocks the blocking the synaptic reuptake of serotonin in the brain.

PRACTICE Active Learning Scenario

A nurse working in a pediatric mental health clinic is caring for a client who has a new prescription for olanzapine for the treatment of OCD. Use the ATI Active Learning Template: Medication to complete this item.

COMPLICATIONS: Identify at least four adverse effects of this medication.

NURSING INTERVENTIONS: Identify at least four nursing interventions to prevent or minimize the adverse effects of this medication.

Application Exercises Key

1. A. **CORRECT:** Seizures are an indication of TCA toxicity.

   B. **CORRECT:** Agitation is an indication of TCA toxicity.

   C. Photophobia is an anticholinergic effect rather than an indication of TCA toxicity.

   D. Dry mouth is an anticholinergic effect rather than an indication of TCA toxicity.

   E. **CORRECT:** Irregular pulse can indicate a dysrhythmia which is an indication of TCA toxicity.

   Ⓝ NCLEX® Connection: Pharmacological and Parenteral Therapies, Adverse Effects/Contraindications/Side Effects/Interactions

2. A. **CORRECT:** Eating a diet high in fiber will decrease constipation, an anticholinergic effect associated with TCA use.

   B. Checking the client's temperature daily is not necessary while taking a TCA.

   C. Taking the medication at bedtime rather than in the morning is appropriate to prevent daytime sleepiness.

   D. Following a well-balanced diet plan rather than adding extra calories as snacks will help prevent weight gain, a common adverse effect of TCAs.

   Ⓝ NCLEX® Connection: Pharmacological and Parenteral Therapies, Medication Administration

3. A. Insomnia, rather than somnolence, is an adverse effect that the client should report to the provider.

   B. **CORRECT:** Yellowing skin is a potential indication of hepatotoxicity that the client should report to the provider.

   C. Decreased appetite with resulting weight loss, rather than increased appetite, is a potential adverse effect that the client should report to the provider.

   D. **CORRECT:** Fever is a potential indication of hepatotoxicity that the client should report to the provider.

   E. **CORRECT:** Malaise is a potential indication of hepatotoxicity that the client should report to the provider.

   Ⓝ NCLEX® Connection: Pharmacological and Parenteral Therapies, Adverse Effects/Contraindications/Side Effects/Interactions

4. A. The transdermal patch is applied once daily in the morning.

   B. For safety when discarding the transdermal preparation, the client should fold the patch and flush it down the toilet to prevent others from using it.

   C. The transdermal patch should be applied to a clean, dry area on the hip, and the waist area should be avoided.

   D. **CORRECT:** The transdermal patch is applied once daily in the morning and is removed after 9 hr.

   Ⓝ NCLEX® Connection: Pharmacological and Parenteral Therapies, Medication Administration

5. A. An adverse effect of fluoxetine is CNS stimulation rather than CNS depression.

   B. **CORRECT:** Fluoxetine should be administered in the morning due to the potential for insomnia.

   C. **CORRECT:** Fluoxetine can result in weight loss.

   D. Fluoxetine takes 4 weeks to fully develop therapeutic effects.

   E. **CORRECT:** Fluoxetine works by blocking the synaptic reuptake of serotonin, allowing more serotonin to stay at the junction of the neurons.

   Ⓝ NCLEX® Connection: Pharmacological and Parenteral Therapies, Medication Administration

---

PRACTICE Answer

Using the ATI Active Learning Template: Medication

COMPLICATIONS

- New onset of diabetes mellitus or loss of glucose control in clients who have diabetes
- Weight gain
- Hypercholesterolemia
- Orthostatic hypotension
- Anticholinergic effects (urinary hesitancy or retention, dry mouth)
- Agitation
- Dizziness
- Sedation
- Sleep disruption
- Tremors

NURSING INTERVENTIONS

- Measure the client's fasting blood glucose prior to and periodically throughout treatment.
- Instruct the client to report indications of diabetes mellitus, including increased thirst, urination, and appetite.
- Advise clients to follow a healthy, well-balanced diet.
- Recommend regular exercise.
- Monitor weight throughout treatment.
- Monitor cholesterol and triglycerides, especially if weight gain is more than 30 lb.
- Monitor blood pressure with first dose, and instruct client to change positions slowly.
- Encourage the client to sip fluids throughout the day.

Ⓝ NCLEX® Connection: Pharmacological and Parenteral Therapies, Medication Administration

UNIT 4   PSYCHOPHARMACOLOGICAL THERAPIES

CHAPTER 26   *Medications for Substance Use Disorders*

Abstinence syndrome occurs when a client abruptly withdraws from a substance on which he is physically dependent.

Clients who have a substance use disorder can experience tolerance and withdrawal. Tolerance is requiring increased amounts of the substance to achieve the desired effect. Withdrawal is the physiological manifestations that occur when the concentration of the substance in the client's bloodstream declines. Withdrawing from a substance that has the potential to cause abstinence syndrome can cause the client to experience distressing manifestations that are potentially life-threatening.

WITHDRAWAL MANIFESTATIONS

Alcohol

- Manifestations usually start within 4 to 12 hr of the last intake of alcohol and can continue 5 to 7 days.
- Common manifestations include nausea; vomiting; tremors; restlessness and inability to sleep; depressed mood or irritability; increased heart rate, blood pressure, respiratory rate, and temperature; diaphoresis; tonic-clonic seizures; and illusions.
- Alcohol withdrawal delirium can occur 2 to 3 days after cessation of alcohol. This is considered a medical emergency. Manifestations include severe disorientation, psychotic effects (hallucinations), severe hypertension, cardiac dysrhythmias, and delirium. This type of withdrawal can progress to death.

Opioids

- Withdrawal manifestations occur within hours to several days after cessation of opioid use.
- Common findings include agitation, insomnia, flu-like manifestations, rhinorrhea, yawning, sweating, and diarrhea.
- Withdrawal manifestations are not life-threatening, but suicidal ideation can occur.

Tobacco (nicotine)

Abstinence syndrome is evidenced by irritability, nervousness, restlessness, insomnia, and difficulty concentrating.

> Other substances associated with substance use disorder include cannabis, hallucinogens, inhalants, sedatives/hypnotics, and stimulants.

Alcohol

WITHDRAWAL

Benzodiazepines

- Chlordiazepoxide
- Diazepam
- Lorazepam
- Oxazepam

INTENDED EFFECTS
- Maintenance of vital signs within expected reference ranges
- Decrease in the risk of seizures
- Decrease in the intensity of withdrawal manifestations
- Substitution therapy during alcohol withdrawal

NURSING CONSIDERATIONS
- Administer around-the-clock or PRN.
- Obtain baseline vital signs.
- Monitor vital signs and neurological status on an ongoing basis.
- Provide for seizure precautions.

Adjunct medications

- Carbamazepine
- Clonidine
- Propranolol
- Atenolol

INTENDED EFFECTS
- Decrease in seizures: Carbamazepine
- Depression of autonomic response (decrease in blood pressure, heart rate): Clonidine, propranolol, atenolol
- Decrease in craving: Propranolol, atenolol

NURSING CONSIDERATIONS
- Provide seizure precautions. Qs
- Obtain baseline vital signs, and continue to monitor on an ongoing basis.
- Check heart rate prior to administration of propranolol, and withhold if less than 60/min.

ABSTINENCE MAINTENANCE

Following withdrawal

Disulfiram

INTENDED EFFECTS
- Disulfiram is a daily oral medication that is a type of aversion (behavioral) therapy.
- Disulfiram used concurrently with alcohol will cause acetaldehyde syndrome to occur. Effects include nausea, vomiting, weakness, sweating, palpitations, and hypotension. Acetaldehyde syndrome can progress to respiratory depression, cardiovascular suppression, seizures, and death.

NURSING CONSIDERATIONS
- Inform the client of the potential dangers of drinking any alcohol.
- Advise the client to avoid any products that contain alcohol (cough syrup, aftershave lotion, mouthwash, hand sanitizer).
- Encourage the client to wear a medical alert bracelet.
- Encourage the client to participate in a 12-step program. Qᴘᴄᴄ
- Advise the client that medication effects, such as the potential for acetaldehyde syndrome with alcohol ingestion, persist for 2 weeks following discontinuation of disulfiram.
- Monitor liver function tests to detect hepatotoxicity.

Naltrexone

INTENDED EFFECTS: Naltrexone is a pure opioid antagonist that suppresses the craving and pleasurable effects of alcohol (also used for opioid withdrawal).

NURSING CONSIDERATIONS
- Assess the client's history to determine whether the client is also dependent on opioids. Concurrent use increases the risk for a client overdose of opiates.
- Advise the client to take naltrexone with meals to decrease gastrointestinal distress.
- Suggest monthly IM injections of depot naltrexone for clients who have difficulty adhering to the medication regimen.

Acamprosate

INTENDED EFFECTS: Acamprosate is taken orally three times a day to reduce the unpleasant effects of abstinence (dysphoria, anxiety, restlessness).

NURSING CONSIDERATIONS
- Inform the client that diarrhea can result. Advise the client to maintain adequate fluid intake to prevent dehydration.
- Advise the client to avoid use in pregnancy.

Opioids

Methadone substitution

INTENDED EFFECTS
- Methadone substitution is an oral opioid agonist that replaces the opioid to which the client is has a physical dependence.
- Methadone administration prevents abstinence syndrome from occurring and removes the need for the client to obtain illegal opioids.
- Methadone substitution is used for withdrawal and long-term maintenance.
- Dependence is transferred from the illegal opioid to methadone.

NURSING CONSIDERATIONS
- Encourage the client to participate in a 12-step program.
- Inform clients that the methadone dose must be slowly tapered to produce detoxification.
- Inform the client that the medication must be administered from an approved treatment center.

Clonidine

INTENDED EFFECTS
- Clonidine assists with withdrawal effects related to autonomic hyperactivity (diarrhea, nausea, vomiting).
- Clonidine therapy does not reduce the craving for opioids.

NURSING CONSIDERATIONS
- Obtain baseline vital signs.
- Advise the client to avoid activities that require mental alertness until drowsiness subsides.
- Encourage the client to chew sugarless gum or suck on hard candy, and to sip on small amounts of water or suck on ice chips to treat dry mouth.

Buprenorphine

INTENDED EFFECTS
- Buprenorphine is an agonist-antagonist opioid used for both withdrawal and maintenance.
- This medication decreases feelings of craving and can be effective in maintaining compliance.

NURSING CONSIDERATIONS
- Unlike methadone, a primary care provider can prescribe and dispense buprenorphine.
- Administer the medication sublingually.

Nicotine

Bupropion

INTENDED EFFECTS: Bupropion decreases nicotine craving and manifestations of withdrawal.

NURSING CONSIDERATIONS

- To treat dry mouth, encourage the client to chew sugarless gum, suck on hard candy, sip on small amounts of water, or suck on ice chips.
- Advise the client to avoid caffeine and other CNS stimulants to control insomnia.

Nicotine replacement therapy

Nicotine gum, nicotine patch, nicotine nasal spray, nicotine lozenges, nicotine inhaler

INTENDED EFFECTS

- Nicotine replacements are pharmaceutical product substitutes for the nicotine in cigarettes or chewing tobacco.
- The rate of tobacco use cessation is nearly doubled with the use of nicotine replacements. Q̲EBP

NURSING CONSIDERATIONS

- Nasal spray provides pleasurable effects of smoking due to rapid rise of the nicotine level in the client's blood.
- Nicotine nasal spray is not recommended for clients who have disorders affecting the upper respiratory system such as chronic sinus problems, allergies, or asthma.
- Avoid the use of nicotine inhalers in clients who have asthma.
- Gradually taper nicotine inhaler use over 2 to 3 months and then discontinue.

CLIENT EDUCATION

- Advise the client to chew nicotine gum slowly and intermittently over 30 min.
- Tell the client to avoid eating or drinking 15 min prior to and while chewing nicotine gum.
- Teach the client that use of nicotine gum is not recommended for longer than 6 months.
- Tell the client to apply a nicotine patch to an area of clean, dry skin each day.
- Advise the client to avoid using any nicotine products while wearing the patch.
- Teach the client to remove the nicotine patch and notify the provider if a local skin reaction occurs.
- Remind the client to remove the nicotine patch prior to magnetic resonance imaging (MRI).
- Tell the client that one spray in each nostril delivers the amount of nicotine in one cigarette.
- Advise client to follow product instructions for dosage of nasal spray frequency.
- Tell the client to avoid oral intake 15 min prior to or during nicotine lozenge use.
- Teach the client to allow nicotine lozenges to slowly dissolve in the mouth (20 to 30 min).
- Teach the client to avoid using any nicotine products while pregnant or breastfeeding.

Varenicline

INTENDED EFFECTS: Varenicline is a nicotinic receptor agonist that promotes the release of dopamine to simulate the pleasurable effects of nicotine.

- Reduces cravings for nicotine as well as the severity of withdrawal manifestations
- Reduces the incidence of relapse by blocking the desired effects of nicotine

NURSING CONSIDERATIONS

- Instruct the client to take medication after a meal.
- Monitor blood pressure during treatment.
- Monitor clients who have diabetes mellitus for loss of glycemic control.
- Follow instructions for titration to minimize adverse effects.
- Can cause neuropsychiatric effects such as unpredictable behavior, mood changes, and thoughts of suicide. Advise the client to notify the provider if nausea, vomiting, insomnia, new-onset depression, or suicidal thoughts occur.
- Due to potential adverse effects, varenicline is banned for use in clients who are commercial truck or bus drivers, air traffic controllers, or airplane pilots. Q̲s

NURSING EVALUATION OF MEDICATION EFFECTIVENESS

Depending on therapeutic intent, effectiveness can be evidenced by the following.

- Absence of injury
- Ongoing abstinence from the substance
- Regular attendance at a 12-step program
- Decreased cravings for substance
- Improved coping skills to replace use of substance

Application Exercises

1. A nurse is providing teaching to a client who has alcohol use disorder and a new prescription for carbamazepine. Which of the following information should the nurse include in the teaching?

   A. "This medication will help prevent seizures during alcohol withdrawal."

   B. "Taking this medication will decrease your cravings for alcohol."

   C. "This medication maintains your blood pressure at a normal level during alcohol withdrawal."

   D. "Taking this medication will improve your ability to maintain abstinence from alcohol."

2. A nurse is assisting in the discharge planning for a client following alcohol detoxification. The nurse should anticipate prescriptions for which of the following medications to promote long-term abstinence from alcohol? (Select all that apply.)

   A. Lorazepam

   B. Diazepam

   C. Disulfiram

   D. Naltrexone

   E. Acamprosate

3. A nurse is evaluating a client's understanding of a new prescription for clonidine for the treatment of opioid use disorder. Which of the following statements by the client indicates an understanding of the teaching?

   A. "Taking this medication will help reduce my craving for heroin."

   B. "While taking this medication, I should keep a pack of sugarless gum."

   C. "I can expect some diarrhea from taking this medicine."

   D. "Each dose of this medication should be placed under my tongue to dissolve."

4. A nurse is teaching a client who has tobacco use disorder about the use of nicotine gum. Which of the following information should the nurse include in the teaching?

   A. Chew the gum for no more than 10 min.

   B. Rinse out the mouth immediately before chewing the gum.

   C. Avoid eating 15 min prior to chewing the gum.

   D. Use of the gum is limited to 90 days.

5. A nurse is discussing the use of methadone with a newly licensed nurse. Which of the following statements by the newly licensed nurse indicates an understanding of the teaching? (Select all that apply.)

   A. "Methadone is a replacement for physical dependence to opioids."

   B. "Methadone reduces the unpleasant effects associated with abstinence syndrome."

   C. "Methadone can be used during opioid withdrawal and to maintain abstinence."

   D. "Methadone increases the risk for acetaldehyde syndrome."

   E. "Methadone must be prescribed and dispensed by an approved treatment center."

PRACTICE Active Learning Scenario

A nurse working in an outpatient clinic is teaching a client who has tobacco use disorder about the use of varenicline. Use the ATI Active Learning Template: Medication to complete this item.

EXPECTED PHARMACOLOGICAL ACTION

THERAPEUTIC USES

NURSING INTERVENTIONS: Identify at least three.

Application Exercises Key

1. A. **CORRECT:** Carbamazepine is used during withdrawal to decrease the risk for seizures.

   B. Carbamazepine is used to promote safe withdrawal rather than to decrease cravings for alcohol.

   C. Clonidine or propranolol is used during withdrawal to depress the autonomic response and its effect on blood pressure.

   D. Carbamazepine is used to promote safe withdrawal rather than abstinence.

   Ⓝ *NCLEX® Connection: Pharmacological and Parenteral Therapies, Medication Administration*

2. A. Lorazepam is prescribed for short-term use during withdrawal.

   B. Diazepam is prescribed for short-term use during withdrawal.

   C. **CORRECT:** Disulfiram promotes abstinence through aversion therapy.

   D. **CORRECT:** Naltrexone promotes abstinence by suppressing the craving and pleasurable effects of alcohol.

   E. **CORRECT:** Acamprosate decreases the unpleasant effects resulting from abstinence.

   Ⓝ *NCLEX® Connection: Psychosocial Integrity, Chemical and Other Dependencies/Substance Use Disorder*

3. A. Clonidine is useful during opioid withdrawal. However, it does not reduce cravings.

   B. **CORRECT:** Clonidine commonly causes clients to experience dry mouth. Chewing sugarless gum is an effective method to address this adverse effect.

   C. Clonidine reduces, rather than causes, diarrhea and other withdrawal manifestations related to autonomic hyperactivity.

   D. Buprenorphine, rather than clonidine, is administered sublingually.

   Ⓝ *NCLEX® Connection: Pharmacological and Parenteral Therapies, Medication Administration*

4. A. The client should chew the gum slowly and intermittently over 30 min.

   B. The client should avoid drinking 15 min prior to chewing the gum.

   C. **CORRECT:** The client should avoid eating or drinking 15 min prior to and while chewing the gum.

   D. Use of nicotine gum is not recommended for longer than 6 months.

   Ⓝ *NCLEX® Connection: Pharmacological and Parenteral Therapies, Medication Administration*

5. A. **CORRECT:** Methadone substitution is an oral opioid agonist that replaces the opioid to which the client has a physical dependence.

   B. **CORRECT:** Methadone administration prevents abstinence syndrome from occurring.

   C. **CORRECT:** Methadone substitution is used for both opioid withdrawal and long-term maintenance.

   D. Disulfiram, rather than methadone, places the client at risk for acetaldehyde syndrome if the client consumes alcohol while taking the medication.

   E. **CORRECT:** Due to the risk for physical dependence, methadone is required to be prescribed and dispensed by an approved treatment center.

   Ⓝ *NCLEX® Connection: Pharmacological and Parenteral Therapies, Medication Administration*

PRACTICE Answer

Using the ATI Active Learning Template: Medication

EXPECTED PHARMACOLOGICAL ACTION: Varenicline is a nicotinic receptor agonist that promotes the release of dopamine to simulate the pleasurable effects of nicotine.

THERAPEUTIC USES: Varenicline is used to reduce cravings for nicotine as well as the severity of withdrawal manifestations. Varenicline also reduces the incidence of relapse by blocking the desired effects of nicotine.

NURSING INTERVENTIONS
- Instruct the client to take medication after a meal.
- Monitor blood pressure during treatment.
- Assess for diabetes mellitus.
- Monitor clients who have diabetes mellitus for loss of glycemic control.
- Advise the client to follow instructions for titration to minimize adverse effects.
- Advise the client to notify the provider if nausea, vomiting, insomnia, new-onset depression, or suicidal thoughts occur.
- Determine if the client is a commercial truck or bus driver, air traffic controller, or airplane pilot.

Ⓝ *NCLEX® Connection: Pharmacological and Parenteral Therapies, Medication Administration*

When reviewing the following chapters, keep in mind the relevant topics and tasks of the NCLEX outline, in particular:

Client Needs: Psychosocial Integrity

END-OF-LIFE CARE
Assist the client in resolution of end–of–life issues.

Identify end of life needs of the client.

GRIEF AND LOSS
Assist the client in coping with suffering, grief, loss, dying, and bereavement.

Inform the client of expected reactions to grief and loss.

MENTAL HEALTH CONCEPTS
Provide care and education for acute and chronic psychosocial health issues.

Evaluate the client's ability to adhere to the treatment plan.

Client Needs: Health Promotion and Maintenance

AGING PROCESS: Provide care and education for the preschool, school age and adolescent client ages 3 through 17 years.

DEVELOPMENTAL STAGES AND TRANSITIONS: Compare client development to expected age/developmental stage and report and deviations.

HIGH RISK BEHAVIORS: Provide information for prevention and treatment of high risk health behaviors.

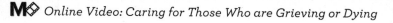
UNIT 5   SPECIFIC POPULATIONS

CHAPTER 27   *Care of Clients Who are Dying and/or Grieving*

Clients experience loss in many aspects of their lives. Grief is the inner emotional response to loss and is exhibited in as many ways as there are individuals.

Bereavement includes both grief and mourning (the outward display of loss) as a person deals with the death of a significant individual. Bereavement can result in depression. A bereavement exclusion was previously used when a client experienced manifestations of depression within the first 2 months after a significant loss. Now, a client can receive a diagnosis of depression during this time so that needed treatment is not delayed.

Palliative, or end-of-life, care is an important aspect of nursing care that attempts to meet the client's physical and psychosocial needs. End-of-life issues include decision-making in a highly stressful time during which the nurse must consider the desires of the client and the family. Qpcc

Any decisions must be shared with other health care personnel for a smooth transition during this time of stress, grief, and bereavement.

TYPES OF LOSS

Necessary loss: Part of the cycle of life; anticipated, but can still be intensely felt

Actual loss: Any loss of a valued person or item

Perceived loss: Any loss defined by a client that is not obvious to others

Maturational loss: Losses normally expected due to the developmental processing of life

Situational loss: Unanticipated loss caused by an external event

THEORIES OF GRIEF

The mental health care nurse should be aware of the various theories of grief. Though multiple theories are present they each tend to identify the same underlying feelings that the client who is grieving experiences.

Kübler-Ross: Five stages of grief

Client might not experience the stages in order, and the length of each stage will vary from person to person. QEBP

Denial: The client has difficulty believing a terminal diagnosis or loss.

Anger: Anger is directed toward self, others, or objects.

Bargaining: The client negotiates for more time or a cure.

Depression: The client mourns and directly confronts feelings related to the loss.

Acceptance: The client accepts what is happening and plans for the future.

Bowlby: Four stages of grief

Identifies behaviors that are observed in clients who are grieving. These stages are present in clients as young as 6 months of age.

Numbness or protest: The client is in denial over the reality of the loss and experiences feelings of shock.

Disequilibrium: The client focuses on the loss and has an intense desire to regain what was lost.

Disorganization and despair: The client feels hopelessness which impacts the client's ability to carry out tasks of daily living.

Reorganization: The client reaches acceptance of the loss.

Engel: Five stages of grief

Shock and disbelief: The client experiences a sense of numbness and denial over the loss.

Developing awareness: The client becomes aware of the reality of the loss resulting in intense feelings of grief. This begins within hours of the loss.

Restitution: The client carries out cultural/religious rituals, such as a funeral, following the loss.

Resolution of the loss: The client is preoccupied with the loss. Over about a 12 month time period this preoccupation gradually decreases.

Recovery: The client moves past the preoccupation and forward with life.

Worden: Four Tasks of Mourning

Completion of all four tasks generally takes about a year, but this can also vary from person to person.

Task I: Accepting the reality of the loss.

Task II: Processing the pain of grief. The client uses coping mechanisms to deal with the emotional pain of the loss.

Task III: Adjusting to a world without the lost entity. The client changes the environment to accommodate the absence of the deceased.

Task IV: Finding an enduring connection with the lost entity in the midst of embarking on a new life. The client finds a way to keep the lost entity a part of her life while at the same time moving forward with life and establishing new relationships.

FACTORS INFLUENCING LOSS, GRIEF, AND COPING ABILITY

- An individual's current stage of development
- Interpersonal relationships and social support network
- Type and significance of the loss
- Culture and ethnicity
- Spiritual and religious beliefs and practices
- Prior experience with loss
- Socioeconomic status

RISK FACTORS FOR MALADAPTIVE GRIEVING

- Being dependent upon the deceased
- Unexpected death at a young age, through violence, or by a socially unacceptable manner
- Inadequate coping skills or lack of social support
- Pre-existing mental health issues, such as depression or substance use disorder

NURSING CONSIDERATIONS

- Clients who are experiencing a maladaptive grief response commonly experience a loss of self-esteem and a sense of worthlessness not associated with normal grief.
- The nurse should assess the client for risk factors and identify a normal versus a maladaptive grief response.

ASSESSMENT

Normal grief

- This grief is considered uncomplicated.
- Emotions can include anger, resentment, withdrawal, hopelessness, and guilt but should change to acceptance with time.
- Client should achieve some acceptance by 6 months after the loss.
- Somatic manifestations can include chest pain, palpitations, headaches, nausea, changes in sleep patterns, or fatigue.
- The nurse should assess the client to identify a normal vs. maladaptive grief response.

Anticipatory grief

- This grief implies the "letting go" of an object or person before the loss, as in the case of a terminal illness.
- Individuals have the opportunity to grieve before the actual loss.

Maladaptive grief

Delayed or inhibited grief

- The client does not demonstrate the expected behaviors of the normal grief process.
- Cultural expectations can influence the development of delayed or inhibited grief.
- Clients can remain in the denial stage of grief for an extended period of time.
- Due to client's inability to progress through the stages/tasks of grief, a subsequent minor loss (even years later) can trigger the grief response.

Distorted or exaggerated grief response

- The client experiences the feelings and somatic manifestations associated with normal grief but to an exaggerated level.
- The client is unable to perform activities of daily living.
- The client can remain in the anger stage of the grief process and can direct the anger towards himself or others.
- The client can develop clinical depression.

Chronic or prolonged grief

- This maladaptive response is difficult to identify due to the varying lengths of time required by clients to work through the stages/tasks of grief.
- Clients can remain in the denial stage of grief and remain unable to accept the reality of the loss.
- Chronic or prolonged grief can result in the client's inability to perform activities of daily living.

NURSING INTERVENTIONS

Facilitating mourning

- Allow time for the grieving process.
- Educate the client and family on the stages and tasks associated with the grieving process.
- Identify expected grieving behaviors, such as crying, somatic manifestations, anxiety.
- Use therapeutic communication. Name the emotion that the client is feeling. For example, a nurse might say, "You sound as though you are angry. Anger is a normal feeling for someone who has lost a loved one. Tell me about how you are feeling." Qpcc
- Avoid communication that inhibits open expression of feelings, such as offering false reassurance, giving advice, changing the subject, and taking the focus away from the individual who is grieving.
- When relating to someone who is bereaved, avoid clichés such as, "She is in a better place now." Rather, encourage the individual to share memories about the deceased.
- Assist the individual to accept the reality of the loss.
- Support the client's efforts to "move on" in the face of the loss.
- Encourage the building of new relationships.
- Provide continuing support. Encourage the support of family and friends.
- Assess for indications of ineffective coping, such as refusing to leave home months after a client's partner has died.
- Share information about mourning and grieving with the client, who might not realize that feelings such as anger toward the deceased are expected.
- Encourage the client who is grieving to attend a bereavement or grief support group.
- Initiate a referral for psychotherapy for a client who is having a maladaptive grief response. Qtc
- Provide information on available community resources.
- Ask the client if contacting a spiritual adviser would be acceptable, or encourage the client to do so.
- Participate in debriefing provided by professional grief or mental health counselors.

Psychosocial care

- Use an interprofessional approach.
- Provide care to the client and the family.
- Discuss specific concerns the client and family can have (financial, role changes). Initiate a social services or other referral as needed.
- Use therapeutic communication to develop and maintain a nurse–client relationship.
- Facilitate communication between the client, family, and provider.
- Encourage the client to participate in religious/spiritual practices that bring comfort and strength, if appropriate.
- Assist the client in clarifying personal values to facilitate effective decision-making.
- Encourage the client to use coping mechanisms that have worked in the past.
- Be sensitive to comments made in the presence of a client who is unconscious, as it is widely accepted that hearing is the last of the senses that is lost. Qebp

Protection against abandonment and isolation

Decrease the fear of dying alone.
- Make presence known by answering call lights in a timely manner and making frequent contact.
- Keep the client informed of procedure/assessment times.
- Allow family members to spend the night and remain with the client as much as possible.
- Determine where the client is most comfortable, such as in a room close to the nurses' station.
- If the client chooses to be at home, move the client's bed to a central location in the home rather than an isolated bedroom. Qpcc

Support for the grieving family

- Suggest that family members plan visits in a manner that promotes client rest.
- Ensure that the family receives appropriate information as the treatment plan changes.
- Provide privacy so family members have the opportunity to communicate and express feelings among themselves.
- Determine family members' desire to provide physical care. Provide instruction as necessary.
- Educate the family about physical changes to expect as the client moves closer to death.

Application Exercises

1. A nurse is caring for a client following the loss of her partner due to a terminal illness. Identify the sequence of Engel's five stages of grief that the nurse should expect the client to experience. (Select the stages of grief in order of occurrence. All steps must be used.)

   A. Developing awareness

   B. Restitution

   C. Shock and disbelief

   D. Recovery

   E. Resolution of the loss

2. A charge nurse is reviewing Kübler-Ross: Five Stages of Grief with a group of newly licensed nurses. Which of the following stages should the charge nurse include in the teaching? (Select all that apply.)

   A. Disequilibrium

   B. Denial

   C. Bargaining

   D. Anger

   E. Depression

3. A nurse is working with a client who has recently lost his mother. The nurse recognizes that which of the following factors influence a client's grief and coping ability? (Select all that apply.)

   A. Interpersonal relationships

   B. Culture

   C. Birth order

   D. Religious beliefs

   E. Prior experience with loss

4. A nurse is discussing normal grief with a client who recently lost a child. Which of the following statements made by the client indicates understanding? (Select all that apply.)

   A. "I may experience feelings of resentment."

   B. "I will probably withdraw from others."

   C. "I can expect to experience changes in sleep."

   D. "It is possible that I will experience suicidal thoughts."

   E. "It is expected that I will have a loss of self-esteem."

5. A nurse is caring for a client who lost his mother to cancer last month. The client states, "I'd still have my mother if the doctor would have diagnosed her sooner." Which of the following responses should the nurse make?

   A. "You sound angry. Anger is a normal feeling associated with loss."

   B. "I think you would feel better if you talked about your feelings with a support group."

   C. "I understand just how you feel. I felt the same when my mother died."

   D. "Do other members of your family also feel this way?"

PRACTICE Active Learning Scenario

A nurse is caring for a client who is dying. Use the ATI Active Learning Template: Basic Concept to complete this item.

UNDERLYING PRINCIPLES
- Define anticipatory grief.
- Identify at least four interventions to provide psychosocial care to the client who is dying

NURSING INTERVENTIONS: Identify at least two interventions to prevent these feeling of abandonment and isolation in the client who is dying.

Application Exercises Key

1. Step 1: C. Shock and disbelief is the first stage in Engel's five stages of grief. In this stage the client experiences a sense of numbness and denial over the loss.

   Step 2: A. Developing awareness is the second stage in Engel's five stages of grief. In this stage the client becomes aware of the reality of the loss resulting in intense feelings of grief. This begins within hours of the loss.

   Step 3: B. Restitution is the third stage in Engel's five stages of grief. In this stage the client carries out cultural/religious rituals, such as a funeral, following the loss.

   Step 4: E. Resolution of the loss is the fourth stage in Engel's five stages of grief. In this stage the client is preoccupied with the loss. This preoccupation gradually decreases over about a 12 month time period.

   Step 5: D. Recovery is the fifth and final stage in Engel's five stages of grief. In this stage the client moves past the preoccupation with the loss and moves forward with life.

   Ⓝ *NCLEX: Psychosocial Integrity, Grief and Loss*

2. A. Disequilibrium is the second stage of Bowlby's four stages of grief.

   B. **CORRECT:** The denial stage is when the client has difficulty believing a terminal diagnosis or loss. This is one of Kübler-Ross Five Stages of Grief.

   C. **CORRECT:** The bargaining stage is when the client negotiates for more time or a cure. This is one of Kübler-Ross Five Stages of Grief.

   D. **CORRECT:** The anger stage is when the client directs anger toward self, others, or objects. This is one of Kübler-Ross Five Stages of Grief.

   E. **CORRECT:** The depression stage is when the client mourns and directly confronts feelings related to the loss. This is one of Kübler-Ross five stages of grief.

   Ⓝ *NCLEX® Connection: Psychosocial Integrity, Grief and Loss*

3. A. **CORRECT:** The client's interpersonal relationships are factors which influence the client's reaction to grief and ability to cope.

   B. **CORRECT:** The client's culture is a factor that influences the client's reaction to grief and ability to cope.

   C. Birth order is not a factor that influences grief and ability to cope.

   D. **CORRECT:** The client's religious beliefs are factors that influences the client's reaction to grief and ability to cope.

   E. **CORRECT:** The client's prior experience with loss is a factor that influences the client's reaction to grief and ability to cope.

   Ⓝ *NCLEX® Connection: Psychosocial Integrity, Religious and Spiritual Influences on Health*

4. A. **CORRECT:** Resentment is an emotion that can be associated with normal grief.

   B. **CORRECT:** Withdrawal is an emotion that can be seen with normal grief.

   C. **CORRECT:** Somatic manifestations such as changes in sleep patterns can be associated with normal grief.

   D. Suicidal ideations are associated with maladaptive grieving. The client who is experiencing a distorted or exaggerated grief response can direct anger towards himself. The nurse should assess and monitor the client for thoughts of suicide or self-injury.

   E. A client who is experiencing a maladaptive grief response commonly experiences a loss of self-esteem and a sense of worthlessness. These findings are not associated with normal grief.

   Ⓝ *NCLEX® Connection: Psychosocial Integrity, Therapeutic Communication*

5. A. **CORRECT:** This is a therapeutic response for the nurse to make. This response acknowledges the client's emotion and provides education on the normal grief response.

   B. This response offers advice, which is a nontherapeutic communication technique.

   C. This response minimizes the client's feelings and takes the focus away from the client ,which are nontherapeutic communication techniques.

   D. This response takes the focus away from the client, which is a nontherapeutic communication technique.

   Ⓝ *NCLEX® Connection: Psychosocial Integrity, Therapeutic Communication*

PRACTICE Answer

Using the ATI Active Learning Template: Basic Concept

UNDERLYING PRINCIPLES

- Anticipatory grief allows the client to work through the grieving process and ideally achieve acceptance prior to her actual death. The client's family can also experience anticipatory grief in preparation for their loss.
- Psychosocial care
  - Use an interprofessional approach.
  - Discuss specific concerns the client and family may have (financial, role changes). Initiate a social services or other referral as needed.
  - Use therapeutic communication to develop and maintain a nurse-client relationship.
  - Facilitate communication between the client, family, and provider.
  - Encourage the client to participate in religious/spiritual practices that bring comfort and strength, if appropriate.
  - Assist the client in clarifying personal values to facilitate effective decision-making.
  - Encourage the client to use coping mechanisms that have worked in the past.
  - Be sensitive to comments made in the presence of a client who is unconscious, as it is widely accepted that hearing is the last of the senses that is lost.

Ⓝ *NCLEX® Connection: Psychosocial Integrity, End of Life Care*

NURSING INTERVENTIONS

- Make presence known by answering call lights in a timely manner and making frequent contact.
- Keep the client informed of procedure/assessment times.
- Allow family members to spend the night and remain with the client as much as possible.
- Determine where the client is most comfortable, such as in a room close to the nurses' station.
- If the client chooses to be at home, move the client's bed to a central location in the home rather than an isolated bedroom.

CHAPTER 28

Mental Health Issues of Children and Adolescents

Mental health and developmental disorders in children and adolescents are not always easily diagnosed, resulting in possible delayed or inadequate treatment interventions.

Childhood and adolescent disorders can have associated comorbid conditions and can meet the criteria for more than one mental health disorder.

A child's behavior is problematic when it interferes with home, school, and interactions with peers.

DISORDERS THAT CAN APPEAR DURING CHILDHOOD AND ADOLESCENCE Qs

Depressive disorders, such as major depressive disorder and dysthymic disorder

Anxiety disorders, including separation anxiety disorder and panic disorder

Trauma- and stressor-related disorders, such as posttraumatic stress disorder (PTSD)

Substance use disorders, such as alcohol use disorder, tobacco use disorder, and cannabis use disorder

Feeding and eating disorders, such as anorexia nervosa, bulimia nervosa, and binge eating disorder

Disruptive, impulse control, and conduct disorders, such as oppositional defiant disorder, disruptive mood dysregulation disorder, and conduct disorder

Neurodevelopmental disorders, including attention deficit/hyperactivity disorder (ADHD), autism spectrum disorder, intellectual developmental disorder, and specific learning disorder

Bipolar and related disorders

Schizophrenia spectrum and other psychotic disorders

Nonsuicidal self-injury and suicidal behavior disorder; suicide is a leading cause of death for youth between the ages of 10 and 24.

Impulse control disorders, such as intermittent explosive disorder

FACTORS IMPEDING DIAGNOSIS

- Children might not have the ability or the necessary skills to describe what is happening.
- Children demonstrate a wide variation of "normal" behaviors, especially in different developmental stages.
- It is difficult to determine whether a child's behavior indicates an emotional problem.

CHARACTERISTICS OF GOOD MENTAL HEALTH

- Ability to appropriately interpret reality, as well as having a correct perception of the surrounding environment
- Positive self-concept
- Ability to cope with stress and anxiety in an age-appropriate way
- Mastery of developmental tasks
- Ability to express oneself spontaneously and creatively
- Ability to develop and maintain satisfying relationships

CHARACTERISTICS OF PATHOLOGIC BEHAVIORS

- Not age-appropriate
- Deviate from cultural norms
- Create deficits or impairments in adaptive functioning

ASSESSMENT

ETIOLOGY AND GENERAL RISK FACTORS

Genetic links or chromosomal abnormalities are associated with some disorders, such as schizophrenia, bipolar disorder, autism spectrum disorder, ADHD, and intellectual developmental disorder.

Biochemical: Alterations in neurotransmitters, including norepinephrine, serotonin, or dopamine, contribute to some mental health disorders.

Social and environmental: Severe marital discord, low socioeconomic status, large families, overcrowding, parental criminality, substance use disorders, maternal psychiatric disorders, parental depression, and foster care placement are all risk factors.

Cultural and ethnic: Difficulty with assimilation, lack of cultural role models, and lack of support from the dominant culture can contribute to mental health issues.

Resiliency: The ability to adapt to changes in the environment, form nurturing relationships, distance oneself from the emotional chaos of the parent or family, model effective coping strategies, and use problem-solving skills can help an at-risk child avoid the development of a mental health disorder.

Witnessing or experiencing traumatic events, such as physical or sexual abuse, during the formative years are risk factors.

DEPRESSIVE DISORDERS

RISK FACTORS
- Family history of depression Q̇EBP
- Physical or sexual abuse or neglect
- Homelessness
- Disputes among parents, conflicts with peers or family, and rejection by peers or family
- Bullying, either as the aggressor or victim, including traditional bullying and cyberbullying behavior
- Engaging in high-risk behaviors
- Learning disabilities
- Chronic illness

EXPECTED FINDINGS
- Feelings of sadness
- Loss of appetite
- Nonspecific complaints related to health
- Engaging in solitary play or work
- Changes in appetite, resulting in weight changes
- Changes in sleeping patterns
- Crying
- Loss of energy
- Irritability
- Aggression
- High-risk behavior
- Poor school performance and/or dropping out of school
- Feelings of hopelessness about the future
- Suicidal ideation or suicide attempts

ANXIETY DISORDERS AND TRAUMA- AND STRESSOR-RELATED DISORDERS

EXPECTED FINDINGS
- The anxiety or level of stress interferes with normal growth and development. Q̇EBP
- The anxiety or level of stress is so serious that the child is unable to function normally at home, in school, and in other areas of life.

Separation anxiety disorder

- This type of disorder is characterized by excessive anxiety when a child is separated from or anticipating separation from home or parents. The anxiety can develop into a school phobia or phobia of being left alone. Depression is also common.
- Anxiety can develop after a specific stressor (death of a relative or pet, illness, move, assault).
- Anxiety can progress to a panic disorder or type of phobia.

Posttraumatic stress disorder

- PTSD is precipitated by experiencing, witnessing, or learning of a traumatic event.
- Children and adolescents who have PTSD exhibit psychological indications of anxiety, depression, phobia, or conversion reactions.
- If the anxiety resulting from PTSD is displayed externally, it is often manifested as irritability and aggression with family and friends, poor academic performance, somatic reports, belief that life will be short, and difficulty sleeping.

DISRUPTIVE, IMPULSE CONTROL, AND CONDUCT DISORDERS

EXPECTED FINDINGS
- Behavioral problems usually occur in school, church, home, and/or recreational activities. Q̇EBP
- In children and adolescents who have disruptive, impulse control, and conduct disorders, manifestations generally worsen in the following.
  - Situations that require sustained attention, such as in the classroom
  - Unstructured group situations, such as the playground

Oppositional defiant disorder

- This disorder is characterized by a recurrent pattern of the following antisocial behaviors.
  - Negativity
  - Disobedience
  - Hostility
  - Defiant behaviors (especially toward authority figures)
  - Stubbornness
  - Argumentativeness
  - Limit testing
  - Unwillingness to compromise
  - Refusal to accept responsibility for misbehavior
- Misbehavior is usually demonstrated at home and directed toward the person best known.
- Children and adolescents who have oppositional defiant disorder do not see themselves as defiant. They view their behavior as a response to unreasonable demands and/or circumstances.
- Clients who have this disorder can exhibit low self-esteem, mood lability, and a low frustration threshold.
- Oppositional defiant disorder can develop into conduct disorder.

Disruptive mood dysregulation disorder

- Clients who have this disorder exhibit recurrent temper outbursts that are severe and do not correlate with situation.
  - Temper outbursts are manifested verbally and/or physically and can include aggression.
  - Temper outbursts are not appropriate for the client's developmental level.
- Temper outbursts are present three or more times per week and are observable by others, such as parents, peers, and teachers, in at least two settings, such as home and school.
- Onset of this disorder is between the ages of 6 and 18 .
- Manifestations are not due to another mental health disorder such as bipolar disorder.

Intermittent explosive disorder

Clients who have this disorder exhibit recurrent episodic violent and aggressive behavior with the possibility of hurting people, property, or animals.
- Occurs in clients 18 years and older
- Includes verbal or physical aggression
- Characterized by aggressive overreaction to normal events followed by feelings of shame and regret
- Prevents the client's ability to have healthy relationships and/or employment. Can lead to the development of chronic disease, such as hypertension or diabetes mellitus.

Conduct disorder (childhood or adolescent onset)

- Clients who have conduct disorder demonstrate a persistent pattern of behavior that violates the rights of others or rules and norms of society. Categories of conduct disorder include the following.
  - Aggression to people and animals
  - Destruction of property
  - Deceitfulness or theft
  - Serious violations of rules
- Childhood-onset develops before the age of 10, with males being more prevalent. Adolescent-onset occurs after the age of 10. The ratio of males-to-females is equal in the adolescent stage. Q EBP

CONTRIBUTING FACTORS
- Parental rejection and neglect
- Difficult infant temperament
- Inconsistent child-rearing practices with harsh discipline
- Physical or sexual abuse
- Lack of supervision
- Early institutionalization
- Frequent changing of caregivers
- Large family size
- Association with delinquent peer groups
- Parent with a history of psychological illness

MANIFESTATIONS
- Demonstrates a lack of remorse or care for the feelings of others
- Bullies, threatens, and intimidates others
- Believes that aggression is justified
- Exhibits low self-esteem, irritability, temper outbursts, reckless behavior
- Can demonstrate signs of suicidal ideation
- Can have concurrent learning disorders or impairments in cognitive functioning
- Demonstrates physical cruelty to others and/or animals
- Has used a weapon that could cause serious injuries
- Destroys property of others
- Has run away from home
- Often lies, shoplifts, and is truant from school

NEURODEVELOPMENTAL DISORDERS

Attention deficit hyperactivity disorder

Involves the inability of a person to control behaviors requiring sustained attention. Q EBP
- Inattention, impulsivity, and hyperactivity are characteristic behaviors of ADHD.
  - **Inattention** is evidenced by a difficulty in paying attention, listening, and focusing.
  - **Hyperactivity** is evidenced by fidgeting, an inability to sit still, running and climbing inappropriately, difficulty with playing quietly, and talking excessively.
  - **Impulsivity** is evidenced by difficulty waiting for turns, constantly interrupting others, and acting without the consideration of consequences.
- Inattentive or impulsive behavior can put the child at risk for injury.
- Behaviors associated with ADHD must be present prior to age 12 and must be present in more than one setting to be diagnosed as ADHD. Behaviors associated with ADHD can receive negative attention from adults and peers.

TYPES OF ADHD
- ADHD predominantly inattentive
- ADHD predominantly hyperactive-impulsive
- Combined type: Client exhibits both inattentive and hyperactive-impulsive behaviors

Autism spectrum disorder

- Autism spectrum disorder is a complex neurodevelopmental disorder thought to be of genetic origin with a wide spectrum of behaviors affecting an individual's ability to communicate and interact with others. Cognitive and language development are typically delayed. Characteristic behaviors include inability to maintain eye contact, repetitive actions, and strict observance of routines.
- This type of disorder is present in early childhood and is more common in boys than girls.
- Physical difficulties experienced by the child who has autism spectrum disorder include sensory integration dysfunction, sleep disorders, digestive disorders, feeding disorders, epilepsy, and/or allergies.
- There is a wide variability in functioning. Abilities can range from poor (inability to perform self-care, inability to communicate and relate to others) to high (ability to function at near normal levels).

Intellectual developmental disorder

- Clients who have intellectual developmental disorder have an onset of deficits and impairments during the developmental period of infancy or childhood.
- The client has intellectual deficits with mental abilities such as reasoning, abstract thinking, academic learning, and learning from prior experiences.
- Clients demonstrate impaired ability to maintain personal independence and social responsibility, including activities of daily living, social participation, and the need for ongoing support at school.
- Deficits in the disorder range from mild to severe.

Specific learning disorder

- Client demonstrates persistent difficulty in acquiring reading, writing, or mathematical skills.
- Performance in one or more academic areas is significantly lower than the expected range for the client's age, level of intelligence, or educational level.
- Clients who have specific learning disorder benefit from an individualized education program (IEP).

PATIENT-CENTERED CARE

NURSING CARE

- Obtain a complete nursing history to include the following.
  - Mother's pregnancy and birth history
  - Sleeping, eating, and elimination patterns
  - Recent weight loss or gain
  - Achievement of developmental milestones
  - Allergies
  - Current medications
  - Peer and family relationships, school performance
  - History of emotional, physical, or sexual abuse
  - Parental perceptions and level of tolerance toward child's behavior
  - Family history, including current members of the household
  - Substance use
    - Tobacco use disorder, such as cigarettes, cigars, snuff, chewing tobacco
    - Alcohol, frequency of use, driving under the influence, and family history of alcohol use disorder
    - Drugs (illegal or prescription) to get high, stay calm, lose weight, or stay awake
  - Safety at home and at school
  - Actual or potential risk for self-injury
  - Presence of depression and suicidal ideation, including a plan, the lethality of that plan, and the means to carry out the plan
  - Availability of weapons in the home
- Perform a complete physical assessment, including a mental status examination.
- Use primary prevention, such as education, peer group discussions, and mentoring to prevent risky behavior and to promote healthy behavior and effective coping.
  - Work with clients to adopt a realistic view of their bodies and to improve overall self-esteem.
  - Identify and reinforce the use of positive coping skills.
  - Employ the use of gun and weapon control strategies.
  - Emphasize the use of seat belts when in motor vehicles.
  - Encourage the use of protective gear for high-impact sports.
  - Provide education on contraceptives and other sexual information, such as the transmission and prevention of HIV and other sexually transmitted infections.
  - Encourage abstinence, but keep the lines of communication open to allow the adolescent to discuss sexual practices.
  - Encourage clients and family members to seek professional help if indicated.

- Intervene for clients who have engaged in high-risk behaviors.
  - Instruct the client and family on factors that contribute to substance use disorders. Make appropriate referrals when indicated.
  - Inform the client and family about support groups in the community for eating disorders, substance use disorders, and general teen support.
  - Instruct the client regarding individuals within the school environment and community to whom concerns can be voiced about personal safety and bullying, such as police officers, school nurses, counselors, teachers.
  - Make referrals to social services when indicated.
  - Discuss the use and availability of support hotlines.
  - Perform a depression and suicide assessment. Make an immediate referral for professional care when indicated. Qs

INTERVENTIONS

For anxiety disorders
- Providing emotional support that is accepting of regression and other defense mechanisms
- Offering protection during panic levels of anxiety by providing for needs
- Implementing methods to increase client self-esteem and feelings of achievement

For trauma- and stressor-related disorders
- Providing assistance with working through traumatic events or losses to reach acceptance
- Encouraging group therapy

For disruptive, impulse control, and conduct disorders, and ADHD
- Use a calm, firm, respectful approach with the child.
- Use modeling to show acceptable behavior.
- Obtain the child's attention before giving directions. Provide short and clear explanations.
- Set clear limits on unacceptable behaviors and be consistent.
- Plan physical activities through which the child can use energy and obtain success.
- Assist parents to develop a reward system using methods, such as a wall chart or tokens. Encourage the child to participate.
- Focus on the family and child's strengths, not just the problems.
- Support the parents' efforts to remain hopeful.
- Provide a safe environment for the child and others.
- Provide the child with specific positive feedback when expectations are met.
- Identify issues that result in power struggles.
- Assist the child in developing effective coping mechanisms.
- Encourage the child to participate in group, individual, and family therapy.
- Administer medications, such as antipsychotics, mood stabilizers, anticonvulsants, and antidepressants; monitor for side effects.

For autism spectrum disorder

- Initiate a referral for early intervention
- Provide for a structured environment.
- Consult with parents to provide consistent and individualized care.
- Encourage parents to participate in the child's care and treatment plan as much as possible.
- Use short, concise, and developmentally appropriate communication.
- Identify desired behaviors and reward them.
- Role-model social skills.
- Role-play situations that involve conflict and conflict resolution strategies.
- Encourage verbal communication.
- Limit self-stimulating and ritualistic behaviors by providing alternative play activities.
- Determine emotional and situational triggers.
- Give plenty of notice before changing routines.
- Carefully monitor the child's behaviors to ensure safety.

MEDICATIONS

ADHD: Psychostimulant drugs (methylphenidate and amphetamine salts) and nonstimulant selective norepinephrine reuptake inhibitor (atomoxetine) Q EBP

Autism spectrum disorders: Selective serotonin reuptake inhibitors and antipsychotic medications (risperidone, olanzapine, quetiapine, and aripiprazole)

Intermittent explosive disorder: Selective serotonin reuptake inhibitors (fluoxetine); mood stabilizers (lithium); antipsychotics (clozapine and haloperidol); beta blockers

Oppositional defiant disorder: Medications not generally prescribed

Conduct disorders: Medications are prescribed to target specific problem behaviors and include second-and third-generation antipsychotic medications (risperidone, olanzapine, quetiapine, ziprasidone, and aripiprazole). Tricyclic antidepressants, antianxiety medications, mood stabilizers, and antipsychotic medications are used to manage aggression.

Anxiety disorders: No FDA approved antianxiety medications for children. Selective serotonin reuptake inhibitors may be prescribed.

PTSD: Medications prescribed to target specific problem areas associated with the disorder such as depression and ADHD.

Disruptive mood dysregulation disorder: Antidepressant therapy

INTERPROFESSIONAL CARE

- Family therapy enables the client and family to address problems. Q EBP
- Cognitive-behavioral therapy is useful to change negative thoughts to positive outcomes when intervening for depressive, and disruptive, impulse control, and conduct disorders.
- Grief and trauma intervention (GTI) for children is effective for clients who have a trauma- and stressor-related disorder. GTI encourages narrative expression, such as drawing, writing, or play regarding the traumatic event.
- Other therapeutic approaches can include group therapy, play or music therapy, and mutual storytelling.

Application Exercises

1. A nurse is assisting the parents of a school-age child who has oppositional defiant disorder in identifying strategies to promote positive behavior. Which of the following is an appropriate strategy for the nurse to recommend? (Select all that apply.)

   A. Allow the child to choose consequences for negative behavior.
   B. Use role-playing to act out unacceptable behavior.
   C. Develop a reward system for acceptable behavior.
   D. Encourage the child to participate in school sports.
   E. Be consistent when addressing unacceptable behavior.

2. A nurse is performing an admission assessment on an adolescent client who has depression. Which of the following manifestations should the nurse expect? (Select all that apply.)

   A. Fear of being alone
   B. Substance use
   C. Weight gain
   D. Irritability
   E. Aggressiveness

3. A nurse is obtaining a health history from the parents of a 12-year-old client who has conduct disorder. Which of the following findings should the nurse expect? (Select all that apply.)

   A. Bullying of others
   B. Threats of suicide
   C. Law-breaking activities
   D. Narcissistic behavior
   E. Flat affect

4. A nurse in a pediatric clinic is caring for a preschool-age child who has a new diagnosis of ADHD. When teaching the parent about this disorder, which of the following statements should the nurse include in the teaching?

   A. "Behaviors associated with ADHD are present prior to age 3."
   B. "This disorder is characterized by argumentativeness."
   C. "Below-average intellectual functioning is associated with ADHD."
   D. "Because of this disorder, your child is at an increased risk for injury."

5. A nurse is assessing a 4-year-old child for indications of autism spectrum disorder. For which of the following manifestations should the nurse assess?

   A. Impulsive behavior
   B. Repetitive counting
   C. Destructiveness
   D. Somatic problems

Application Exercises Key

1. A. The parents should set clear limits on unacceptable behavior.

   B. The parents should focus on acceptable behavior and demonstrate this through modeling.

   C. **CORRECT:** The parents should have a method to reward the child for acceptable behavior.

   D. **CORRECT:** The parents should encourage physical activity through which the child can use energy and obtain success.

   E. **CORRECT:** The parents should set clear limits on unacceptable behavior and should be consistent.

   Ⓝ *NCLEX® Connection: Psychosocial Integrity, Behavioral Interventions*

2. A. Solitary play or work, rather than the fear of being alone, is an expected finding associated with depression.

   B. **CORRECT:** Substance use is an expected finding associated with depression.

   C. Loss of appetite and weight loss, not weight gain, are expected findings associated with depression.

   D. **CORRECT:** Irritability is an expected finding associated with depression.

   E. **CORRECT:** Aggressiveness is an expected finding associated with depression.

   Ⓝ *NCLEX® Connection: Psychosocial Integrity, Mental Health Concepts*

3. A. **CORRECT:** Bullying behavior is an expected finding of conduct disorder.

   B. **CORRECT:** Suicidal ideation is an expected finding of conduct disorder.

   C. **CORRECT:** Law- and/or rule-breaking behavior is an expected finding of conduct disorder.

   D. Low self-esteem, rather than narcissism, is an expected finding of conduct disorder.

   E. Irritability and temper outbursts, rather than a flat affect, are expected findings of conduct disorder.

   Ⓝ *NCLEX® Connection: Psychosocial Integrity, Mental Health Concepts*

4. A. Behaviors associated with ADHD are present before the age of 12.

   B. Argumentativeness is associated with oppositional defiant disorder rather than ADHD.

   C. Below-average intellectual functioning is associated with intellectual developmental disorder rather than ADHD.

   D. **CORRECT:** Inattentive or impulsive behavior increases the risk for injury in a child who has ADHD.

   Ⓝ *NCLEX® Connection: Psychosocial Integrity, Mental Health Concepts*

5. A. Impulsive behavior is an indication of ADHD rather than autism spectrum disorder.

   B. **CORRECT:** Repetitive actions and strict routines are an indication of autism spectrum disorder.

   C. Destructiveness is an indication of conduct disorder rather than autism spectrum disorder.

   D. Somatic problems are an indication of posttraumatic stress disorder rather than autism spectrum disorder.

   Ⓝ *NCLEX® Connection: Psychosocial Integrity, Mental Health Concepts*

PRACTICE Active Learning Scenario

A nurse is conducting a peer group discussion with a group of high school students about primary prevention. Use the ATI Active Learning Template: Basic Concept to complete this item.

UNDERLYING PRINCIPLES: Identify the purpose of primary prevention.

NURSING INTERVENTIONS: Identify at least four primary prevention interventions.

PRACTICE Answer

Using ATI Active Learning Template: Basic Concept

UNDERLYING PRINCIPLES: The purpose of primary prevention is to help the adolescent avoid risky behavior and to promote healthy behavior and effective coping.

NURSING INTERVENTIONS:
- Assist clients in adopting a realistic view of their bodies.
- Promote positive self-esteem.
- Identify and reinforce the use of positive coping skills.
- Teach the use of gun and weapon control strategies.
- Emphasize the use of seat belts when in motor vehicles.
- Encourage the use of protective gear for high-impact sports.
- Provide education on contraceptives and the prevention of sexually transmitted infections.

Ⓝ *NCLEX® Connection: Health Promotion and Maintenance, Health Promotion/Disease Prevention*

When reviewing the following chapters, keep in mind the relevant topics and tasks of the NCLEX outline, in particular:

Client Needs: Psychosocial Integrity

ABUSE/NEGLECT

Assess client for abuse or neglect and intervene as appropriate.

Identify risk factors for domestic, child, elder abuse/neglect and sexual abuse.

Plan interventions for victims/suspected victims of abuse.

BEHAVIORAL INTERVENTIONS

Assist the client with achieving and maintaining self-control of behavior.

Incorporate behavioral management techniques when caring for a client.

COPING MECHANISMS: Assess the client's support systems and available resources.

CRISIS INTERVENTION

Assess the potential for violence and use safety precautions.

Identify a client in crisis.

Use crisis intervention techniques to assist the client in coping.

Apply knowledge of client psychopathology to crisis intervention.

CHAPTER 29

CHAPTER 29 *Crisis Management*

A crisis is an acute, time-limited (usually lasting 4 to 6 weeks) event during which a client experiences an emotional response that cannot be managed with the client's normal coping mechanisms.

Everyone experiences crises. A crisis is not pathological, but represents a struggle for equilibrium and adaptation. Crises are also personal in nature. What might be considered a crisis for one person might not be so for another.

COMMON CRISIS CHARACTERISTICS

- Experiencing a sudden event with little or no time to prepare
- Perception of the event as overwhelming or life-threatening
- Loss or decrease in communication with significant others
- Sense of displacement from the familiar
- An actual or perceived loss

TYPES OF CRISES

Situational/external: Often unanticipated loss or change experienced in everyday, often unanticipated, life events

Maturational/internal: Achieving new developmental stages, which requires learning additional coping mechanisms

Adventitious
- The occurrence of natural disasters, crimes, or national disasters
- People in communities with large-scale psychological trauma caused by natural disasters

ASSESSMENT

RISK FACTORS

- Accumulation of unresolved losses
- Current life stressors
- Concurrent mental and physical health issues
- Excessive fatigue or pain
- Age and developmental stage

PROTECTIVE FACTORS

- Support system
- Prior experience with stress/crisis

EXPECTED FINDINGS

The nursing history should include the following.
- Presence of suicidal or homicidal ideation requiring hospitalization **Qs**
- The client's perception of the precipitating event
- Cultural or religious needs of the client
- Support system
- Present coping skills

Phases of a crisis

PHASE 1: Escalating anxiety from a threat activates increased defense responses.

PHASE 2: Anxiety continues escalating as defense responses fail, functioning becomes disorganized, and the client resorts to trial-and-error attempts to resolve anxiety.

PHASE 3: Trial-and-error methods of resolution fail, and the client's anxiety escalates to severe or panic levels, leading to flight or withdrawal behaviors.

PHASE 4: The client experiences overwhelming anxiety that can lead to anguish and apprehension, feelings of powerlessness and being overwhelmed, dissociative symptoms (depersonalization, detachment from reality), depression, confusion, and/or violence against others or self.

PATIENT-CENTERED CARE

NURSING CARE

- Crisis intervention is designed to provide rapid assistance for individuals or groups who have an urgent need.
- The initial task of the nurse is to promote a sense of safety by assessing the client's potential for suicide or homicide.
- Initial interventions include the following.
  - Identifying the current problem and directing interventions for resolution
  - Taking an active, directive role with the client.
  - Helping the client to set realistic, attainable goals
- Critical Incident Stress Debriefing is a group approach that can be used with a group of people who have been exposed to a crisis situation.
- Provide for client safety. **Qs**
  - Initiate hospitalization to protect clients who have suicidal or homicidal thoughts.
  - Prioritize interventions to address the client's physical needs first.
- Use strategies to decrease anxiety.
  - Develop a therapeutic nurse–client relationship.
  - Remain with the client.
  - Listen and observe.
  - Make eye contact.
  - Ask questions related to the client's feelings.
  - Ask questions related to the event.
  - Demonstrate genuineness and caring.
  - Communicate clearly and, if needed, with clear directives.
  - Avoid false reassurance and other nontherapeutic responses.

- Teach relaxation techniques.
- Identify and teach coping skills (assertiveness training and parenting skills).
- Assist the client with the development of the following type of action plan.
  - Short-term, no longer than 24 to 72 hr
  - Focused on the crisis
  - Realistic and manageable

MEDICATIONS

Administer antianxiety and/or antidepressant medication as prescribed.

PSYCHOTHERAPEUTIC INTERVENTIONS

Primary care: Collaborate with client to identify potential problems; instruct on coping mechanisms; and assist in lifestyle changes.

Secondary care: Collaborate with client to identify interventions while in an acute crisis that promote safety.

Tertiary care: Collaborate with client to provide support during recovery from a severe crisis that include outpatient clinics, rehabilitation centers, and workshops.

CLIENT EDUCATION

- Identify and coordinate with support agencies and other resources. Qℝℂ
- Plan and provide for follow-up care.

Application Exercises

1. A nurse is conducting chart reviews of multiple clients at a community mental health facility. Which of the following events is an example of client experiencing a maturational crisis?

   A. Rape

   B. Marriage

   C. Severe physical illness

   D. Job loss

2. A nurse is caring for a client who is experiencing a crisis. Which of the following medications might the provider prescribe? (Select all that apply.)

   A. Lithium carbonate

   B. Paroxetine

   C. Risperidone

   D. Haloperidol

   E. Lorazepam

> **PRACTICE Active Learning Scenario**
>
> A nurse manager is conducting an in-service on crisis management for a group of newly licensed emergency care nurses. Use the ATI Active Learning Template: Basic Concept to complete this item.
>
> **NURSING INTERVENTIONS:** Identify three that the nurse can use to assist the client who is experiencing a crisis.

Application Exercises Key

1. A. Rape is an example of an adventitious crisis. It is not a part of everyday life.

   B. **CORRECT:** Marriage is an example of a maturational crisis, which is a naturally occurring event during the life span.

   C. Severe physical illness is an example of a situational crisis.

   D. Loss of a job is an example of a situational crisis.

   Ⓝ NCLEX® Connection: Psychosocial Integrity, Crisis Intervention

2. A. Mood stabilizers, such as lithium carbonate, are prescribed for bipolar disorder and are not indicated in a short-term crisis situation.

   B. **CORRECT:** SSRI antidepressants, such as paroxetine, may be prescribed to decrease the anxiety and depression of a client who is experiencing a crisis.

   C. Antipsychotic medications, such as risperidone, may be prescribed for disturbed thought processes, usually when accompanied by other psychotic symptoms (hallucinations, delusions, blunt affect). Antipsychotics are not indicated in a short-term crisis situation.

   D. Antipsychotic medications, such as haloperidol, may be prescribed for disturbed thought processes, usually when accompanied by other psychotic symptoms (hallucinations, delusions, blunt affect). Antipsychotics are not indicated in a short-term crisis situation.

   E. **CORRECT:** Benzodiazepines, such as lorazepam, may be prescribed to decrease the anxiety of a client who is experiencing a crisis.

   Ⓝ NCLEX® Connection: Psychosocial Integrity, Crisis Intervention

> **PRACTICE Answer**
>
> *Using the ATI Active Learning Template: Basic Concept*
>
> **NURSING INTERVENTIONS**
> - Identify the current problem, and direct interventions for resolution.
> - Take an active, directive role with the client.
> - Help the client to set realistic, attainable goals.
> - Provide for client safety.
> - Initiate hospitalization to protect clients who have suicidal or homicidal thoughts.
> - Prioritize interventions to address the client's physical needs first.
> - Use strategies to decrease anxiety.
> - Develop a therapeutic nurse-client relationship.
> - Teach relaxation techniques.
> - Teach coping skills.
> - Administer prescribed antianxiety and/ or antidepressant medications.
>
> Ⓝ NCLEX® Connection: Psychosocial Integrity, Crisis Intervention

UNIT 6   PSYCHIATRIC EMERGENCIES

CHAPTER 30 *Suicide*

Suicide is the intentional act of killing oneself. A client who is suicidal can be ambivalent about death; interventions can make a difference. A client contemplating suicide believes that the act is the end to problems. Little concern is given to the aftermath or the ramifications to those left behind. Long-term therapy is needed for the survivors.

Suicidal ideation occurs when a client is having thoughts about committing suicide.

MYTHS REGARDING SUICIDE

- People who talk about suicide never commit it.
- People who are suicidal only want to hurt themselves, not others.
- There is no way to help someone who really wants to kill himself.
- Mention of the word suicide will cause the suicidal individual to actually commit suicide.
- Ignoring verbal threats of suicide, or challenging a person to carry out suicide plans, will reduce the individual's use of these behaviors.
- People who talk about suicide are only trying to get attention.

ASSESSMENT

RISK FACTORS

While females are more likely to attempt suicide, adolescent, middle, and older adult males are more likely to have a completed suicide. Other individuals at increased risk for suicide include active military personnel/veterans; those who are lesbian, gay, bisexual, or transgender; and people who have a comorbid mental illness, such as depressive disorders, substance use disorders, schizophrenia, bipolar disorder, and personality disorders.

OLDER ADULT CLIENTS Ⓒ
- Untreated depression
- Loss of employment and finances
- Feelings of isolation, powerlessness
- Prior attempts at suicide (older adult clients are more likely to succeed)
- Change in functional ability
- Alcohol or other substance use disorder
- Loss of loved ones

BIOLOGICAL FACTORS
- Family history of suicide
- Physical disorders, such as AIDS, cancer, cardiovascular disease, stroke, chronic kidney disease, cirrhosis, dementia, epilepsy, head injury, Huntington's disease, and multiple sclerosis

PSYCHOSOCIAL FACTORS
- Sense of hopelessness
- Intense emotions, such as rage, anger, or guilt
- Poor interpersonal relationships at home, school, and work
- Developmental stressors, such as those experienced by adolescents

CULTURAL FACTORS
- American Indian and Alaskan Native ethnic groups have the highest rate of suicide.

ENVIRONMENTAL FACTORS
- Access to lethal methods, such as firearms
- Lack of access to adequate mental health care
- Unemployment

PROTECTIVE FACTORS

- Feelings of responsibility toward partner and children
- Current pregnancy
- Religious and cultural beliefs
- Overall satisfaction with life
- Presence of adequate social support
- Effective coping and problem–solving skills
- Access to adequate medical care

EXPECTED FINDINGS

- Assess carefully for verbal and nonverbal clues. It is essential to ask the client if he is thinking of suicide. This will not give the client the idea to commit suicide. Q͟s
- Suicidal comments usually are made to someone that the client perceives as supportive.
- Assess for potential suicide risk using a standardized assessment tool, such as the SAD PERSONS scale. Q͟EBP
- Comments or signals can be overt (direct) or covert (indirect).
    ○ **Overt comment:** "There is just no reason for me to go on living."
    ○ **Covert comment:** "Everything is looking pretty grim for me."
- Assess the client's suicide plan. Q͟s
    ○ Does the client have a plan?
    ○ How lethal is the plan?
    ○ Can the client describe the plan exactly?
    ○ Does the client have access to the intended method?
    ○ Has the client's mood changed? A sudden change in mood from sad and depressed to happy and peaceful can indicate a client's intention to commit suicide.

PHYSICAL ASSESSMENT FINDINGS: Lacerations, scratches, and scars that could indicate previous attempts at self-harm.

PATIENT-CENTERED CARE

NURSING CARE

Nursing care consists of primary, secondary, and tertiary interventions.

- **Primary interventions** focus on suicide prevention through the use of community education and screenings to identify individuals at risk.
- **Secondary interventions** focus on suicide prevention for an individual client who is having an acute suicidal crisis. Suicide precautions are included in this level of intervention.
- **Tertiary interventions** focus on providing support and assistance to survivors of a client who completed suicide.

Suicide precautions

Suicide precautions include milieu therapy within the facility.

- Initiate one-on-one constant supervision around the clock, always having the client in sight and close. Documentation should indicate which staff member is accountable for the client, with specific start and stop times. There is an increased risk for suicide during staff rotation times.
- Document the client's location, mood, quoted statements, and behavior every 15 min or per facility protocol.
- Search the client's belongings with the client present. Remove all glass, metal silverware, electrical cords, vases, belts, shoelaces, metal nail files, tweezers, matches, razors, perfume, shampoo, plastic bags, and other potentially harmful items from the client's room and vicinity.
- Allow the client to use only plastic eating utensils. Count utensils when brought into and out of the client's room.
- Check the environment for possible hazards (such as windows that open, overhead pipes that are easily accessible, non-breakaway shower rods, non-recessed shower nozzles).
- Ensure that the client's hands are always visible, even when sleeping.
- Do not assign to a private room and keep door open at all times.
- Ensure that the client swallows all medications. Clients can try to hoard medication until there is enough for a suicide attempt.
- Identify whether the client's current medications can be lethal with overdose. If so, collaborate with the provider to have less dangerous medications substituted if possible.
- Restrict visitors from bringing possibly harmful items to the client.

Self-assessment

- The nurse must determine how she feels personally about suicide.
- The nurse must become comfortable asking personal questions about suicidal ideation and following up on client's answers.
- Death of a client by suicide can cause health care professionals to experience hopelessness, helplessness, ambivalence, anger, anxiety, avoidance, and denial.
- Nurses who work with clients who have suicidal ideation can benefit personally by debriefing, sharing, and collaborating with other health professionals.

MEDICATIONS

Classifications of medications to prevent suicide include the following.

Antidepressants: Selective serotonin reuptake inhibitors

- Citalopram
- Fluoxetine
- Sertraline

NURSING CONSIDERATIONS

- Decreased risk of lethal overdose compared to other categories of antidepressants.
- Do not stop taking medication suddenly.
- Medications can take 1 to 3 weeks for therapeutic effects for initial response with up to 2 months for maximal response.
- Avoid hazardous activities (driving, operating heavy equipment/machinery) until medication adverse effects are known. Adverse effects can include nausea, headache, and central nervous system (CNS) stimulation (agitation, insomnia, anxiety).
- Sexual dysfunction can occur. Notify the provider if effects are intolerable.
- Follow a healthy diet, as weight gain can occur with long-term use.
- Monitor for indications of increased depression and intent of suicide.

Sedative hypnotic anxiolytics (benzodiazepines)

- Diazepam
- Lorazepam

NURSING CONSIDERATIONS

- Observe for CNS depression, such as sedation, lightheadedness, ataxia, and decreased cognitive function.
- Avoid the use of other CNS depressants, such as alcohol.
- Avoid hazardous activities (driving, operating heavy equipment/machinery).
- Caffeine interferes with the desired effects of the medication.
- Advise the client who wants to discontinue a benzodiazepine to seek the advice of a provider. The client should not abruptly discontinue these medications. The provider should gradually taper the dosage over several weeks.

Mood stabilizers

Lithium carbonate

NURSING CONSIDERATIONS
- The client can minimize gastrointestinal effects by taking medication with food or milk.
- Maintain a healthy diet, and exercise regularly to minimize weight gain.
- Maintain fluid intake of 2 to 3 L/day from food and beverage sources.
- Maintain adequate sodium intake.
- Encourage the client to comply with laboratory appointments needed to monitor lithium effectiveness and adverse effects.

Second-generation antipsychotics

- Risperidone
- Olanzapine

NURSING CONSIDERATIONS
- Preferred over first-generation antipsychotics due to decreased adverse effects.
- To minimize weight gain, advise the client to maintain a healthy diet and exercise regularly.
- Instruct the client to report clinical findings of agitation, dizziness, sedation, and sleep disruption to the provider, as the medication might need to be changed.

THERAPEUTIC PROCEDURES

Therapeutic communication

- When questioning the client about suicide, always use a follow-up question if the first answer is negative. For example, the client says, "I'm feeling completely hopeless." The nurse says, "Are you thinking of suicide?" Client: "No, I'm just sad." Nurse: "I can see you're very sad. Are you thinking about hurting yourself?" Client: "Well, I've thought about it a lot." Qs
- Establish a trusting therapeutic relationship.
- Limit the amount of time an at-risk client spends alone.
- Involve significant others in the treatment plan.
- Carry out treatment plans for the client who has a comorbid disorder, such as a dual diagnosis of substance use disorder.

Electroconvulsive therapy (ECT)

ECT is effective in decreasing suicidal ideation in clients who have a depressive or psychotic disorder.

CLIENT EDUCATION

Assist the client to develop a support-system list with specific names, agencies, and telephone numbers that the client can call in case of an emergency.

CARE AFTER DISCHARGE
Ask the client to agree to a no-suicide contract, which is a verbal or written agreement that the client makes to not harm himself, but instead to seek help. Qpcc
- A no-suicide contract is not legally binding and should only be used according to facility policy.
- A no-suicide contract can be beneficial, but it should not replace other suicide prevention strategies.
- A no-suicide contract can be used as a tool to develop and maintain trust between the nurse and the client.
- A no-suicide contract is discouraged for clients who are in crisis, under the influence of substances, psychotic, very impulsive, and/or very angry/agitated.

Application Exercises

1. A nurse is assessing a client who has major depressive disorder. The nurse should identify which of the following client statements as an overt comment about suicide? (Select all that apply.)

   A. "My family will be better off if I'm dead."

   B. "The stress in my life is too much to handle."

   C. "I wish my life was over."

   D. "I don't feel like I can ever be happy again."

   E. "If I kill myself then my problems will go away."

2. A nurse is caring for a client who states, "I plan to commit suicide." Which of the following assessments should the nurse identify as the priority?

   A. Client's educational and economic background

   B. Lethality of the method and availability of means

   C. Quality of the client's social support

   D. Client's insight into the reasons for the decision

3. A nurse is assisting with the development of protocols to address the increasing number of suicide attempts in the community. Which of the following interventions should the nurse include as a primary intervention? (Select all that apply.)

   A. Conducting a suicide risk screening on all new clients

   B. Creating a support group for family members of clients who completed suicide

   C. Educating high school teens about suicide prevention

   D. Initiating one-on-one observation for a client who has current suicidal ideation

   E. Teaching middle-school educators about warning indicators of suicide

4. A nurse is caring for a client who is on suicide precautions. Which of the following interventions should the nurse include in the plan of care?

   A. Assign the client to a private room.

   B. Document the client's behavior every hour.

   C. Allow the client to keep perfume in her room.

   D. Ensure that the client swallows medication.

5. A nurse is conducting a class for a group of newly licensed nurses on caring for clients who are at risk for suicide. Which of the following information should the nurse include in the teaching?

   A. A client's verbal threat of suicide is attention-seeking behavior.

   B. Interventions are ineffective for clients who really want to commit suicide.

   C. Using the term suicide increases the client's risk for a suicide attempt.

   D. A no-suicide contract decreases the client's risk for suicide.

PRACTICE Active Learning Scenario

A nurse is caring for a client who has a new prescription for sertraline. Use the ATI Active Learning Template: Medication to complete this item.

COMPLICATIONS: Identify four.

CLIENT EDUCATION: Describe at least three teaching points.

Application Exercises Key

1. A. **CORRECT:** This statement is an overt comment about suicide in which the client directly talks about his perception of an outcome of his death. The nurse should assess the client further for a suicide plan.

   B. This statement is a covert comment in which the client identifies a problem but does not directly talk about suicide. The nurse should assess the client further for suicidal ideation.

   C. **CORRECT:** This statement is an overt comment about suicide in which the client directly talks about his wish to no longer be alive. The nurse should assess the client further for a suicide plan.

   D. This statement is a covert comment in which the client identifies a problem but does not directly talk about suicide. The nurse should assess the client further for suicidal ideation.

   E. **CORRECT:** This statement is an overt comment about suicide in which the client directly talks about his perception of an outcome of his completed suicide. The nurse should assess the client further for a suicide plan.

   Ⓝ *NCLEX® Connection: Psychosocial Integrity, Crisis Intervention*

2. A. This is an appropriate assessment for the nurse to include. However, it is not the priority.

   B. **CORRECT:** The greatest risk to the client is self-harm as a result of carrying out a suicide plan. The priority assessment is to determine how lethal the method is, how available the method is, and how detailed the plan is.

   C. This is an appropriate assessment for the nurse to include. However, it is not the priority.

   D. This is an appropriate assessment for the nurse to include. However, it is not the priority.

   Ⓝ *NCLEX® Connection: Psychosocial Integrity, Crisis Intervention*

3. A. **CORRECT:** Primary interventions include suicide prevention through the use of screenings to identify individuals at risk. Conducting a suicide risk screening on all new clients is an example of a primary intervention.

   B. Creating a support group for family members of clients who completed suicide is an example of a tertiary intervention.

   C. **CORRECT:** Primary interventions include suicide prevention through the use community education. Educating high school teens about suicide prevention is an example of a primary intervention.

   D. Initiating one-on-one observation for a client who has current suicidal ideation is an example of a secondary intervention.

   E. **CORRECT:** Primary interventions include suicide prevention through the use community education. Educating middle-school teachers to recognize the warning indicators of suicide is an example of a primary intervention.

   Ⓝ *NCLEX® Connection: Psychosocial Integrity, Crisis Intervention*

4. A. Clients who are suicidal should not be assigned a private room.

   B. Client's behavior should be documented every 15 min or according to facility policy.

   C. Remove perfume from the client's room.

   D. **CORRECT:** Ensure that the client swallows medication to prevent hoarding of medication for an attempted overdose.

   Ⓝ *NCLEX® Connection: Psychosocial Integrity, Crisis Intervention*

5. A. It is a myth that a threat of suicide or suicide attempt is attention-seeking behavior.

   B. It is a myth that interventions are ineffective for clients who really want to commit suicide. Suicide precautions are shown to be effective in reducing the risk of a completed suicide.

   C. It is a myth that using the term suicide increases the client's risk for a suicide attempt. The nurse should discuss suicide openly with the client.

   D. **CORRECT:** The use of a no-suicide contract decreases the client's risk for suicide by promoting and maintaining trust between the nurse and the client. However, it should not replace other suicide prevention strategies.

   Ⓝ *NCLEX® Connection: Health Promotion and Maintenance, Health Promotion/Disease Prevention*

PRACTICE Answer

Using the ATI Active Learning Template: Medication

SIDE/ADVERSE EFFECTS
- Nausea
- Headache
- Central nervous system stimulation (agitation, insomnia, anxiety)
- Sexual dysfunction

CLIENT EDUCATION
- Do not stop taking medication suddenly.
- Medications can take 1 to 3 weeks for therapeutic effects for initial response with up to 2 months for maximal response.
- Avoid hazardous activities (driving, operating heavy equipment/machinery) until medication adverse effects are known.
- Follow a healthy diet, as weight gain can occur with long-term use.
- Monitor for indications of increased depression and intent of suicide.

Ⓝ *NCLEX® Connection: Pharmacological and Parenteral Therapies, Medication Administration*

UNIT 6   PSYCHIATRIC EMERGENCIES

CHAPTER 31 *Anger Management*

Anger, a normal feeling, is an emotional response to frustration as perceived by the individual. It can be positive if there is truly an unfair or wrong situation that needs to be righted. Anger becomes negative when it is denied, suppressed, or expressed inappropriately, such as by using aggressive behavior. Denied or suppressed anger can manifest as physical or psychological findings, such as headaches, coronary artery disease, hypertension, gastric ulcers, depression, or low self-esteem.

Aggression, unlike anger, is typically goal-directed with the intent of harming a specific person or object. Inappropriately expressed anger can become hostility or aggression. Aggression includes physical or verbal responses that indicate rage and potential harm to self, others, or property. A client who is often angry and aggressive can have underlying feelings of inadequacy, insecurity, guilt, fear, and rejection.

Despite the potential for anger and aggression among individuals who have mental illness, it is important to know that clients who have mentally illness are more likely to hurt themselves than to express aggression against others.

COMORBIDITIES

- Depressive disorders
- Posttraumatic stress disorder
- Alzheimer's disease
- Personality and psychotic disorders

CATEGORIES/TAXONOMIES OF DISORDER

Preassaultive: The client begins to become angry and exhibits increasing anxiety, hyperactivity, and verbal abuse.

Assaultive: The client commits an act of violence. Seclusion and physical restraints can be required.

Postassaultive: Staff reviews the incident with the client during this stage.

SECLUSION AND RESTRAINTS

Seclusion and restraint must be used only according to legal guidelines and should be the interventions of last resort after other less restrictive options have been tried.

- New initiatives are being proposed to reduce or eliminate the use of mechanical restraints. National, state, and local initiatives advocate for restraint elimination. There is also heightened awareness of the damaging effects restraints can have on clients, health care professionals, and caretakers. **Q**EBP
- Seclusion and restraint do not usually lead to positive behavior change. Seclusion and restraint can keep individuals safe during a violent outburst, but the use of restraint itself can be dangerous and has, on rare occasions, led to the death of clients due to reasons such as suffocation and strangulation.
- Intramuscular medication can need to be given if aggression is threatening and if no medications were previously administered.
- When it is deemed essential to use restraints, remove the client from seclusion or restraint as soon as the crisis is over and when the client attempts reconciliation and is no longer aggressive.

ASSESSMENT

RISK FACTORS

- Past history of aggression, poor impulse control, and violence
- Poor coping skills, limited support systems
- Comorbidity that leads to acts of violence (psychotic delusions, command hallucinations, violent angry reactions with cognitive disorders)
- Living in a violent environment
- Limit setting by the nurse within the therapeutic milieu

EXPECTED FINDINGS

- Hyperactivity such as pacing, restlessness
- Defensive response when criticized, easily offended
- Eye contact that is intense, or no eye contact at all
- Facial expressions, such as frowning or grimacing
- Body language, such as clenching fists, waving arms
- Rapid breathing
- Aggressive postures, such as leaning forward, appearing tense
- Verbal clues, such as loud, rapid talking
- Drug or alcohol intoxication

PATIENT-CENTERED CARE

NURSING CARE

- Provide a safe environment for the client who is aggressive, as well as for the other clients and staff on the unit.
- Follow policies of the mental health setting when working with clients who demonstrate aggression.
- Assess for triggers or preconditions that escalate client emotions.

STEPS TO HANDLE AGGRESSIVE BEHAVIOR
Steps to handle aggressive and/or escalating behavior in a mental health setting include the following. Qs
- Responding quickly
- Remaining calm and in control
- Encouraging the client to express feelings verbally, using therapeutic communication techniques (reflective techniques, silence, active listening)
- Allowing the client as much personal space as possible
- Maintaining eye contact and sitting or standing at the same level as the client
- Communicating with honesty, sincerity, and nonaggressive stance
- Avoiding accusatory or threatening statements
- Describing options clearly and offering choices
- Reassuring the client that staff members are present to help prevent loss of control
- Setting limits for the client
  - Tell the client calmly and directly what he must do in a particular situation, such as, "I need you to stop yelling and walk with me to the day room where we can talk."
  - Use physical activity, such as walking, to deescalate anger and behaviors.
  - Inform the client of the consequences of his behavior, such as loss of privileges.
  - Use pharmacological interventions if the client does not respond to calm limit-setting.
  - Plan for four to six staff members to be available and in sight of the client as a "show of force" if appropriate.

FOLLOWING AN AGGRESSIVE/VIOLENT EPISODE
- Discuss ways for the client to keep control during the aggression cycle.
- Encourage the client to talk about the incident, and what triggered and escalated the aggression from the client's perspective.
- Debrief the staff to evaluate the effectiveness of actions.
- Document the entire incident completely by including the following.
  - Behaviors leading up to, as well as those observed throughout the critical incident
  - Nursing interventions implemented, and the client's response

MEDICATIONS

Olanzapine, ziprasidone

CLASSIFICATION: Atypical antipsychotics

THERAPEUTIC INTENT: Olanzapine and ziprasidone are used to control aggressive and impulsive behaviors. These are used more commonly than haloperidol because of the severity of adverse effects of haloperidol.

Haloperidol

CLASSIFICATION: Antipsychotic agent

THERAPEUTIC INTENT: Haloperidol is an used to control aggressive and impulsive behavior.

NURSING CONSIDERATIONS
- Monitor for clinical findings of parkinsonian and anticholinergic adverse effects.
- Keep client hydrated, check vital signs, and test for muscle rigidity due to the risk of neuroleptic malignant syndrome.

Other medications

Other medications may be used to prevent violent behavior by treating the underlying disorder. These include antidepressants, such as selective serotonin reuptake inhibitors; mood stabilizers, such as lithium; and sedative/hypnotic medications, such as benzodiazepines. Qs

CLIENT EDUCATION

- Encourage clients to return for follow up.
- Encourage clients to attend a support group.

CARE AFTER DISCHARGE
- Teach clients how to manage medications.
- Assist clients to develop problem-solving skills.

Application Exercises

1. A nurse is conducting group therapy with a group of clients. Which of the following statements made by a client is an example of aggressive communication?

   A. "I wish you would not make me angry."

   B. "I feel angry when you leave me."

   C. "It makes me angry when you interrupt me."

   D. "You'd better listen to me."

2. A nurse is caring for a client who is speaking in a loud voice with clenched fists. Which of the following actions should the nurse take?

   A. Insist that the client stop yelling.

   B. Request that other staff members remain close by.

   C. Move as close to the client as possible.

   D. Walk away from the client.

3. A nurse is assessing a client in an inpatient mental health unit. Which of the following findings should the nurse expect if the client is in the preassaultive stage of violence? (Select all that apply.)

   A. Lethargy

   B. Defensive responses to questions

   C. Disorientation

   D. Facial grimacing

   E. Agitation

4. A nurse is caring for a client in an inpatient mental health facility who gets up from a chair and throws it across the day room. Which of the following is the priority nursing action?

   A. Encourage the client to express her feelings.

   B. Maintain eye contact with the client.

   C. Move the client away from others.

   D. Tell the client that the behavior is not acceptable.

5. A nurse is caring for a client who is screaming at staff members and other clients. Which of the following is a therapeutic response by the nurse to the client?

   A. "Stop screaming, and walk with me outside."

   B. "Why are you so angry and screaming at everyone?"

   C. "You will not get your way by screaming."

   D. "What was going through your mind when you started screaming?

PRACTICE Active Learning Scenario

A nurse is caring for a client who hit another client. The nurse is preparing to administer haloperidol. Use the ATI Active Learning Template: Medication and the ATI Pharmacology Review Module to complete this item.

EXPECTED PHARMACOLOGICAL ACTION

COMPLICATIONS: Identify at least four adverse effects.

CLIENT EDUCATION: Describe at least four teaching points.

1. A. This statement does not imply a threat, nor does it indicate a lack of respect for another individual.

   B. This statement does not imply a threat, nor does it indicate a lack of respect for another individual.

   C. This statement does not imply a threat, nor does it indicate a lack of respect for another individual.

   D. **CORRECT:** This statement implies a threat and a lack of respect for another individual.

   Ⓝ *NCLEX® Connection: Psychosocial Integrity, Therapeutic Communication*

2. A. The nurse should not make demands of the client by insisting that he stop yelling.

   B. **CORRECT:** The nurse should request that other staff members remain close by to assist if necessary.

   C. Clients who are angry need a large personal space.

   D. The nurse should never walk away from a client who is angry. It is the nurse's responsibility to intervene as appropriate.

   Ⓝ *NCLEX® Connection: Psychosocial Integrity, Crisis Intervention*

3. A. Lethargy is more likely to be observed in a client who has depression.

   B. **CORRECT:** Defensive responses to questions are an assessment finding that can indicate that a client is in the preassaultive stage of violence.

   C. Disorientation is more likely to be assessed in a client who has a cognitive disorder.

   D. **CORRECT:** Facial grimacing is an assessment finding that can indicate that a client is in the preassaultive stage of violence.

   E. **CORRECT:** Agitation is an assessment finding that can indicate that a client is in the preassaultive stage of violence.

   Ⓝ *NCLEX® Connection: Psychosocial Integrity, Crisis Intervention*

4. A. Encouraging the client to express her feelings is appropriate. However, it is not the priority action.

   B. Maintaining eye contact with the client is appropriate. However, it is not the priority action.

   C. **CORRECT:** The client's behavior indicates that he is at greatest risk for harming others. The priority action for the nurse is to move the client away from others.

   D. It is appropriate to tell the client that the behavior is not acceptable. However, it is not the priority action.

   Ⓝ *NCLEX® Connection: Psychosocial Integrity, Crisis Intervention*

5. A. **CORRECT:** This is an appropriate therapeutic response. Setting limits and the use of physical activity, such as walking, to deescalate anger is an appropriate intervention.

   B. "Why" questions imply criticism and will often cause the client to become defensive.

   C. This is a closed-ended, nontherapeutic statement.

   D. The client is not ready to discuss this issue.

   Ⓝ *NCLEX® Connection: Psychosocial Integrity, Therapeutic Communication*

PRACTICE Answer

Using the ATI Active Learning Template: Medication

EXPECTED PHARMACOLOGICAL ACTION: Haloperidol is an antipsychotic agent used to control aggressive and impulsive behavior.

ADVERSE EFFECTS
- Parkinsonian and anticholinergic side effects
- Photosensitivity
- Shuffling gait
- Dry mouth
- Blurred vision
- Orthostatic hypotension
- Extrapyramidal symptoms
- Sedation
- Constipation

CLIENT EDUCATION
- Encourage the client to drink frequent sips of water.
- Instruct the client to increase fiber intake and that a stool softener can be needed.
- Instruct the client to limit sunlight exposure.
- Encourage the client to wear sunscreen and sunglasses.

Ⓝ *NCLEX® Connection: Pharmacological and Parenteral Therapies, Medication Administration*

UNIT 6   PSYCHIATRIC EMERGENCIES

CHAPTER 32   *Family and Community Violence*

Violence from one person toward another is a social act involving a serious abuse of power. Usually, a relatively stronger person controls or injures another, typically the least powerful person accessible to the abuser. This includes acts of violence that a partner commits against the other partner, a parent against a child, or a child against a parent.

TYPES OF VIOLENCE

A nurse must prepare to deal with various types of violence and the mental health consequences.
- Violence can be directed toward a family member, stranger, or acquaintance. Or, it can come from a human-made mass-casualty incident, such as a terrorist attack.
- Natural disasters, such as hurricanes and earthquakes, can cause mental health effects comparable to those caused by human-made violence.
- Violence against a person who has a mental illness is more likely to occur when factors such as poverty, transient lifestyle, or a substance use disorder are present.
- A person who has a mental illness is no more likely to harm strangers than anyone else.
- The factor most likely to predict violence between strangers is a past history of violence and criminal activity.

ASSESSMENT

RISK FACTORS

Cultural differences can influence whether the nursing assessment data is valid, how the client responds to interventions, and the appropriateness of nursing interactions with the client. Qᴘᴄᴄ
- **A female partner** is the vulnerable person in the majority of family violence, but the male partner can also be a vulnerable person.
- Vulnerable persons are at the greatest risk for violence when they try to leave the relationship.
- **Pregnancy** tends to increase the likelihood of violence toward the intimate partner. The reason for this is unclear.
- **Older adults** or other adults who are vulnerable within the home can suffer abuse because they are in poor health, exhibit disruptive behavior, or are dependent on a caregiver. The potential for violence against an older adult is highest in families where violence has already occurred. Ⓖ

FAMILY GROUPS

Violence is most common within family groups, and most is aimed at family and friends rather than strangers.
- Family violence occurs across all economic and educational backgrounds and racial and ethnic groups in the U.S. It's often termed "maltreatment."
- Family violence or maltreatment can occur against children, intimate partners, or vulnerable adult family members.
- Within the family, a cycle of violence can occur between intimate partners.
  - **Tension-building phase:** The abuser has minor episodes of anger and can be verbally abusive and responsible for some minor physical violence. The vulnerable person is tense during this stage and tends to accept the blame for what is happening.
  - **Acute battering phase:** The tension becomes too much to bear, and serious abuse takes place. The vulnerable person can try to cover up the injury or try to get help.
  - **Honeymoon phase:** The situation is defused for a while after the violent episode. The abuser becomes loving, promises to change, and is sorry for the behavior. The vulnerable person wants to believe this and hopes for a change. Eventually, the cycle begins again.
  - **Periods of escalation and deescalation** usually continue with shorter and shorter periods of time between the two. Emotions for the abuser and vulnerable person, such as fear or anger, increase in intensity. Repeated episodes of violence lead to feelings of powerlessness.

RISK FACTORS FOR ABUSE TOWARD A CHILD
- The child is under 3 years of age.
- A perpetrator perceives the child as being different (the child is the result of an unwanted pregnancy, is physically disabled, or has some other trait that makes him particularly vulnerable).

TYPES OF VIOLENCE

PHYSICAL VIOLENCE occurs when physical pain or harm is directed toward the following.
- An infant or child, as is the case with shaken baby syndrome (caused by violent shaking of young infants).
- An intimate partner, such as striking or strangling the partner.
- A vulnerable adult in the home, such as pushing an older adult parent and causing her to fall.

SEXUAL VIOLENCE occurs when sexual contact takes place without consent, whether the vulnerable person is able or unable to give that consent.

EMOTIONAL VIOLENCE includes behavior that minimizes an individual's feelings of self-worth or humiliates, threatens, or intimidates a family member.

NEGLECT, which includes the failure to provide the following.
- Physical care, such as feeding
- Emotional care, such as interacting with a child, or stimulation necessary for a child to develop normally
- Education, such as enrolling a young child in school
- Necessary health or dental care

ECONOMIC MALTREATMENT

- Failure to provide for the needs of a vulnerable person when adequate funds are available
- Unpaid bills, resulting in disconnection of heat or electricity

VULNERABLE PERSON CHARACTERISTICS

- Demonstration of low self-esteem and feelings of helplessness, hopelessness, powerlessness, guilt, and shame
- Attempts to protect the perpetrator and accept responsibility for the abuse
- Possible denial of the severity of the situation and feelings of anger and terror

PERPETRATOR CHARACTERISTICS

- Possible use of threats and intimidation to control the vulnerable person
- Usually an extreme disciplinarian who believes in physical punishment
- Poor impulse control
- Perceives the child as bad
- Violent outbursts
- Poor coping skills
- Low self-esteem
- Feelings of worthlessness
- Possible history of substance use disorder
- Difficulty assuming typical adult roles
- Likely to have experienced family violence as a child

AGE-SPECIFIC ASSESSMENTS

INFANTS

- Shaken baby syndrome: Shaking can cause intracranial hemorrhage. Assess for respiratory distress, bulging fontanels, and an increase in head circumference. Retinal hemorrhage can be present.
- Any bruising on an infant before age 6 months is suspicious.

PRESCHOOLERS TO ADOLESCENTS

- Assess for unusual bruising, such as on abdomen, back, or buttocks. Bruising is common on arms and legs in these age groups.
- Assess the mechanism of injury, which might not be congruent with the physical appearance of the injury. Numerous bruises at different stages of healing can indicate ongoing beatings. Be suspicious of bruises or welts that resemble the shape of a belt buckle or other object.
- Assess for burns. Burns covering "glove" or "stocking" areas of the hands or feet can indicate forced immersion into boiling water. Small, round burns can be from lit cigarettes.
- Assess for fractures with unusual features, such as forearm spiral fractures, which could be a result of twisting the extremity forcefully. The presence of multiple fractures is suspicious.
- Assess for human bite marks.
- Assess for head injuries: level of consciousness, equal and reactive pupils, and nausea or vomiting.

OLDER AND OTHER VULNERABLE ADULTS Ⓒ

Assess for any bruises, lacerations, abrasions, or fractures in which the physical appearance does not match the history or mechanism of injury.

PATIENT-CENTERED CARE

NURSING CARE

All states have mandatory reporting laws that require nurses to report suspected abuse; there are civil and criminal penalties for not reporting suspicions of abuse.

- Nursing interventions for child or vulnerable adult abuse must include the following.
  - Mandatory reporting of suspected or actual cases of child or vulnerable adult abuse Qs
  - Complete and accurate documentation of subjective and objective data obtained during assessment
- A forensic nurse has advanced training in the collection of evidence for suspected or actual cases of sexual assault or other forms of physical abuse.
- Conduct a nursing history.
  - Provide privacy when conducting interviews about family abuse.
  - Be direct, honest, and professional.
  - Use language the client understands.
  - Be understanding and attentive.
  - Use therapeutic techniques that demonstrate understanding.
  - Use open-ended questions to elicit descriptive responses.
  - Inform the client if a referral must be made to child or adult protective services. And, be sure to explain the process.
- Provide basic care to treat injuries.
- Make appropriate referrals.

Interventions

Nursing interventions for community-wide or mass casualty incidents, such as a school shooting or gang violence

EARLY INTERVENTION

- Provide psychological first aid.
- Make sure clients are physically and psychologically safe from harm.
- Reduce stress-related manifestations, such as using techniques to alleviate a panic attack.
- Provide interventions to restore rest and sleep, and provide links to social supports and information about critical resources.
- Depending on their level of expertise and training, mental health nurses can provide assessment, consultation, therapeutic communication and support, triage, and psychological and physical care.

CRITICAL INCIDENT STRESS DEBRIEFING

This is a crisis intervention strategy that assists individuals who have experienced a traumatic event, usually involving violence (staff experiencing client violence, school children and personnel experiencing the violent death of a student, rescue workers after an earthquake) in a safe environment.

- Debriefing can take place in group meetings with a facilitator who promotes a safe environment where there can be expression of thoughts and feelings. Qtc
- The facilitator will acknowledge reactions, provide anticipatory guidance for manifestations that can still occur, teach stress management techniques, and provide referrals.
- The group can choose to meet on an ongoing basis or disband after resolution of the crisis.

CLIENT EDUCATION

- Instruct clients regarding normal growth and development.
- Teach clients self-care and empowerment skills.
- Teach clients ways to manage stress.

CARE AFTER DISCHARGE

- Help client develop a safety plan, identify behaviors and situations that might trigger violence, and provide information regarding safe places to live. Qs
- Encourage participation in support groups.
- Use case management to coordinate community, medical, criminal justice, and social services.
- Use crisis intervention techniques to help resolve family or community situations where violence has been devastating.

PRACTICE Active Learning Scenario

A nurse is discussing intimate partner abuse with a newly licensed nurse. Use the ATI Active Learning Template: Basic Concept to complete this item.

UNDERLYING PRINCIPLES
- Discuss the three phases in the cycle of violence.
- Identify at least three characteristics of a vulnerable person.
- Identify at least three characteristics of a perpetrator.

NURSING INTERVENTIONS: Identify at least four nursing actions when conducting a nursing history.

Application Exercises

1. A charge nurse is leading a peer group discussion about family and community violence. Which of the following statements by a member of the group indicates an understanding of teaching?

    A. "Children older than 3 are at greater risk for abuse"

    B. "Substance use disorder does not increase the risk for violence."

    C. "Entering an intimate relationship increases the risk for violence."

    D. "Pregnancy increases the risk for violence toward the intimate partner."

2. A nurse is preparing to assess an infant who has shaken baby syndrome. Which of the following is an expected finding? (Select all that apply.)

    A. Sunken fontanels

    B. Respiratory distress

    C. Retinal hemorrhage

    D. Altered level of consciousness

    E. Increase in head circumference

3. A nurse working in an emergency department is assessing a preschool-age child who reports abdominal pain. When conducting a head-to-toe assessment, which of the following findings should alert the nurse to possible abuse? (Select all that apply.)

    A. Abrasions on knees

    B. Round burn marks on forearms

    C. Mismatched clothing

    D. Abdominal rebound tenderness

    E. Areas of ecchymosis on torso

4. A nurse is preparing a community education seminar about family violence. When discussing types of violence, the nurse should include which of the following?

    A. Refusing to pay bills for a dependent, even when funds are available, is neglect.

    B. Intentionally causing an older adult to fall is an example of physical violence.

    C. Striking an intimate partner is an example of sexual violence.

    D. Failure to provide a stimulating environment for normal development is emotional abuse.

5. A nurse is caring for an adult client who has injuries resulting from intimate partner abuse. The client does not wish to report the violence to law enforcement authorities. Which of the following nursing actions is the highest priority?

    A. Advise the client about the location of women's shelters.

    B. Encourage the client to participate in a support group for survivors of abuse.

    C. Implement case management to coordinate community and social services.

    D. Educate the client about the use of stress management techniques.

Application Exercises Key

1. A. Children younger than 3 years of age are at an increased risk for abuse.

   B. Substance use disorder increases the risk for violence.

   C. Vulnerable persons are an increased risk for violence when they try to leave the relationship.

   D. **CORRECT:** Pregnancy tends to increase the likelihood of violence toward the intimate partner.

   ⓝ *NCLEX® Connection: Psychosocial Integrity, Crisis Intervention*

2. A. Bulging, rather than sunken, fontanels are an expected finding of shaken baby syndrome.

   B. **CORRECT:** Respiratory distress is an expected finding of shaken baby syndrome.

   C. **CORRECT:** Retinal hemorrhage is an expected finding of shaken baby syndrome.

   D. **CORRECT:** An altered level of consciousness is an expected finding of shaken baby syndrome due to intracranial trauma or hemorrhage.

   E. **CORRECT:** An increase in head circumference is an expected finding of shaken baby syndrome.

   ⓝ *NCLEX® Connection: Psychosocial Integrity, Abuse/Neglect*

3. A. Minor injuries, such as abrasions, on the arms and legs are common in this age group.

   B. **CORRECT:** Round burn marks anywhere on the child's body can indicate cigarette burns and should alert the nurse to possible abuse.

   C. Mismatched clothing is consistent with the child's developmental age.

   D. Abdominal rebound tenderness is a possible indication of appendicitis rather than abuse.

   E. **CORRECT:** Areas of ecchymosis on the torso, back, or buttocks should alert the nurse to possible abuse.

   ⓝ *NCLEX® Connection: Psychosocial Integrity, Abuse/Neglect*

4. A. Refusing to pay bills for a dependent is economic maltreatment, rather than neglect.

   B. **CORRECT:** Physical violence occurs when physical pain or harm is directed toward another individual.

   C. Striking an intimate partner or other individual is an example of physical, rather than sexual, violence. Sexual violence occurs when sexual contact takes place without consent.

   D. Failure to provide a stimulating environment for normal development is neglect, rather than emotional abuse.

   ⓝ *NCLEX® Connection: Psychosocial Integrity, Abuse/Neglect*

5. A. **CORRECT:** The greatest risk to this client is injury from intimate partner abuse; therefore, the priority action the nurse should take is to assist the client with the development of a safety plan that includes the identification of safe places to live.

   B. The nurse should encourage participation in a support group. However, this does not address the greatest risk to the client and is therefore not the priority nursing action.

   C. The nurse should implement case management. However, this does not address the greatest risk to the client and is therefore not the priority nursing action.

   D. The nurse should educate the client about the use of stress management techniques. However, this does not address the greatest risk to the client and is therefore not the priority nursing action.

   ⓝ *NCLEX® Connection: Psychosocial Integrity, Abuse/Neglect*

PRACTICE Answer

Using the ATI Active Learning Template: Basic Concept

UNDERLYING PRINCIPLES

Cycle of violence
- Tension-building phase: The initial phase when the perpetrator has minor episodes of anger and can inflict verbal abuse or minor physical violence. The vulnerable person is tense and can accept the blame for what is happening.
- Acute battering phase: The tension reaches a peak, and a serious battering incident occurs. The vulnerable person can try to cover up the injury or seek help.
- Honeymoon phase: The abuser is sorry for the behavior and promises to change. The vulnerable person wants to believe the abuser and hopes for a change.
- Periods of escalation and deescalation usually continue with shorter and shorter periods of time between the two. Emotions for the abuser and vulnerable person, such as fear or anger, increase in intensity. Repeated episodes of violence lead to feelings of powerlessness.

Characteristics of a vulnerable person
- Feelings of low self-esteem, helplessness, hopelessness, powerlessness, guilt, and shame
- Attempts to protect the perpetrator and accept responsibility for the abuse
- Possible denial of the severity of the situation
- Feelings of anger and terror

Characteristics of a perpetrator
- Uses threats and intimidation to control the vulnerable individual
- Extreme disciplinarian who uses physical punishment
- Possible history of substance use disorder
- Possible history of family violence as a child
- Difficulty assuming adult roles

NURSING INTERVENTIONS
- Provide a safe and private environment to conduct the interview.
- Be direct, honest, and professional.
- Use language that the client understands.
- Be understanding and attentive.
- Use therapeutic communication.

ⓝ *NCLEX® Connection: Psychosocial Integrity, Crisis Intervention*

UNIT 6   PSYCHIATRIC EMERGENCIES

CHAPTER 33 *Sexual Assault*

Sexual assault is defined as pressured or forced sexual contact, including sexually stimulated talk or actions, inappropriate touching or intercourse, incest, human sex trafficking, female genital mutilation, and rape (forced sexual penetration). Sexual violence also refers to the denial of emergency contraception or measures to prevent sexually transmitted infections, organized rape during war or conflict, and sexual homicide.

Most survivors of sexual assault suffer long-term, severe emotional trauma. Rape-trauma syndrome, which is similar to posttraumatic stress disorder, can occur after a rape.

RAPE

Rape is defined as nonconsensual sexual activity involving any penetration of the vagina or anus with any body part or object, or the oral penetration by a sex organ of someone else. It is a crime of violence, aggression, anger, and power.

- Types of rape include stranger, marital, date, and acquaintance. The majority of perpetrators are known to the person who is raped. Acquaintance rape and spousal (or marital) rape specify the relationship between the perpetrator and vulnerable person. Date rape is a form of acquaintance rape in which the parties agreed upon a social engagement.
- Alcohol and other substances are often associated with date or acquaintance rape. These substances produce a sedative and amnesic effect on the vulnerable person.

SPECIFIC SUBSTANCES
- Gamma-hydroxybutyrate: Street names include "G" and "liquid ecstasy."
- Flunitrazepam: Street names include "roofies," "club drug," and "roachies."
- Ketamine: Street names include "black hole," "kit kat," and "special K."

ASSESSMENT

RISK FACTORS

- There is no "typical" description of a person who is vulnerable to rape. Individuals of all ages are affected by sexual assault and can be male or female.
- There is no "typical" rape survivor. Individuals can experience a variety of physical and emotional injuries and effects.

EXPECTED FINDINGS

Rape-trauma syndrome

Sustained and maladaptive response to a forced, violent sexual penetration against the individual's will and consent.
- Initial emotional (or impact) reaction
  - An **expressed reaction** is overt and consists of emotional outbursts, including crying, laughing, hysteria, anger, and incoherence.
  - A **controlled reaction** is ambiguous. The survivor can appear calm and have blunted affect, but can also be confused, have difficulty making decisions, and feel numb.
- Following the initial emotional response, clients can experience a variety of emotional reactions, including embarrassment, a desire for revenge, guilt, anger, fear, anxiety, and denial. These reactions can persist and become sustained and maladaptive.
- A **somatic reaction** can occur later in which the client can have a variety of physical manifestations
  - Muscle tension, headaches, and sleep disturbances
  - Gastrointestinal manifestations (nausea, anorexia, diarrhea, abdominal pain)
  - Genitourinary manifestations (vaginal pain or discomfort)

Posttraumatic stress disorder

Can occur beyond 1 month after the attack. Long-term psychological effects of sexual assault include the following.
- Reliving the event, such as flashbacks, recurrent dreams, and other intrusive thoughts about the assault
- Increased activity, such as visiting friends frequently or moving residence, due to a fear that the assault will reoccur
- Hyperarousal and increased emotional responses (easily startled, anxiety, angry outbursts, difficulty falling asleep or concentrating)
- Avoidance, fears, and phobias (fear of being alone, fear of sexual encounters, avoiding triggers of the event, memory problems about the trauma, emotional numbness, guilt, and depression)
- Difficulties with daily functioning, low self-esteem, depression, sexual dysfunction, and somatic reports, such as headache or fatigue

Compound rape reaction

Some survivors of rape can experience additional disorders as a result of the sexual assault.
- Mental health disorders, such as depression or substance use disorder
- Physical disorders, such as manifestations of a prior physical illness

Silent rape reaction

The survivor does not report or tell anyone of the sexual assault, including family, friends, or the authorities.
- Abrupt changes in relationships with partners
- Nightmares
- Increased anxiety during interview
- Marked changes in sexual behavior
- Sudden onset of phobic reactions
- No verbalization of the occurrence of sexual assault

LABORATORY TESTS

- Obtain blood for laboratory tests (HIV, hepatitis B and C).
- Collect samples for legal evidence (hair, skin, semen).

PATIENT-CENTERED CARE

NURSING CARE

- Perform a self-assessment. It is vital that the nurse who works with the client who has been sexually assaulted be empathetic, objective, and nonjudgmental. If the nurse feels emotional about the assault due to some event or person in his own past, it can be better to allow another nurse to care for the client.
- Perform an initial and ongoing assessment of the client's level of anxiety, coping mechanisms, and available support systems. The nurse should also assess for indications of emotional and/or physical trauma.
- Provide a private environment for an examination with a specially trained nurse-advocate, if available. A sexual assault nurse examiner (SANE) is a specially trained nurse who performs such examinations and collects forensic evidence. Qᴛᴄ
- Follow national standard protocol for the assessment, which includes client information, examination, documentation of biological and physical findings, collection of evidence, and follow-up as needed to document additional evidence.
- Provide for client safety. Qs
- Provide nonjudgmental and empathetic care.
- Obtain informed consent to collect data that can be used as legal evidence (photos, pelvic exam). The rape survivor has the right to refuse either a medical examination or a legal exam, which provides forensic evidence for the police.
- Treat any injuries, and document care given.

- Assist the SANE with the physical examination and the collection, documentation, and preservation of forensic evidence. Sexual assault evidence collection kits are used for collecting blood, oral swabs, hair samples, nail swabs, or scrapings, and genital, anal, or penile swabs. Document physical injuries in narrative and pictorial form, using body maps or photographs. Also document subjective data, using the client's verbatim statements.
- Support the client while legal evidence is being collected (samples of hair, skin, semen). Avoid minimizing the client's level of emotional suffering, as psychological responses can be subtle or not easily identifiable. Refrain from asking "Why" questions.
- Assess for suicidal ideation.
- Administer prophylactic treatment for sexually transmitted infections as outlined by the Centers for Disease Control and Prevention. This can include prophylactic treatment of syphilis, chlamydia, gonorrhea, HIV, and hepatitis exposure. Qs
- Evaluate for pregnancy risk and provide for prevention (emergency contraception).
- Call the client's available personal support system, such as a partner or parents, if the client gives permission.
- Assist the client during the acute phase of rape-trauma syndrome to prepare for thoughts, manifestations, and emotions that can occur during the long-term phase of the syndrome.
  - Encourage the client to verbalize her story and emotions.
  - Listen and let the client talk. Use therapeutic techniques of reflection, open-ended questions, and active listening.

CLIENT EDUCATION

CARE AFTER DISCHARGE
- Provide phone numbers for 24-hr hotlines for rape survivors.
- Promote self-care activities. Give follow-up instructions in writing, because the client might be unable to comprehend or remember verbal instructions.
- Initiate referrals for needed resources and support services. Individual psychotherapy and group therapy can be helpful to increase coping skills and prevent long-term disability, such as depression, or suicidal ideation.
- Schedule follow-up calls or visits at prescribed intervals after the assault.
- Emphasize importance of after care, as sexual assault clients historically have a poor compliance rate with follow-up visits.

1. A nurse is discussing silent rape reaction with a newly licensed nurse. The nurse should identify which of the following characteristics as expected for this type of reaction? (Select all that apply.)

    A. Sudden development of phobias

    B. Development of substance use disorder

    C. Increased level of anxiety during interview

    D. Reactivation of a prior physical disorder

    E. Unwillingness to discuss the sexual assault

2. A nurse is assessing a client who experienced sexual assault. Which of the following findings indicate the client is experiencing an emotional reaction of rape-trauma syndrome? (Select all that apply.)

    A. Genitourinary soreness

    B. Difficulties with low self-esteem

    C. Sleep disturbances

    D. Emotional outbursts

    E. Difficulty making decisions

3. A nurse is discussing the care of a client following a sexual assault with a newly licensed nurse. Which of the following statements by the newly licensed nurse indicates an understanding of teaching?

    A. "I will administer prophylactic treatment for sexually transmitted infections, like chlamydia."

    B. "I am not required to obtain informed consent before the sexual assault nurse examiner collects forensic evidence."

    C. "I can expect manifestations of rape-trauma syndrome to be similar to bipolar disorder."

    D. "I should use narrative documentation when documenting subjective data."

4. A nurse is caring for a client who was recently raped. The client states, "I never should have been out on the street alone at night." Which of the following responses should the nurse make?

    A. "Your actions had nothing to do with what happened."

    B. "You should focus on recovery rather than blaming yourself for what happened."

    C. "You believe this wouldn't have happened if you hadn't been out alone?"

    D. "Why do feel that you should not have been alone on the street at night?"

5. A community health nurse is leading a discussion about rape with a neighborhood task force. Which of the following statements by a neighborhood citizen indicates an understanding of the teaching?

    A. "Rape is a crime of passion."

    B. "Acquaintance rape often involves alcohol."

    C. "Young adults are the typical victims of sexual assault."

    D. "The majority of rapists are unknown to the victims."

PRACTICE Active Learning Scenario

A nurse in the emergency department is caring for a client who is a survivor of date rape after being given a substance. Use the ATI Active Learning Template: Basic Concept to complete this item.

RELATED CONTENT: Identify at least two substances, other than alcohol, commonly associated with date rape. Include the street names for these substances.

UNDERLYING PRINCIPLES: Compare and contrast rape and date rape.

NURSING INTERVENTIONS: Identify at least four interventions that are appropriate during the physical examination.

Application Exercises Key

1. A. **CORRECT:** Sudden onset of phobic reactions is a characteristic of a silent rape reaction.

   B. Development of substance use disorder is a characteristic rape reaction.

   C. **CORRECT:** Increased anxiety during interview is a characteristic of a silent rape reaction.

   D. Reactivation of a prior physical disorder is a characteristic of a compound rape reaction.

   E. **CORRECT:** No verbalization of the sexual assault is a characteristic of a silent rape reaction.

   Ⓝ *NCLEX® Connection: Psychosocial Integrity, Abuse/Neglect*

2. A. Genitourinary soreness indicates a somatic reaction.

   B. Difficulties with low self-esteem are an indication of a sustained and maladaptive emotional response beyond the initial reaction.

   C. Sleep disturbances indicates a somatic reaction.

   D. **CORRECT:** Emotional outbursts indicate an expressed initial reaction of rape-trauma syndrome.

   E. **CORRECT:** Difficulty making decisions indicates a controlled initial reaction of rape-trauma syndrome.

   Ⓝ *NCLEX® Connection: Psychosocial Integrity, Abuse/Neglect*

3. A. **CORRECT:** The nurse should administer prophylactic treatment for infections such as chlamydia according to the Centers for Disease Control and Prevention.

   B. The nurse must obtain informed consent to collect data that can be used as legal evidence.

   C. Manifestations of rape-trauma syndrome are similar to posttraumatic stress disorder.

   D. The nurse should document subjective data, using the client's verbatim statements.

   Ⓝ *NCLEX® Connection: Psychosocial Integrity, Abuse/Neglect*

4. A. This response offers the nurse's opinion, which is a nontherapeutic communication technique.

   B. This responses indicates disapproval, which is a nontherapeutic communication technique.

   C. **CORRECT:** This response uses the therapeutic communication technique of restating, which promotes reflection and verbalization of feelings.

   D. This responses asks a "why" question, which is a nontherapeutic communication technique.

   Ⓝ *NCLEX® Connection: Psychosocial Integrity, Therapeutic Communication*

5. A. Rape is a crime of violence, aggression, anger, and power.

   B. **CORRECT:** Alcohol and other substances are often associated with date or acquaintance rape.

   C. Individuals of all ages are affected by sexual assault and can be male or female.

   D. The majority of perpetrators are known to the vulnerable persons.

   Ⓝ *NCLEX® Connection: Psychosocial Integrity, Abuse/Neglect*

PRACTICE Answer

Using the ATI Active Learning Template: Basic Concept

RELATED CONTENT

- Gamma-hydroxybutyrate: Street names "G," "liquid ecstasy"
- Flunitrazepam: Street names "roofies," "club drug," "roachies"
- Ketamine: Street names "black hole," "kit kat," "special K"

UNDERLYING PRINCIPLES:

Both rape and date rape are forced sexual penetration and a form of sexual assault. However, date rape specifically refers to rape by a known acquaintance during a mutually agreed upon social engagement.

NURSING INTERVENTIONS

- Provide a private, secure environment.
- Provide nonjudgmental and empathetic care.
- Assist the sexual assault nurse examiner with obtaining, documenting, and preserving legal evidence.
- Treat any injuries, and document care given.
- Administer prophylactic treatment for the prevention of STIs.
- Evaluate the client for pregnancy risk and provide prevention if indicated.
- Call the client's available personal support system, if the client gives permission.
- Encourage the client to verbalize her story and emotions.
- Use therapeutic communication techniques.

Ⓝ *NCLEX® Connection: Psychosocial Integrity, Abuse/Neglect*

References

Berman, A., Snyder, S., & Frandsen, G. (2016). *Kozier & Erb's fundamentals of nursing: Concepts, process, and practice* (10th ed.). Upper Saddle River, NJ: Prentice-Hall.

Burchum, J. R., & Rosenthal, L. D. (2016). *Lehne's pharmacology for nursing care* (9th ed.). St. Louis: Elsevier.

Eliopoulos, C. (2014). *Gerontological nursing* (8th ed.). Philadelphia: Lippincott Williams & Wilkins.

Halter, M. J. (2014). *Varcarolis' foundations of psychiatric mental health nursing: A clinical approach* (7th ed.). St. Louis, MO: Saunders.

Hockenberry, M. J., & Wilson, D. (2015) *Wong's nursing care of infants and children* (10th ed.). St. Louis, MO: Mosby.

Ignatavicius, D. D., & Workman, M. L. (2016). *Medical-surgical nursing* (8th ed.). St. Louis, MO: Elsevier.

Pagana, K. D. & Pagana, T. J. (2014). *Mosby's manual of diagnostic and laboratory tests* (5th ed.). St. Louis, MO: Elsevier.

Potter, P. A., Perry, A. G., Stockert, P., & Hall, A. (2013). *Fundamentals of nursing* (8th ed.). St. Louis, MO: Mosby.

Skidmore-Roth, L. (2016). *Mosby's 2016 nursing drug reference* (29th ed.). St. Louis, MO: Elsevier.

Taketomo, C. K., Hodding, J. H., & Kraus D. M. (2014). *Lexi-Comp's pediatric & neonatal dosage handbook: A comprehensive resource for all clinicians treating pediatric and neonatal patients (pediatric dosage handbook)* (21st ed.). Hudson, Ohio: Lexi-Comp.

Townsend, M. C. (2014). *Essentials of psychiatric mental health nursing: Concepts of care in evidence-based practice* (6th ed.). Philadelphia: F. A. Davis.

Touhy, T. A., & Jett, K. F. (2012) *Ebersole & Hess' toward healthy aging: Human needs and nursing response* (8th ed.). St. Lois, MO: Mosby.

STUDENT NAME _____

CONCEPT_____   REVIEW MODULE CHAPTER_____

Related Content

(E.G., DELEGATION, LEVELS OF PREVENTION, ADVANCE DIRECTIVES)

Underlying Principles

Nursing Interventions

WHO? WHEN? WHY? HOW?

STUDENT NAME _____

PROCEDURE NAME _____ REVIEW MODULE CHAPTER_____

Description of Procedure

Indications

CONSIDERATIONS

Nursing Interventions (pre, intra, post)

Interpretation of Findings

Client Education

Potential Complications

Nursing Interventions

Growth and Development

STUDENT NAME _____

DEVELOPMENTAL STAGE _____ REVIEW MODULE CHAPTER_____

EXPECTED GROWTH AND DEVELOPMENT

Physical Development	Cognitive Development	Psychosocial Development	Age-Appropriate Activities

Health Promotion

Immunizations	Health Screening	Nutrition	Injury Prevention

STUDENT NAME _____

MEDICATION _____ REVIEW MODULE CHAPTER_____

CATEGORY CLASS_____

PURPOSE OF MEDICATION

Expected Pharmacological Action

Therapeutic Use

Complications

Medication Administration

Contraindications/Precautions

Nursing Interventions

Interactions

Client Education

Evaluation of Medication Effectiveness

STUDENT NAME _____

SKILL NAME_____ REVIEW MODULE CHAPTER_____

Description of Skill

Indications

CONSIDERATIONS

Nursing Interventions (pre, intra, post)

Outcomes/Evaluation

Client Education

Potential Complications

Nursing Interventions

System Disorder

STUDENT NAME _____

DISORDER/DISEASE PROCESS _____ REVIEW MODULE CHAPTER_____

Alterations in Health (Diagnosis)

Pathophysiology Related to Client Problem

Health Promotion and Disease Prevention

ASSESSMENT

Risk Factors

Expected Findings

Laboratory Tests

Diagnostic Procedures

SAFETY CONSIDERATIONS

PATIENT-CENTERED CARE

Nursing Care

Medications

Client Education

Therapeutic Procedures

Interprofessional Care

Complications

STUDENT NAME _____

PROCEDURE NAME _____ REVIEW MODULE CHAPTER_____

Description of Procedure

Indications

CONSIDERATIONS

Nursing Interventions (pre, intra, post)

Outcomes/Evaluation

Client Education

Potential Complications

Nursing Interventions